This journal belongs to

....

SISTERHOOD

The Journal

SISTERHOOD: THE JOURNAL

Men's and women's bodies are fundamentally different; however, modern medicine, healthcare, technology and let's face it... the world, have been slow to adapt to the specific needs of women. From the horrendous, excruciating experiments of the early 19th century, conducted on enslaved women to the more recent pelvic mesh scandal, even the history of gynaecology is chequered. We believe the time has come for healthcare solutions that are tailored and designed for women.

The full power of our menstrual cycles, of our hormones and how they impact our minds, bodies and wellbeing are still unknown to many of us. We learn from an early age to put up with a range of symptoms, only to discover much later (if at all!), that they are not only linked to our cycles and our hormones, but that something can be done about them.

Sisterhood has been designed to support you in your quest for optimal female health and happiness. With this journal we want to demystify the menstrual cycle. We want to help you better understand your symptoms, and gather personal insights more easily, so you can get what you want and what you need. We have created this journal, with you in mind, so you can unlock, and live, your life to its fullest.

We hope you enjoy using this journal as much as we have enjoyed creating it.

Team Hood x

WHO IS THIS FOR?

Sisterhood: The Journal has been designed to support you on your journey to achieving improved health and happiness outcomes. It is worth noting that if you are currently on hormonal contraception, your cycle is being generated by synthetic hormones and you are therefore not experiencing a menstrual cycle (more on this in the Hormonal contraceptive section). While you can practise cycle tracking using this journal, or look to identify any symptoms related to hormonal contraceptive use, this journal will be most useful to those not currently using hormonal contraception.

HOW TO USE

Information and resources
Understand more about your menstrual cycle, your hormones and how to make them work for you. Discover resources to help you on your journey.

Period and cycle trackers
Your period can be a key indicator of your overall health. Track details of your cycle, identify patterns and get to know your body better.

3 month daily cycle tracker
Your menstrual cycle is more than your period. Gather insights over 3 cycles to better understand the link with mind and body. Share with your doctor to help them differentiate between chronic and hormonal issues.

All-in-one monthly cycle tracker
Once you have a sense of your rhythm, track your entire cycle on a page. Easily compare one cycle to the next. Nurture and develop healthy habits.

Space for notes and creativity
Personalise your journal by colouring in any or all of the illustrations on the pages of this journal. There is also plenty of free space for making notes.

Body literacy*

noun [c]

1. Learning to read and understand the language of the body.
2. Learning to observe, chart and interpret an ovulatory menstrual cycle.

Most women learn about the menstrual cycle from family, friends or school. But few young women are guided through the early years of puberty with a comprehensive understanding of their cycle and the role it plays as part of their overall female health. There is also an absence of this education later on in life, with few expanding upon that initial learning as they grow and their bodies change.

What's worse is that some women may have been given incorrect or outdated information to start with, which then leads to a lifetime of unnecessary worry and discomfort.

The first path to female body literacy (learning to read and understand the language of our body), is to ensure we have a good understanding of our reproductive system and the important role it has to play in our lives. Only then do we believe women will be able to make fully informed choices about their female health.

> *'Men do not have this warning system and we do. And so if we can start to maybe see our periods as information versus being just a pain in the ass, then we will start to change the dialogue that we have with our health and our bodies.'*
>
> ***– Nicole Jardim, The Period Girl, Fix Your Period.***

**The creator of the term was veteran menstrual advocate Laura Wershler who, along with her colleagues Geraldine Matus and Megan Lalonde, introduced the concept in the Fall 2005 issue of 'Femme Fertile'.*

THE UTERUS

The uterus or womb sits just behind your bladder and in front of your rectum. It houses your fallopian tubes, ovaries and cervix and is shaped like an upside-down pear.

Not all uteruses are the same and depending on our physicality, family history, or even lifestyle, the position of our uterus can be different. Most tilt forwards, but they can also be retroverted or 'tipped'. This means that the uterus tilts backward towards your bum and base of your spine. This can have a negative effect on period pain and blood flow, and can change how we carry children during pregnancy. The uterus is also incredibly dynamic, changing and responding to hormonal signals from our bodies.

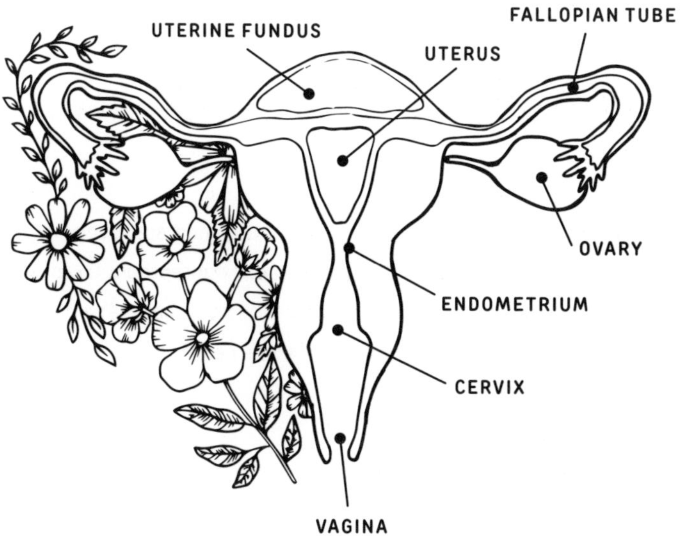

The innermost layer of the uterus is called the endometrium, which is also known as the lining of the womb. This layer builds up throughout your cycle ready for implantation of a fertilised egg or to shed if no pregnancy has occurred. This shedding is most commonly known as your period.

THE CERVIX

The cervix is a cylinder-shaped neck of tissue that connects the vagina and uterus. Located at the lowermost portion of the uterus, the cervix is composed primarily of fibromuscular tissue. The cervix acts as the door to the uterus, which sperm can travel through to fertilise eggs. When your body is not carrying a child, your cervix helps keep unhealthy things travelling too far into your body, like tampons and bath water.

Cervical screening helps to check the health of your cervix. During the test, a sample is collected and then checked for certain types of human papillomavirus (HPV) that can cause changes to the cells of your cervix. These 'high risk' types of HPV and can be treated before they get a chance to develop into cervical cancer.

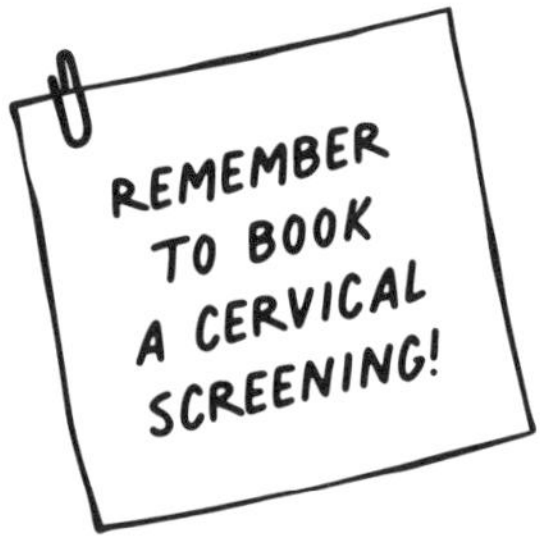

WHILE WE ARE HERE ... LET'S TALK ABOUT CERVICAL FLUID

Cervical fluid (aka cervical mucus) is a core component of vaginal discharge. It changes in consistency throughout your cycle and can be yellow, white or cloudy. Tracking changes to your cervical fluid gives you a better indication of where you are in your cycle and also what hormonal changes are occurring.

> *'Egg white CM, or EWCM as it's often termed, is your most fertile mucus and this type of mucus indicates that you are either ovulating or about to ovulate. It is actually your MOST reliable indicator. Once you know what to look for, and importantly, get to know what's normal for you, then observing your CM can become pretty simple. CM is important to assist the passage of sperm to the egg. Sperm LOVE fertile CM!'*
>
> ***– Kate Davies, Your Fertility Journey***

Check out our cervical fluid and temperature trackers on our website if you need help pin-pointing when you ovulate.

THE OVARIES

The are two ovaries within the female reproductive system, one on the left and one on the right. Both contain ovarian follicles, which are small fluid-filled sacs that each house an immature egg designed to mature and be released each cycle. They produce hormones which influence stages of the menstrual cycle and women begin puberty with about 300,000 to 400,000 of them . The corpus luteum (which is the casing of the follicle that ruptures to release the egg) dies off, (hence corpus luteum), and as a result creates progesterone, the dominant hormone in the Luteal phase.

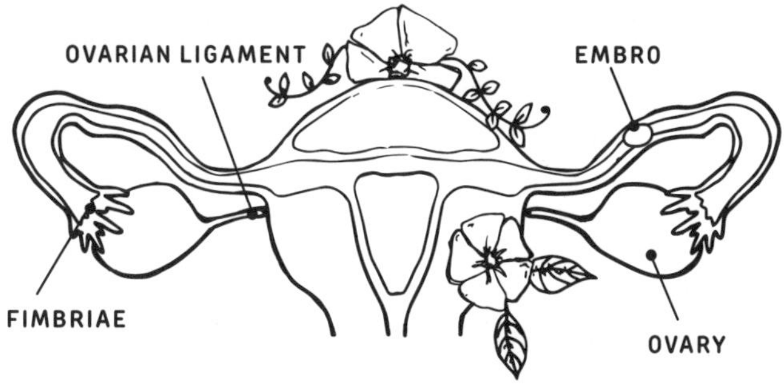

VULVA AND VAGINA ... WHAT'S THE DIFFERENCE?

In 2016, the Eve Appeal conducted research that showed only 44% of women surveyed could accurately label the vagina, with 60% unable to label the vulva correctly.

The vagina is the name for the internal tube that connects your vulva to your womb. The vulva is the external genitalia which includes your mons pubis, labia minora and majora, the clitoris, and your urethra (where you urinate from). If you are as fascinated with this body part as we are, check out The Vulva Gallery on Insta for lots of different illustrations!

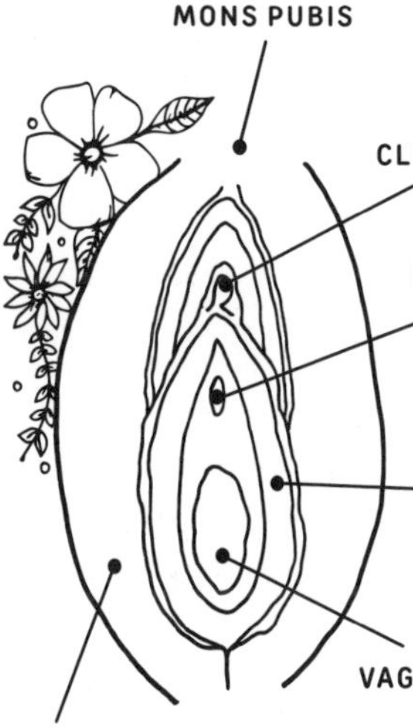

THE CLITORIS

Our favourite part! Unlike a penis, which has several functions, the clitoris is the only human organ designed specifically to give pleasure ... lucky us. Packed with over 8,000 nerve endings in the tip alone (double the number in a penis), it's best to think of the clitoris like an iceberg. The visible 'button' is just the head and it can actually extend up to 3 inches into every part of your vagina, including the G spot. The clitoris can range from 7–12 cm in length and, when aroused, becomes engorged, swelling by 50–300 per cent.

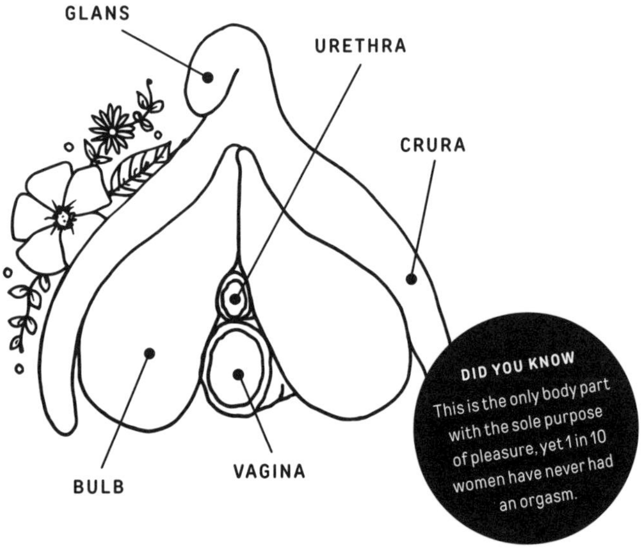

'When they are conceived, all babies initially have exactly the same genital tissue. At 12 weeks, developments start to happen to this tissue, which later leads to the formation of either a penis or the labia. In reality, the clitoris and penis are actually both made up of the same things: erectile tissue, a foreskin (the clitoral hood), glans, and even a small shaft! Interesting that they don't receive the same amount of education and attention.'

– Maisie Hill, Period Power

COMMON MISCONCEPTIONS

Excerpt from interview with Billie Quinlan, Co-founder and CEO at Ferly – a business focused on improving sexual wellbeing. Visit our blog for the full interview.

There are plenty [of common misconceptions about the female body] but I'm going to share two: the clitoris and desire. For centuries we've believed that men are more sexual than women, that they get more pleasure from sex and have a higher level of desire than women. These two things aren't true. They come from a fundamental lack of knowledge about the female body. Firstly, let's address the misconceptions about the clitoris. We sent a man to the moon before we fully understood the shape and size of the clitoris. It wasn't until the 90s that scientists discovered it was shaped like a wishbone and had 8,000 nerve endings! Now we need to re-educate ourselves on how to give that girl some love! Secondly, let's set some things straight regarding female desire. There are two different drive systems: spontaneous and situational. Spontaneous desire is triggered when we see something we like, e.g. a beautiful woman walks into a bar. This type of desire is most often experienced by men, which is why we have this myth that men are more sexual. Conversely, the majority of women experience situational desire, e.g. you've been taken out on a nice date, you feel really good in your body and the person you're with has made you laugh all night. This lovely situation is what triggers situational desire. It takes a little more effort and requires a deeper understanding of what situations arouse you as an individual. It certainly doesn't mean those with a situational drive system are less sexual!

> 'Body literacy is especially powerful when it comes to pleasure. It empowers you to explore your erogenous zones and unlock different sensations, which in turn provides you with a lexicon to communicate with your partner(s). There is a beautiful practice on the Ferly app called 'Body Mapping'. If you're struggling to explore on your own, tune into this practice and be guided through the exploration.'
>
> ***– Billie Quinlan, CEO Ferly***

YOUR HORMONES

The menstrual cycle is controlled by the hormones your body produces, which act as the body's chemical messengers. They travel around your bloodstream, telling your tissues and organs what to do and when. Hormones help to control and maintain balance within the body, affecting key bodily functions such as your metabolism, reproduction, mood and sleep cycles.

Hundreds of hormones circulate in your bloodstream at any one time. Insulin, oestrogen, testosterone, and cortisol are examples of key hormones in the body. You will find that the level and concentration of many hormones will fluctuate depending on where you are in your menstrual cycle, the time of day, or even the seasons of the year.

The menstrual cycle is regulated by the interaction of key hormones including:

- **Follicle stimulating hormone (FSH)**, causing maturation of an egg in the ovary.
- **Luteinising hormone (LH)**, stimulating the release of the egg.
- **Oestrogen and progesterone,** involved in maintaining the uterus lining.

In the first phase of your cycle (the Follicular phase), increasing levels of oestrogen and follicle stimulating hormone cause one of the ovaries to develop an egg while your luteinising hormone stimulates the release of it (ovulation). At the same time, the womb lining also starts to thicken ready to house the egg if conception occurs.

In the second half of the cycle (your Luteal phase), the hormone progesterone helps the womb to prepare for the implantation of a developing embryo. The egg makes its journey down the fallopian tubes and if pregnancy doesn't occur, it will disintegrate after about 12 to 24 hours and either get reabsorbed into the body or pass out with your period. This is then followed by a drop in oestrogen and progesterone levels, which is the signal for the womb lining to break down and leave the body.

All hormones work together like an orchestra. If an instrument is played too quickly or too slowly, or if it is not played at all, it can affect the whole musical piece. In the same way, if any of your key hormones are out of sync, this tends to show in your reproductive cycle. Developing an understanding of your reproductive cycle therefore has benefits that go beyond monitoring fertility. It can be a key way of picking up if there is an imbalance somewhere in your body.

HORMONE IMBALANCES

Hormones work best when balanced. However, stress, synthetic hormones, poor nutrition and a lack of exercise or regular sleep can disrupt this balance, leading to side effects across the body.

It can be helpful to consider a hormone hierarchy, as championed by Dr. Anna Cabeca, with oxytocin (love and bonding hormone) at the top of the pyramid, followed by cortisol (stress hormone) on the next level, insulin on the next and then progesterone, oestrogen and testosterone at the base.

Hormone hierarchy

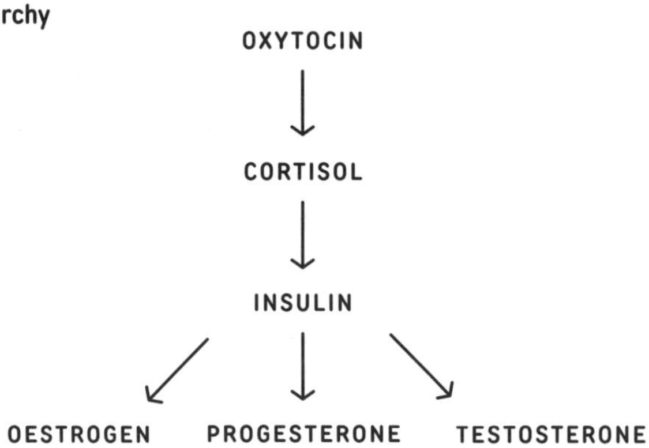

Imbalances in oxytocin, cortisol and insulin can have a detrimental, knock-on effect on the balance of the other three hormones. Common conditions linked to hormonal imbalances include PCOS, endometriosis, heavy periods (menorrhagia), irregular periods and fibroids.

PCOS

Polycystic Ovary Syndrome is a hormone imbalance usually caused by excessively high levels of Luteinising hormone / LH or insulin (from the pancreas), which in turn causes the ovaries to produce extra amounts of testosterone. Although everyone produces testosterone, having PCOS means that your ovaries make more testosterone than they are meant to.

PCOS is so called due to the presence of tiny cysts inside the ovaries. Some people have many cysts while some only have a few. These cysts are unharmful and do not require removal.

Due to the hormonal imbalance, the ovaries do not receive the right signals and therefore may not produce an egg (ovulation) every month. This means that your period may be irregular or may not occur at all. In some cases, PCOS can contribute to difficulty conceiving / getting pregnant.

Endometriosis

Endometriosis is a condition in which tissue like that found in the lining of the womb (uterus) is found in other parts of the body. This endometrial tissue can be found behind the uterus, on the ovaries, the fallopian tubes, on or near the bladder and on the rectum. Although endometrial tissue is located outside the womb, it continues to respond to oestrogen – the hormone that tells the lining of your womb to thicken, break down and then bleed every menstrual cycle. However, unlike tissue in the womb that leaves the body as a period, blood from endometrial tissue has no way to exit the body. This may cause inflammation, pain and the formation of scar tissue.

Fibroids

Fibroids are non-cancerous growths that form in or around the uterus / womb. Varied in size and made up of fibrous tissue and muscle, they are often symptomless.

Although the exact cause of fibroids is unknown, they have been linked to high levels of oestrogen and they do tend to shrink when oestrogen levels are low (e.g. after the menopause). Possible treatments include medication, surgery and managing symptoms through diet and exercise.

PMS/PMDD

Premenstrual syndrome (PMS) relates to physical and emotional symptoms that usually start approximately a week before your period. Symptoms include headaches, bloating, anxiety and sudden mood changes. Premenstrual dysphoric disorder (PMDD) is considered to be similar to PMS; however, its associated symptoms are so severe they often interfere with your quality of life. The exact causes of PMS/PMDD are unknown; however, experts believe they are linked to hormonal changes in the second part of your cycle.

If you have a hormone imbalance, there are various ways to manage your symptoms and restore your hormones to appropriate levels. It's best to seek advice from a medical practitioner with any concerns you may have. Check out our blog at wearethehood.com/blog, for information on these conditions and others.

There are other factors that contribute to hormonal imbalances. Two of these, which are less known but fairly common, are covered in this section.

HORMONE DISRUPTORS

Stress

Adrenaline and cortisol are the two main hormones involved in the body's natural response to stress – fight-or-flight mode. In response to a perceived threat, cortisol suppresses non-essential functions in the body such as the digestion, immune responses and the reproductive system. Stressors can be psychological, physical, environmental and nutritional such as:

- Too much sugar, flour, caffeine or alcohol
- Over-exercising (cardio in particular)
- Not enough sleep
- Too much screen time
- Commitments and life events (e.g. weddings, changing jobs)

If your body's stress response system is working properly, your levels of adrenaline and cortisol return to normal once the perceived threat is gone. If it isn't, your body can remain constantly in fight-or-flight mode, turning into chronic stress (associated with heavy or irregular periods, infertility and PMS).

Health risks associated with chronic stress include weight gain (especially around the abdomen), digestive problems, depression, anxiety, low libido, heavy or irregular periods, infertility and PMS.

Here are a few steps you can take to improve your relationship with stress, many of which work to boost oxytocin, the love and bonding hormone, as well:

- Be active, eat healthily, be kind to yourself
- Connect with people, laugh, play, hug
- Work smart not hard, help others
- Meditation, mindfulness
- Orgasm!
- Keep a gratitude journal
- Seek support from a doctor or therapist

Hormonal contraceptives

While contraception is typically perceived as a method of pregnancy prevention, some forms of contraception, such as the pill, are often prescribed in the management of period symptoms.

The contraceptive pill is described as containing Progesterone and Oestrogen (the combined pill) or just Progesterone. This is not entirely accurate as the pill actually contains synthetic versions of these hormones, built to imitate the naturally occurring ones.

The contraceptive pill works by:

- Halting the functioning of the ovaries
- Thickening the mucus in the cervix to stop sperm reaching an egg

As a result, the pill also thins the lining of the endometrium. The desogestrel progestogen-only pill can also stop ovulation in some cases.

Other forms of hormonal contraception include the contraceptive patch, vaginal ring, injection and the IUD. If you are using hormonal contraceptives, you should be aware that you are not currently experiencing a menstrual cycle.

Whatever form of contraception you choose is up to you. It's important, however, to do your research and to be aware of how your body and menstrual cycle might be affected today and in the future.

Did you know

During early trials of the pill, participants did not have a monthly bleed, which made some worry that they were pregnant. To build trust, the pill was altered to force monthly artificial bleeding. This means that any bleeding on the pill is not actually a period at all and is known as a withdrawal bleed.

THINKING ABOUT YOUR FERTILITY

Interview with Kate Davies, RN BSc (HONS) FP Cert, Fertility Nurse Consultant and IVF Coach. Co-Host of The Fertility Podcast

What fertility advice would you give to your younger self?

This is a great question! We spend so much time trying NOT to get pregnant, and clearly that's important when getting pregnant would be disastrous. However, we just don't give enough thought to how our lifestyle and environment, and the things we do or don't do, can impact on our fertility in the future. Protecting your future fertility is vital.

I'm currently on hormonal contraception and planning to come off it. What do I need to be thinking about?

If you're thinking about coming off contraception before you start trying to conceive, then you're making the right decision. After stopping hormonal contraception it can take a number of months for your fertility to return to normal and therefore you can use this time to get pregnancy ready and importantly start taking daily folic acid supplementation.

What can I do to increase my chances of conceiving?

One of the things that will make the biggest difference is to start tracking your cycles. Research tells us that fertility awareness education can reduce your time to conception significantly. Having an awareness of when you're fertile and when you ovulate is so empowering and Mother Nature has given us a super way of doing this. Start observing your natural fertility indicators – your waking temperature, cervical mucus and, if you wish, the changes in your cervix, throughout the month. With practice, you'll get to understand your body better and what your menstrual cycle is telling you, and from this information you'll be able to tell exactly when your fertile window is and when ovulation occurs, and make the most of this time!

What can I do in terms of habits, practices or lifestyle changes to boost my fertility?

There is SO much you can do. Eat a healthy diet – protein is your building block for good fertility – and keep your refined carbohydrates low. Take a daily folic acid and Vitamin D supplement. Reduce alcohol, don't smoke or take drugs. Enjoy moderate exercise and keep a healthy weight. Lastly, and importantly, make sure you're having regular sex – every 2–3 days through the cycle is perfect.

SPACE FOR NOTES

ENDOCRINE DISRUPTORS - WHAT'S IN YOUR VAGINA?

Because the vaginal walls are incredibly absorbent, it is important to note that any chemicals used in period products can make it into the bloodstream. Even a small amount can be damaging given the significant use of these products over a person's lifetime, and repeated exposure to chemicals found in period products, such as dioxin, can have a compounded effect over time.

'A woman uses approximately 11,400 tampons in her menstrual life, that's exposure to dioxins 11,400 times,' says Philip Tierno, a clinical microbiology and pathology professor at New York University. Chronic exposure increases our risk of cancer, causes oxidative stress and can disrupt our endocrine system.

So what's in a tampon?
In most cases, tampons are constructed from cotton and rayon. Rayon is a form of plastic which is usually treated with chemicals such as dioxin and phthalates and while cotton is a natural material, it is typically grown using pesticides and herbicides. These tampons are then bleached with chlorine. In addition to this, the bulk of tampons you will find in the supermarket have been treated with odour neutralisers and fragrances. So just like additives in our foods, we should be equally mindful about avoiding them when it comes to other areas of our bodies.

TOXIC CHEMICALS IN PADS AND TAMPONS

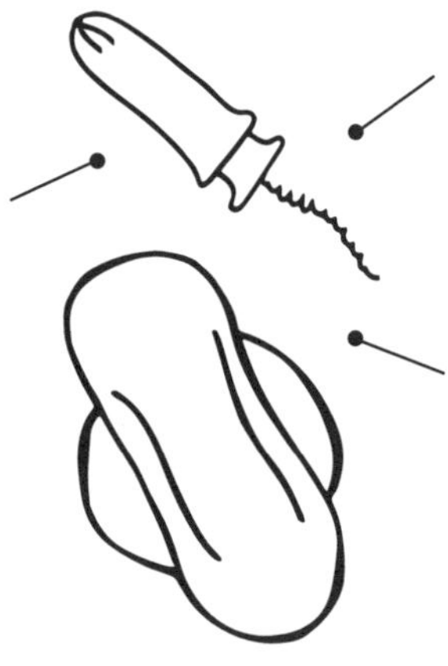

'Tampons and pads are bleached and contain a harmful chemical known as dioxin. Because our vaginal tissue is super sensitive, these chemicals can be absorbed. I have repeatedly found that women with heavy and painful periods see symptoms reduce and even disappear when they switch to 100% organic products or use menstrual cups or period underwear.'

– Nicole Jardim, The Period Girl, Fix Your Period.

Looking for a more natural approach to your period products? Try out the following:

Organic period products

90 per cent of a traditional period pad is made of plastic and that is the equivalent to 4 plastic bags in each pad. We now have access to 100% organic cotton period products (MyFreda, TOTM, HeyGirls, & Ohne to name a few) so shifting away from toxic chemicals and synthetic materials has never been easier.

Period underwear

The average woman throws away anywhere between 10,000 and 15,000 pads and tampons in her lifetime. Period underwear is a great reusable option allowing the wearer to free-bleed; then pop them in the wash just like their other clothes. You'll need between two and five pairs for the duration of your period, but they could last for years.

Menstrual cups

Menstrual cups are reusable and each one can last up to 10 years! A menstrual cup is a flexible silicone cup that can be folded up and inserted inside your vagina. The cup will collect your menstrual blood and needs to be emptied every 4–6 hours, depending on your flow.

Reusable pads

Reusable pads are an easy choice for people who are like the comfort and coverage of a conventional pad. The only difference with these is that they're reusable and can be washed, unlike traditional 'throw away' products.

IMPROVING HORMONE HEALTH

It can be daunting to think how interconnected our hormones and overall health can be. But if we look at this information as a form of empowerment, we can make choices that positively affect both our physical and mental wellbeing.

Hormones control nearly every aspect of how we feel and how our bodies function. While we can't identify or avoid everything that might disrupt this balance, we can focus on changes that are within our control.

A great place to start is with our diet and nutritional habits. In the next section of this journal, we will examine the relationship between our hormones and nutrition, and hear from experts on how we can easily improve the way we feel through what we eat.

Food and nutrition are just two pieces of the puzzle when it comes to reproductive health, but important ones nonetheless. You are unique and there isn't one diet that will work for everyone, but we will cover some core principals that can be of benefit and simple changes you might wish to try.

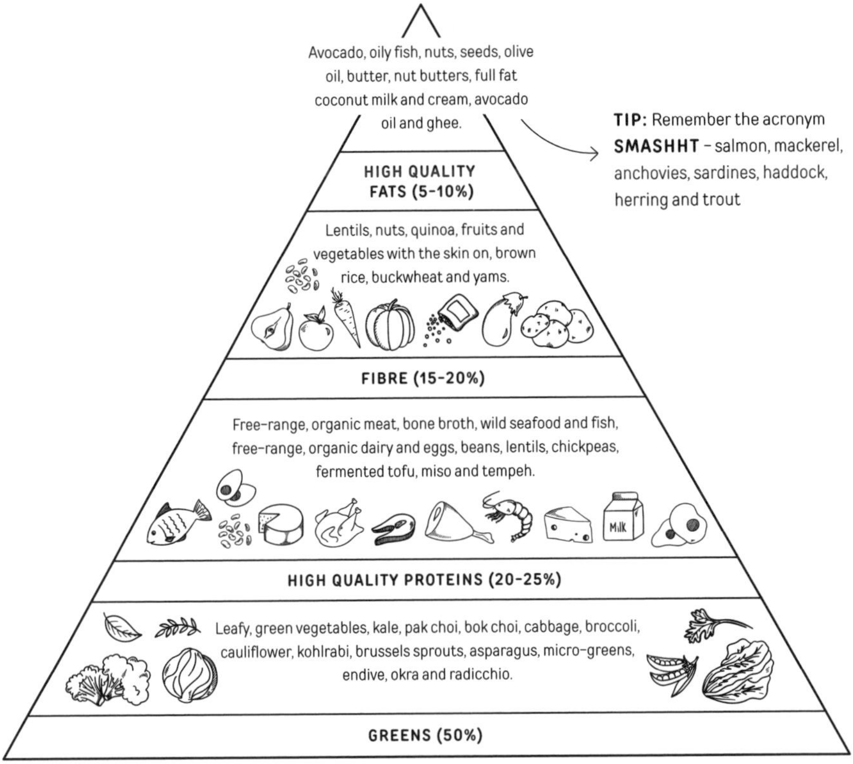

High quality fats: Support steroid hormone (oestrogen, testosterone, progesterone, cortisol) production and support egg quality in the ovaries.

Fibre: Supports the gut microbiome in breaking down oestrogen that the body has already used. Supports healthy digestion and daily bowel movements (removing hormones that our bodies have already used from our system). Slow carbohydrates support blood sugar balance and energy levels.

High quality proteins: Supports liver function, thyroid hormone conversion (important for ovulation!) and blood sugar balance.

Greens: Supports oestrogen detoxification in the gut, liver and overall immune health.

By Le'nise Brothers, Registered Nutritional Therapist @eatlovemove

BEST FOODS FOR EACH PHASE OF THE MENSTRUAL CYCLE

By Le'nise Brothers, Registered Nutritional Therapist @eatlovemove

Menstrual phase

The start of our menstrual cycle is when our bodies need extra support from the food we eat, more rest and more intentional movement. Being mindful about what we include in our meals during our periods can help during this time of shedding and letting go.

Adding in iron foods such as free-range, organic (or the highest quality in your budget!) red meat, the dark meat from poultry, clams and liver can help improve energy levels and support your body as it rebuilds the blood that has been lost during menstruation. If you tend towards plant-based options, try chickpeas, lentils, kidney beans, chard, kale and mustard greens instead. Make sure you eat these plant-based sources of iron with foods rich in Vitamin C like berries, citrus, peppers and broccoli which help increase iron absorption. Remember that spinach is not a great source of iron because it contains oxalic acid, which blocks most iron absorption.

Magnesium-rich foods such as dark, leafy greens, nuts and seeds can help even out moods and reduce menstrual cramps because of the relaxing nature of this mineral. Our oestrogen levels start to rise again midway through our menstrual cycle so adding phyto-oestrogen foods such as flaxseed, miso, fermented tofu and chickpeas can help.

Follicular phase

After our periods end, we move into our follicular phase, a time of growth and renewed energy. We can use food to support our rising oestrogen and testosterone levels and support our growing eggs. Pumpkin seeds, seafood and free-range, organic red meat all include zinc, which is brilliant for our immune system and healthy testosterone levels. Brightly coloured fruits and vegetables are full of antioxidants and fibre that keep us regular and balance out oestrogen in the body. Eggs (eat the yolks!) and liver are great sources of choline, a nutrient that supports the quality of the maturing eggs that are released from our ovaries each cycle.

Ovulation and Luteal phase

During ovulation and the early part of the Luteal phase, our energy levels peak and this is the time when many of us feel like our best and brightest selves! We're riding the wave of oestrogen and the peak of progesterone and the foods we eat now will have a beneficial effect on our menstrual and hormone health. Try adding in slow-releasing carbohydrates such as sweet potatoes, carrots, yams, quinoa and brown rice to manage rising energy levels (great for the cardiovascular workouts you might feel drawn to!). Fermented foods such as kimchi, sauerkraut, pickled vegetables, kefir and kvass are great to support gut health (when we support our gut health, we support our hormone, immune and mental health!) and brassicas (think cauliflower, broccoli, cabbage and asparagus) and dark leafy greens (kale, chard, spinach, watercress and collard greens) which are full of the fibre that keep us regular and get the hormones that our gut and liver have broken down out of our systems.

Late Luteal phase

We want to be really gentle with ourselves during this time, especially if we experience any of the symptoms of PMS: bloating, anxiety, pain, depression or cravings. The food we eat can really give us a helping hand now. Omega-3 foods like oily fish, seeds and algae help support mood and skin health. Wild salmon, organic poultry and almonds contain tryptophan, an amino acid that supports serotonin and melatonin production, i.e. it helps balance our moods and improves sleep.

NUTRIENTS TO HELP SUPPORT YOUR CYCLE

By Monica Grohne, Founder and CEO of Marea Wellness

In addition to being mindful of eating a Mediterranean, anti-inflammatory diet (let's not forget our healthy carbs and fats), supplementing commonly deficient and crucial nutrients can go a long way for menstruators. Let's take a look at some of these nutrients. Remember always consult your doctor before starting a new supplement regimen.

Magnesium

Magnesium is a magic mineral that helps to achieve the ultimate hormone balance between progesterone and oestrogen. Many find it necessary to supplement their diets with magnesium as it is depleted by the natural stress response and our modern diet can't always keep up with replenishing this mineral. Experiencing cramping, headaches or bowel issues? Magnesium can also help with these symptoms.

Zinc

Our bodies don't store zinc and yet it is a crucial mineral to produce, synthesize and transport our cycle hormones (FSH, LH, oestrogen, progesterone). [1] By supporting our ovarian follicles, zinc helps to support ovulation, which we know is crucial to a healthy cycle. Due to our bodies not storing zinc, it's key to nourish your body with this mineral daily.

Vitamin D

Many of us know the importance of Vit D has for our mood – but it also helps regulate our immune and hormone function making it a crucial nutrient for period health. Vit D also has a correlation to calcium absorption and is affected by magnesium deficiency. Our primary source of Vit D is the sun which many of us don't see enough of in our modern lifestyle.

[1] Jamilian M, Foroozanfard F, Bahmani F, Talaee R, Monavari M, Asemi Z. Effects of Zinc Supplementation on Endocrine Outcomes in Women with Polycystic Ovary Syndrome: a Randomized, Double-Blind, Placebo-Controlled Trial. Biol Trace Elem Res. 2016 Apr;170(2):271-8. doi: 10.1007/s12011-015-0480-7. Epub 2015 Aug 28. PMID: 26315303.

B Vitamins

Stress is a common theme and B vitamins can assist in reducing stress and supporting the regulation of our HPA axis (the central response system between hypothalamus, pituitary gland, and adrenal glands). These nutrients boost serotonin and GABA, known as the calming neurotransmitters. B12 can also help with fatigue as it delivers more oxygen to cells, boosting red blood cell count and increasing energy.

SEED CYCLING

Seed cycling (also known as seed rotation) simply means eating different types of seeds at key times in the menstrual cycle to boost the right hormones at the right time of the cycle.

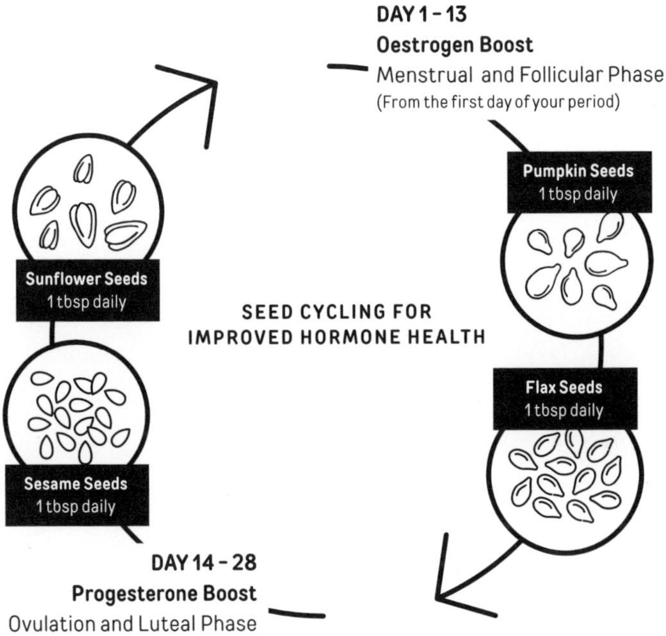

> 'I mix my seeds up in two tubs so they are ready to sprinkle on my food; I can then bung them in a smoothie or my porridge.'
>
> ***– Gemma Brown, The WellWoman project***

Water tracker

The fluid in our lymphatic system is 96% water and keeps everything running smoothly. It flows through the body, helping to flush out toxins and to deliver vital nutrients. Keep track of your daily water intake (recommended 8 glasses a day) by colouring in the tracker below.

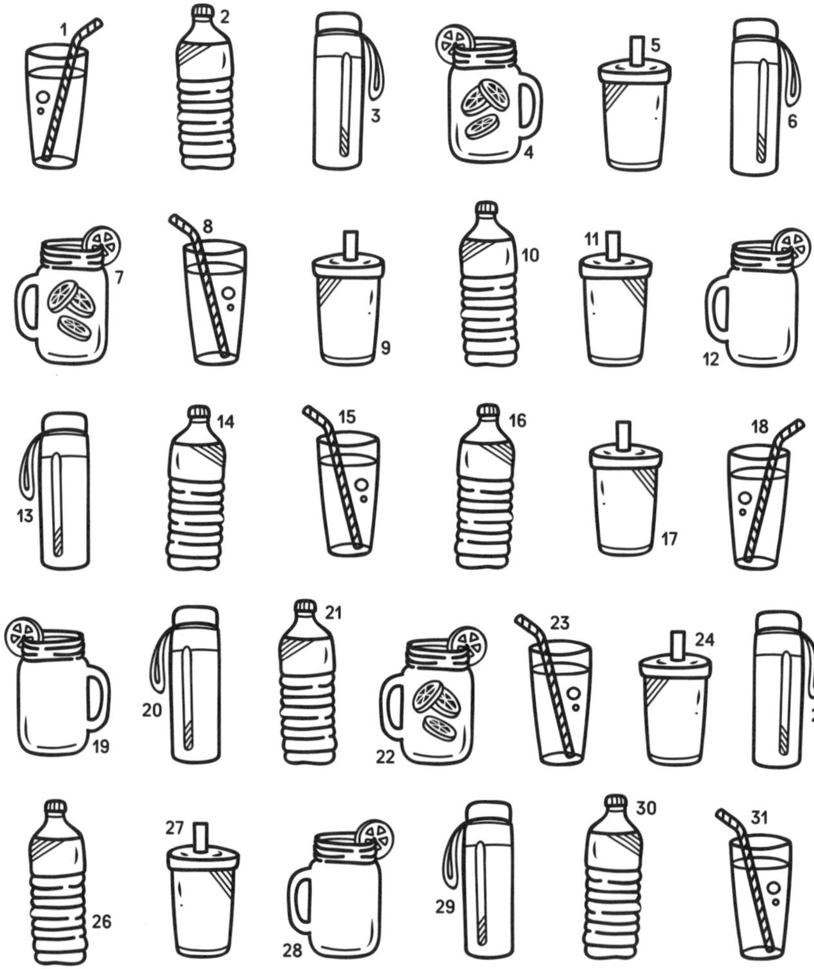

SPACE FOR NOTES

You and your cycle

'Active tracking helps everyone with a cycle to understand their bodies and to be empowered by that knowledge. To live in tune with their biology, not in spite of it. Clue helps people to understand their bodies and as a result, feel empowered to ask questions and seek answers. It also helps them advocate for their own health and notice when something is off.'

– Ida Tin, CEO of Clue

WHY TRACK AND THE BENEFITS

To truly understand your menstrual cycle will give you a clearer picture of your overall health and (as everyone is unique) what is normal for you. If you are practising cycle awareness, you are uniquely positioned to take control of how you manage your period and any symptoms, as well as to notice any changes that might require further investigation.

From a diagnostic point of view, having a consistent log of your cycle makes it easier to discuss patterns with your practitioner should you have any worries. It also helps you to optimise life choices around nutrition, exercise and managing stress.

There are additional benefits, such as avoiding or planning for pregnancy, as tracking important events, such as your period and ovulation, can help with identifying when you are most fertile. Whilst this journal will help you to identify these types of indicators, it is primarily focused on body literacy and menstrual cycle awareness. For information on tracking your cycle for fertility or as a natural form of contraception, we recommend checking out naturalcycles.com, which is a Fertility awareness-based mobile app designed specifically for contraception.

How?

The best place to start is logging the first day of your period, as this marks Day 1 of your cycle. To begin with, you may just want to track the duration of your period in the yearly Period Tracker and then advance to adding symptoms such as cramps, appetite, bloating, etc. into the daily reflection section of your journal, and then advance to using the All-in-One Cycle Tracker to capture symptoms. We would suggest logging three cycles of information, to help spot clear trends or patterns.

What?

While building a clear picture of your period is incredibly useful (and helps you prepare for your next period), it is just one part of your menstrual cycle. We encourage you to continue tracking outside of your period to better understand the changes that occur throughout the month. A good way to do this is to expand your tracking to other areas such as mood, diet and energy levels. These can all be good indicators of your hormonal fluctuations and how you respond to things like stress, exercise and food choices.

YOUR CYCLE

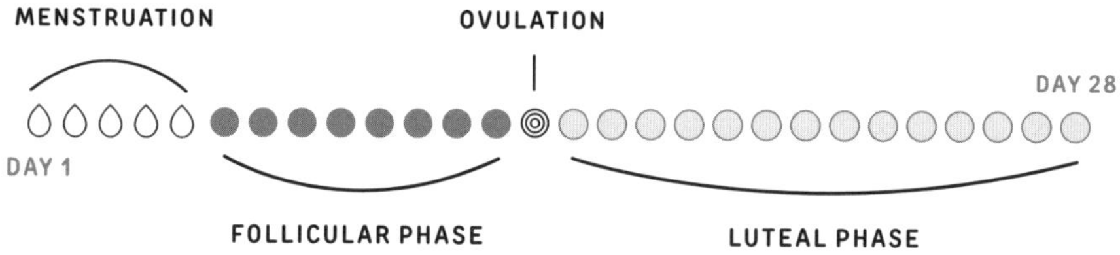

If you menstruate, you will (on average) have 350–400 periods in your lifetime starting from your first period (menarche) right through to menopause, over a period of about 35 years. Interestingly, our ancestors had far fewer periods, as on average women were pregnant for more of their fertile years and also entered menopause much earlier (40 versus the average age of 50 at present).

The average cycle is 28 days long with Day One being on the first day of real bleeding. It's worth noting that spotting doesn't actually class as your period.

Your menstrual cycle is made up of two phases. The first is the Follicular phase, menstruation and the preparation for ovulation. The second is known as the Luteal phase. This is the time from ovulation to menstruation and is when the body either houses a successful pregnancy or doesn't become pregnant and starts to shed the lining of the womb in preparation for menstruation.

The two main events of your cycle are your period and ovulation. Usually, it takes between 10 to 16 days from the release of an egg to the start of a period.

Please don't feel discouraged if your cycle is longer or shorter than the standard 28-day cycle. Cycle lengths can vary from person to person and can run for anywhere between 21–34 days.

AN INTRODUCTION TO CYCLE AWARENESS

In simple terms, cycle awareness is the process of tracking your period, but also your feelings and physiological changes throughout each of your monthly cycles. Although it can be seen as more of a nuisance, it's helpful to view your menstrual cycle as a natural diagnostic tool that takes place every month. Your period can be viewed as another one of your body's vital signs that can be an important indicator of your health and wellbeing.

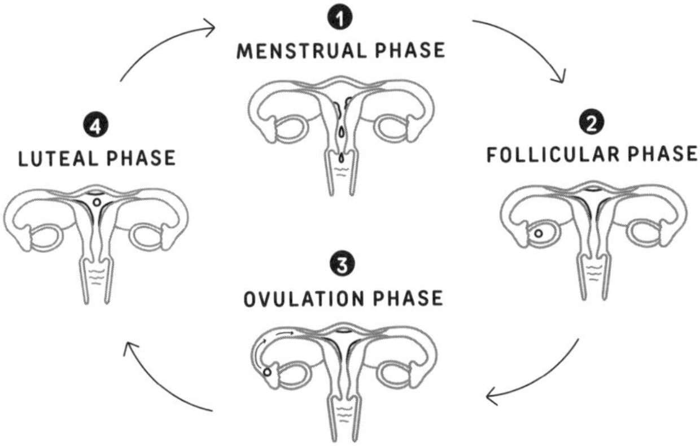

Most people think of their menstrual cycle only through the lens of their period but as you can see, this is just one part (albeit very important). With the changing phases, we should look to adapt our different activities and recognise the shifts in ourselves to promote our wellbeing and optimum health.

You may already be familiar with how your circadian rhythm affects your energy levels during the day and also how you feel with changing seasons of the year. Taking the same approach with your menstrual cycle will ground you in a form of body literacy that can be a firm foundation for your female health.

Let's take a closer look at the different seasons and what you can expect from each of them.

YOUR FLOW

A 'normal' amount of menstrual fluid loss during your period is understood to be between 5–80 ml. As a guide:

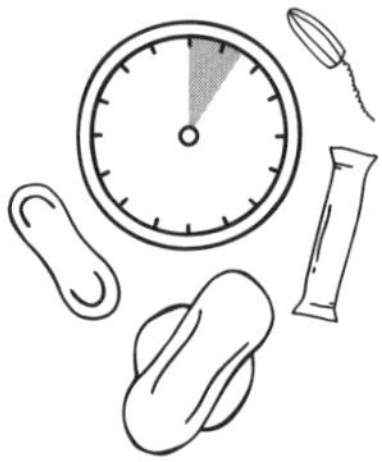

Severe vaginal bleeding means that you are soaking 1 or 2 pads or tampons in 1 or 2 hours.

Moderate bleeding means that you are soaking more than 1 pad or tampon in 3 hours.

Mild bleeding indicates that you are soaking less than 1 pad or tampon in more than 3 hours.

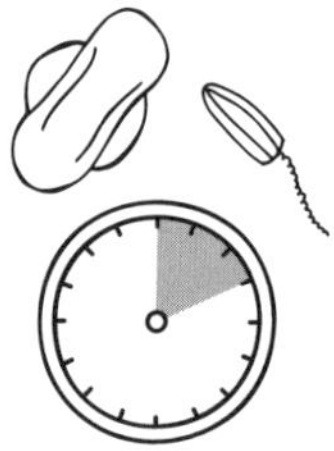

HOW DO I MEASURE BLOOD LOSS?

It can be hard to estimate how much menstrual fluid you produce during your period. One of the perks of a menstrual cup is that you are more accurately able to measure and also check on consistency, colour etc.

WHAT ARE HEAVY PERIODS? (MENORRHAGIA)

Heavy periods, or Menorrhagia as they are technically known, can interfere with your quality of life from an emotional, social, physical and psychological point of view.

- Over 6 tablespoons (80 ml) of blood loss in one cycle
- A duration longer than 7 days
- Passing of large clots of blood (bigger than 2.5 cm or a 10p coin)

It is not usually necessary to measure blood loss precisely, but if you are using a menstrual cup, that can work as a handy guide as most come with measurement indicators on the side. Some further signs that you might have heavy periods include:

- Having to change period products every 1 to 2 hours
- Needing to use 2 types of period products at the same time (e.g. pads and tampons)
- Bleeding into your clothes or bedding

Heavy periods are not always an indication that something serious is going on, but it is worth further investigation, as they can be a sign of:

- High levels of oestrogen or progesterone in the body
- Endometriosis
- PCOS
- Fibroids
- Pelvic inflammatory disease
- Insertion of an intrauterine contraceptive device (IUD)

In rarer cases, heavy periods can be due to thyroid problems, kidney or liver disease, endometrial cancer or blood clotting disorders. When severe, heavy periods can cause an iron deficiency (anaemia) in your body. You should consult with your doctor or medical health practitioner if you:

- Feel tired all the time
- Feel dizzy, faint or light-headed
- Feel breathless
- Aren't sleeping well
- Bleed after sex
- Bleed between periods
- Have periods that last longer than half the month

SPOTTING / MID CYCLE

Keeping track of any bleeding that occurs outside of your period, can be extremely important. Also referred to as spotting, this can have a variety of causes including (but not limited to) hormonal imbalance, pregnancy, infections or gynaecological cancers.

LIGHT OR NO BLEEDING

It is worth noting that many people experience lighter bleeding and some don't bleed at all while using hormonal birth control. Hormonal contraceptives work by thinning the lining of your uterus. This typically results in lighter, shorter periods or occasionally the complete absence of one.

If you are not taking any form of hormonal contraceptive and you experience infrequent or absent periods you should discuss this with your healthcare provider. From there, together you can explore a potential pregnancy or look at addressing causes such as stress, excessive exercising or diet.

Infrequent or absent periods is a common feature of with PCOS, see more on page 12.

COLOUR

Changes in the colour or consistency of your period blood are to be expected. The range in colours can tell you anything from the age of the blood to deficiencies or underlying conditions that you may be experiencing.

Bright red
This is indicative of a healthy period. A healthy blood colour ranges from bright red to dark red or brown depending on when the blood was shed from the uterus.

Light pink
It is common to see pink to light pink blood at the beginning or end of each cycle, and this is usually connected to a lower level of blood loss at these times. However, consistent light bleeding over multiple periods can be an indication of possible low oestrogen levels. Another symptom of low oestrogen levels is vaginal dryness so you may want to check in with your health provider if you notice both symptoms together.

Dark purple
This can be a sign of high oestrogen levels. Watch out for other symptoms associated with endometriosis, PCOS or ovarian cysts.

Brown/maroon

If found on your first day, this can be a sign of low progesterone levels. However, it could also be left-over blood from your last cycle and it's normal to see this at the beginning or end of your cycle.

Grey or orange

This could be a sign of infection or just your blood mixed with cervical fluid. Other signs of infection include irritation, pain, fever or a foul odour and shouldn't be left unchecked.

CLOTS

Do not be alarmed by clots in your menstrual blood. This is completely normal and more common around the heavier days of your period. In most cases, this involves darker period blood which has had time to build up, compared with faster-flowing, new blood.

You should talk with your healthcare provider if you notice the clots are larger than usual (golf ball size or bigger) or consistently around the size of a UK 10p coin or a US quarter (2.5 cm).

YOUR PERIOD WHILST ON HORMONAL BIRTH CONTROL

Contrary to popular belief, the bleed you experience while using hormonal birth control is not a real period and is actually what is known as a withdrawal bleed. Bleeding is triggered by the withdrawal of reproductive hormones delivered by your pill, patch or ring.

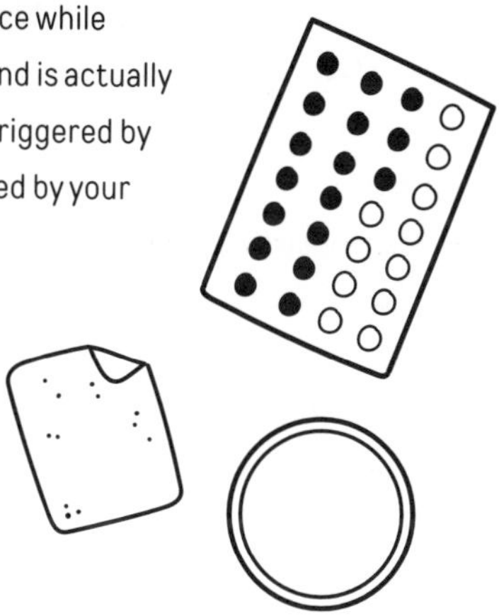

Tuning in to your period ♡

When did you start your first period?

How did you feel about it?

Who did you speak to about your period when you were younger?

Who do you speak to now about your period?

How do you feel when you get your period?

How does your mood evolve during menstruation?

What would your ideal period be like?

How would you describe your period?

Not quite sure how to answer some of these questions? Get more in tune with your period by using the Period Tracker in this journal.

Period Tracker

	Jan	Feb	Mar	Apr	May	Jun
1						
2						
3						
4						
5						
6						
7						
8						
9						
10						
11						
12						
13						
14						
15						
16						
17						
18						
19						
20						
21						
22						
23						
24						
25						
26						
27						
28						
29						
30						
31						

Notes

TIP: Shades of red will make it easier to note flow changes at a glance.

KEY

Add a colour code

- Heavy
- Medium
- Light
- Spotting

	Jul	Aug	Sep	Oct	Nov	Dec
1						
2						
3						
4						
5						
6						
7						
8						
9						
10						
11						
12						
13						
14						
15						
16						
17						
18						
19						
20						
21						
22						
23						
24						
25						
26						
27						
28						
29						
30						
31						

How to use the period tracker

Your period can be a key indicator of your overall health and wellbeing. The more intimately you get to know your body's patterns, by logging details of your cycle, the more familiar you will get with your own rhythm and the more easily you can recognise any trends or changes. You can get started by shading/colouring in this tracker with your period start date, blood flow, frequency and length. See the Your Flow section for more tips on what to note and how.

Notes

SISTERHOOD
The Journal

TRACKING YOUR

Cycle days

By knowing your cycle more intimately, you can get in sync with your body's individual rhythm and more deeply understand how your mind and body are impacted by your cycle. It also becomes easier to notice when something is amiss, which is vital because changes to the menstrual cycle are often the first indicator of an underlying health issue (even health issues that seem unconnected with the reproductive organs).

At a minimum, tracking the first day of your period will help you to spot irregularities with your cycle rhythm. However, by noting insights about your cycle over a 3-month timeframe, you can gather enough information to spot patterns, helping you to make your cycle work better for you. For instance, the more you know about how your moods and energy levels evolve within a cycle, the more easily you can prepare for them.

Tracking in this way will also help you to gather information about your symptoms, which you can share with your doctor, helping them to more easily differentiate between chronic issues and hormonal ones.

This 3-Month Daily Cycle Tracker is divided into the 4 seasons of the menstrual cycle – Winter, Spring, Summer and Autumn (see section on Menstrual Awareness for more details). It is best to start tracking on day 1 of your cycle – the first day of full period flow (i.e. spotting not included). There is enough space for you to make notes over 34 days for 3 full cycles.

As a typical cycle can run for up to 34 days, you may find that you require more space for your notes, in which case you can download additional tracking pages from our website.

Once you get your next period, you are at the start of your next cycle and should loop back to the beginning of this section (Winter) to start making notes on this new cycle. Set some time aside every day to make notes about your experiences. It might feel like a big commitment initially but you will soon get into the swing of it. It can be worth tracking with a friend so you can keep one another motivated and share what you are discovering with each other.

Some examples of things to track include:

- Blood flow and colour
- Mood evolution through your cycle
- Appetite
- Energy levels
- Spatial awareness / balance
- Your skin and hair
- Headaches
- Pain
- Digestive and respiratory issues

Once you have tracked for 3 full cycles, you can use the Reflection section at the end of each season to look back and identify key observations, patterns and learnings. When you have finished the 3-Month Daily Cycle Tracker, you can progress to the All-In-One Monthly Cycle Tracker section. Use these trackers to monitor your entire cycle on a single page, making it easier to compare one cycle with the next at a glance.

MENSTRUATION

Winter

‘Our winter serves us by allowing us to mourn what hasn’t gone our way and no longer serves us, as well as connecting us to our deepest, most authentic needs and desires. Set an intention to allow everything that arises during this season and ease into it over several cycles. Know that you need to feel it, to heal it. If you’re craving more clarity and purpose: embracing the depths and ebb of winter are key.’

– Pia Stanchina, Life and Business Coach @piastanchina

Winter starts a couple of days before the first day of your period and marks the beginning of your cycle. Winter is a time for you to nurture yourself, prioritise self-care, and ultimately rest and repair. This is when your oestrogen and progesterone levels are at their lowest and this may manifest as extreme fatigue, anxiety, tearfulness. In order to prepare for this season, you should know roughly when you are due for your period and make sure you have created space in your schedule for that time. Even if you can't get away with doing absolutely nothing, planning some 'downtime' will still be beneficial. Taking a break from exercising or going for gentler forms such as light cardio, yoga or walking can help you to conserve energy.

In the later stages of your period or Winter, your oestrogen levels start to increase. You might notice your energy levels lifting and that you feel more upbeat. Winter presents a great opportunity for general reflection, including looking back at your menstrual cycle notes and comparing them to previous cycles for similarities and differences.

Tasks

- [ ] Make sure you are stocked up with food and meals. Batch cooking and freezing meals in your Autumn is a good way to prep for when you don't feel up to it in Winter.

- [ ] Relax in a luxuriously warm scented bubble bath.

- [ ] Burn some scented candles, read a book and turn off your devices. Escape from the pressures of the world to focus on yourself.

CYCLE DAY *one*

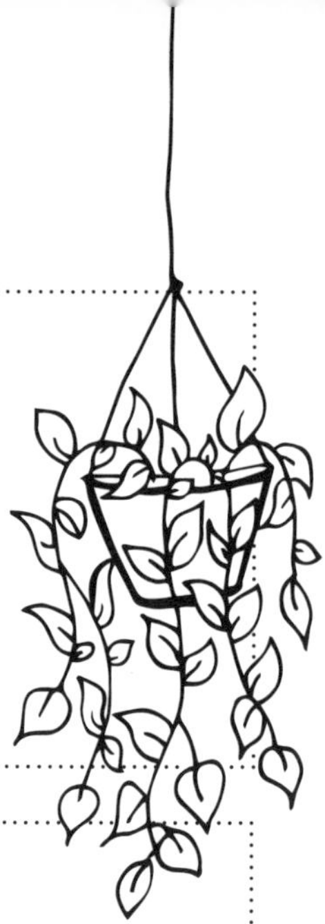

Date: / /

It's common to lack energy on day 1 as your oestrogen levels will be at their lowest. If your energy is low and you feel more vulnerable, lean into that feeling and don't push yourself. You may find your sensitivity makes you more aware of details that may have gone unnoticed previously. Replenish with iron-rich food and stock up on anti-inflammatory food such as ginger, turmeric, berries and oily fish.

Date: / /

Date: / /

CYCLE DAY *two*

The second day usually yields the heaviest flow. But even if this is the case, you still may feel a bit more relaxed as oestrogen levels start climbing again and PMS symptoms subside. If you are passing small clots, don't worry. That's perfectly normal for this point in your cycle.

Date: / /

Date: / /

Date: / /

CYCLE DAY *three*

A vaginal pH of 3.5 – 4.5 is a sign of a good balance between good and bad bacteria. However, blood has a pH of 7.4, so during your period, vaginal pH can become elevated. With all those tampons and extra blood flow, this can lead to increased vulnerability to yeast infections. Make sure to change your pad, tampon or period pants regularly or opt for a menstrual cup instead. An over-the-counter probiotic or foods such as yoghurt or sauerkraut, and avoiding high sugar foods can also help.

Date: / /

Date: / /

Date: / /

CYCLE DAY *four*

Date: / /

From day 4, your period usually starts to lighten up and may change in colour from bright red to brown. You may want to get back out there and get on with life, as it can be hard to allow ourselves to rest. Try to ignore the FOMO and take time for some self-care. A goddess bath with essential oils and candles is the perfect way to rest and renew!

Date: / /

Date: / /

CYCLE DAY *five*

Date: / /

This is a good time to focus on creative projects or connect with loved ones. Sleep might be a bit off in the first week of your cycle too; try lavender oil or limit screen time to help you switch off at night.

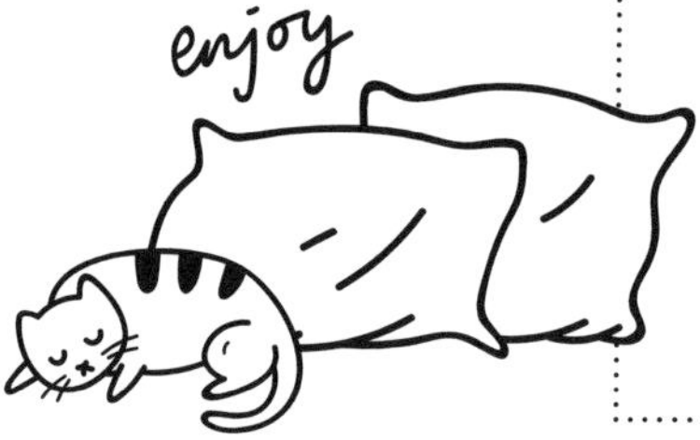

Date: / /

Date: / /

CYCLE DAY *six*

Your mood should be starting to lift as your oestrogen levels increase. Your flow may start to ease off now if it hasn't already.

> 'When you bleed, take the time to slow down and get a little self-indulgent while your body does its magic. Drench yourself in love. I can't remember exactly when it changed, but I found that when I started thinking of my period in a more appreciative way, it became kinder to me. Try it.'
>
> ***– Dominique Tipper, Actress***

Date: / /

Date: / /

Date: / /

CYCLE DAY *seven*

You should be starting to feel like your normal self now and possibly a bit more optimistic than usual. You can thank the increasing levels of oestrogen for newly found energy or motivation.

Date: / /

Date: / /

Date: / /

CYCLE DAY *eight*

Date: / /

Energy might be on the up but your body is still getting over menstruation. We are so used to being irritated by our periods that when they stop, we launch straight back into our hectic schedules. You are prone to injury and burnout around this time, so stretch out and pace yourself!

Date: / /

Date: / /

WINTER REFLECTION

Look back over each day of your cycle.

What similarities and differences do you notice month to month?

What do you notice about your mood, feelings and energy levels?

What did you struggle with?

What did you enjoy or do you want more of?

ABOUT YOUR PERIOD

How much blood do you lose each period?

What do you notice about the colour and consistency of your blood?

What might it look like to love having your period?

Self-care checklist

- ☐ Tried something new
- ☐ Gave someone a hug
- ☐ Treated myself
- ☐ Did some exercise
- ☐ Laughed a lot
- ☐ Wrote a gratitude list
- ☐ Had a long soak in the bath
- ☐ Had a manicure/pedicure
- ☐ Drank lots of water
- ☐ Listened to music
- ☐ Had some nourishing veg
- ☐ Went for a walk
- ☐ Messaged a friend
- ☐ Went to bed on time
- ☐ Read a book
- ☐ Applied a face mask
- ☐ Gave myself a compliment
- ☐ Watched a film

'Self-care, ultimately, is about taking the time to be comfortable and know yourself. In order for your self-care strategy to be tailor-made for you, work out what brings you peace. What gives you comfort? Start from there. For me, it's a solo trip to an art gallery. Time with my thoughts amongst beautiful art.'

– Ann Akin, Actress

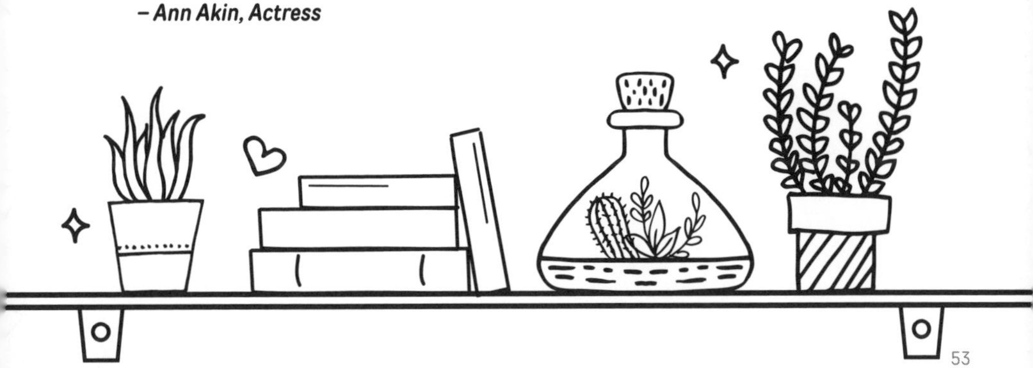

PRE-OVULATION

Spring

‘Aiming for results and outcome is premature and shuts down all the potential and possibility of this spring phase.’

– Alexandra Pope and Sjanie Hugo Wurlitzer, Wild Power

You will start to enter Spring around the time your period comes to an end. For most, this is around day 6 or 7, but this may differ if you have a shorter or longer period. Spring is pre-ovulation, during which the body starts to produce more oestrogen, to prepare for a potential pregnancy.

Your testosterone levels also begin to increase and you may notice that you feel more positive, energised and motivated, and like taking initiative. Your oestrogen levels peak in the later stages of Spring, usually Day 10 onwards. This is when you feel at your sexiest and most fertile. Your orgasms may also be at their most intense and attainable.

Spring is a time of 'build-up' and you may notice that you are more in tune with the practical parts of your life and also the bigger plans you may have for the future. It's important to note that the move from Winter (menstruation) to Spring (pre-ovulation) can leave you vulnerable and prone to burn out. If you start to find yourself becoming overwhelmed or losing focus, it could be a sign to pull back a bit.

Tasks

☐ Now is a great time to explore any ideas you've been having. You'll be naturally curious at this point in the cycle and you'll be in your element writing your journal or creating some to-do lists.

☐ Anaerobic exercise, such as running, spinning, weights, HIIT and swimming, is a good fit for this season.

CYCLE DAY *nine*

Those follicles are gearing back up and preparing to release an egg. As the egg develops, it produce oestrogen. While oestrogen levels starts to rise, testosterone and progesterone levels will stay the same. Take advantage of the extra energy you will be experiencing now.

Date: / /

Date: / /

Date: / /

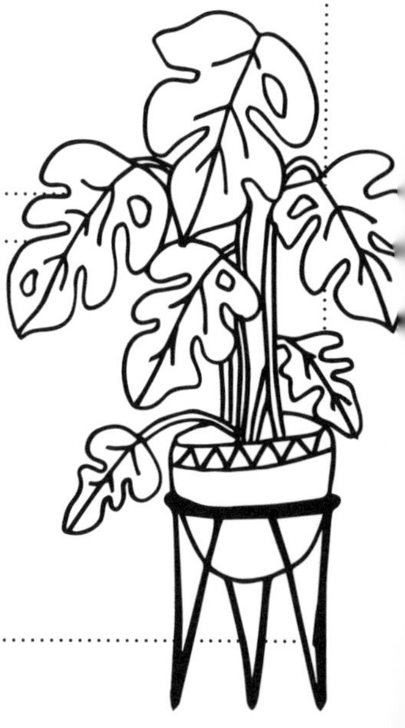

CYCLE DAY *ten*

Your spring phase is a great time to learn something new. The increased level of oestrogen energises your brain, piques your interest, and helps to keep your memory extra sharp.

Date: / /

Date: / /

Date: / /

CYCLE DAY *eleven*

Date: / /

If you're trying to conceive, now's the time to kick your efforts into high gear, since you're either ovulating or getting close to ovulation. Your cervical mucus is flowing and stretchy! It's a great time for some batch cooking whilst you are feeling more productive and creative. That way you will benefit from healthy, homemade food waiting in the freezer for when your next period arrives.

Date: / /

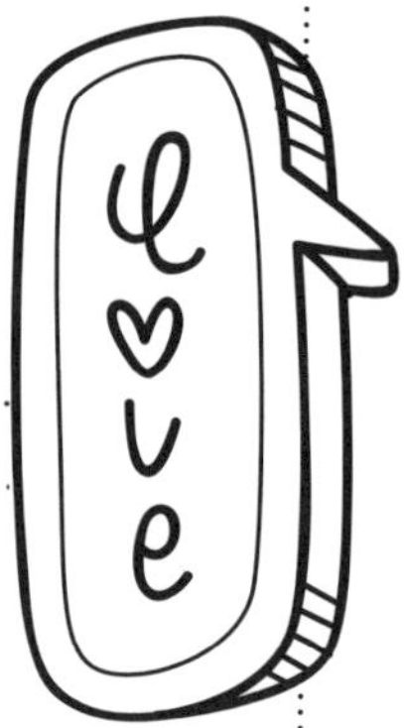

Date: / /

CYCLE DAY *twelve*

Date: / /

Feeling loved up? You may notice increased libido around this time, as testosterone levels are surging. You're also extra chatty and social, so grab some mates or get out on a date. If you are an athlete, you may notice an improvement in performance around this time of your cycle.

Date: / /

Date: / /

CYCLE DAY *thirteen*

Our oestrogen levels peak just before ovulation and then drop suddenly just after. Take this as your last day to tackle any difficult or complex tasks. Cervical fluid is most favourable for conceiving. Be warned, the spike of oestrogen can mean a lot of energy and lead to anxiety if not monitored. Maintain intentional breath work and try not to overwork yourself.

Date: / /

Date: / /

Date: / /

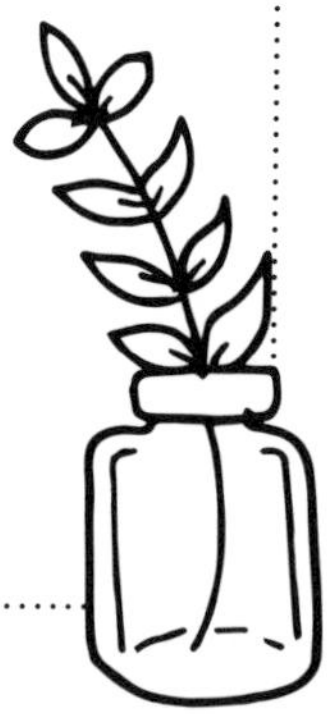

SPRING REFLECTION

Look back over each day of your cycle.

What similarities and differences do you notice month to month?

What do you notice about your mood, feelings and energy levels?

What did you struggle with?

What did you enjoy or do you want more of?

OVULATION

Summer

'Right before ovulation, your estrogen levels are going to rise and peak. And that means increased collagen production, so prepare to shine! You might want to get your hands on a gentle exfoliant because this phase really emphasizes cell turnover and skin renewal.'

– Isabel Ho, beautywithinofficial.com

You are approaching the halfway point and oestrogen should peak (around day 12 in a 28-day cycle), combining with testosterone and the luteinising hormone to trigger ovulation. You may notice that you feel and look good, and now is the perfect time to socialise or put yourself out there. Your confidence and communication skills will be at their highest, thanks to testosterone, which plays a role at this time.

Now is when you may lean more into your inner extrovert before you feel more like retreating, in Autumn and Winter. After the natural high of ovulation (around day 12), hormone levels will start to dip again, and mood and energy levels usually follow. However, testosterone and progesterone continue to surge, so you might notice an increase in appetite and excess oil on the skin, which can lead to breakouts and higher sensitivity.

Tasks

- ☐ Meet up with some friends and plan something a little different. Now is when you feel your most adventurous, so take advantage!

- ☐ Got an important meeting or interview? Try to schedule it in your Summer period when you'll be feeling your best.

- ☐ Towards the end of summer, you may want to take specific notice of how you feel during your transition into Autumn, as this can be a sensitive time.

CYCLE DAY *fourteen*

Date: / /

The dominant follicle releases the egg for its journey down the fallopian tube. The egg will live for 12 to 24 hours, while sperm can survive for 3 to 5 days. Cervical fluid should be stretchy like egg whites. You may feel a twinge of pain or have a little spotting, which is perfectly normal.

Date: / /

Date: / /

CYCLE DAY *fifteen*

Hello, progesterone. Goodbye, oestrogen. Oestrogen levels plummet as progesterone begins to take its place. You may be a bit irritable, but don't worry – oestrogen will be back soon.

Date: / /

Date: / /

Date: / /

CYCLE DAY *sixteen*

It's getting hot in here. With increased amounts of progesterone, you may notice your body temperature sits a little higher than usual.

Date: / /

Date: / /

Date: / /

CYCLE DAY *seventeen*

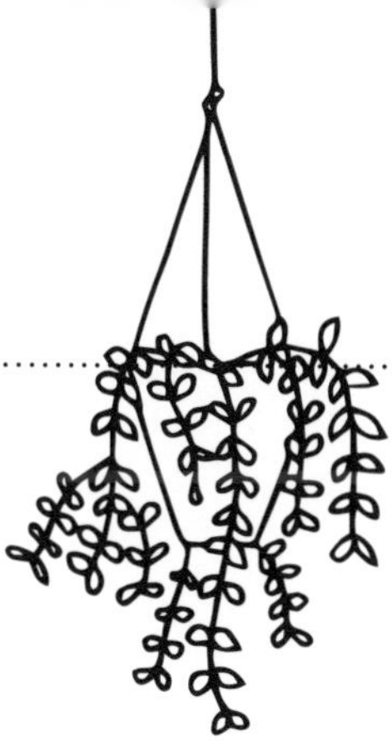

Date: / /

The lining of the uterus is getting thick. If the egg has successfully united with sperm, it will soon make its home there. If conception hasn't taken place within 24 hours of ovulation, the egg will die. Oestrogen levels are on the way down, while progesterone levels are sky-high.

Date: / /

Date: / /

CYCLE DAY *eighteen*

Date: / /

Now oestrogen will start to make its comeback. Progesterone levels are still up there. It is worth noting that during the Luteal phase, the body is not best primed for high-intensity training.

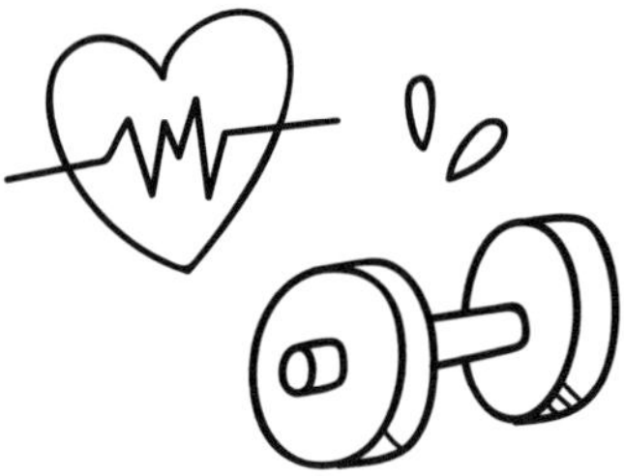

Date: / /

Date: / /

CYCLE DAY *nineteen*

Easy with the girls. The hormones in your system increase blood flow to your breasts and may cause them to be fuller but extra sensitive.

Date: / /

Date: / /

Date: / /

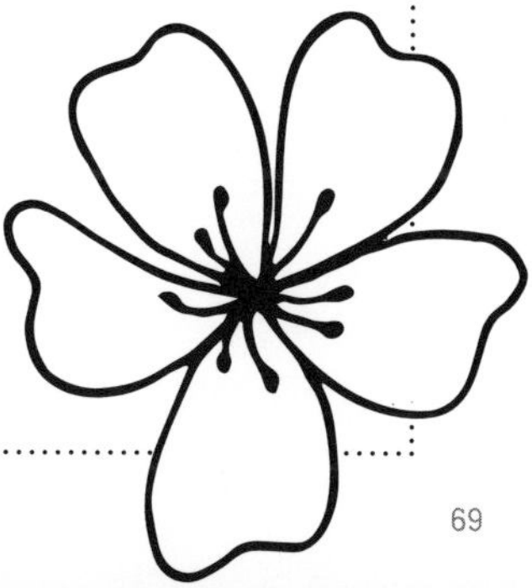

CYCLE DAY *twenty*

Date: / /

If your egg hasn't been fertilised, then your body will call it quits on producing oestrogen. This is when PMS comes into play.

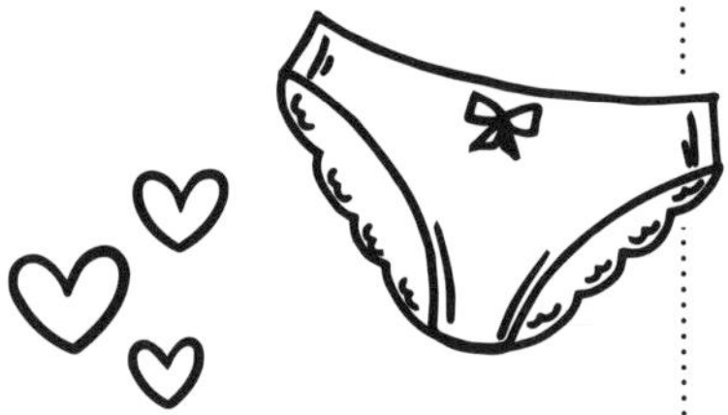

Date: / /

Date: / /

CYCLE DAY *twenty one*

Try to start planning for your upcoming period. Now is the time to clear the diary, stock up on nutritious food and tie up any loose ends.

Date: / /

Date: / /

Date: / /

SUMMER REFLECTION

Look back over each day of your cycle.

What similarities and differences do you notice month to month?

What do you notice about your mood, feelings and energy levels?

What did you struggle with?

What did you enjoy or do you want more of?

SPACE FOR NOTES

PREMENSTRUAL

Autumn

'The premenstrual phase often gets a bad reputation (think PMS, bloating, mood swings). But what if we looked at it as a teacher? You'll notice it is a fertile ground to learn to trust your instinct, let go of what no longer serves you and stand your ground.'

– Maria Carmen Punzi, Menstrual Health Researcher @periodswithmariacarmen

The transition from Summer to Autumn occurs after ovulation, but how long after ovulation varies from person to person. In the middle of the Luteal phase (which is the second half of your cycle), progesterone starts to take over and there will be a peak around Day 21. With progesterone dominating in this phase, you might experience a drop in energy and a shift in mood. In contrast to how sociable you felt in Spring and Summer, you might feel more like retreating. On the plus side, this need to be alone can manifest itself as a sense of productivity or extreme focus. Whether it's finishing up a project or finally getting around to sorting through your bills, doing this ahead of entering your Winter season will make you feel like a productivity pro!

Whilst you may be busy being busy, emotions can creep up on you, making you feel out of sorts. Mood swings, teary outbursts or complete meltdowns can be the result of hormone fluctuations, as can bloating and low libido at this time. It is important, though, not to be dismissive about how you are feeling just because you might be approaching 'that time of the month'.

Tasks

- ☐ Have a good declutter! This can be therapeutic as you cleanse and clear your space, but can also set you up perfectly to relax, reducing anxiety and stress in the run-up to your period.

- ☐ It is important to stay hydrated, to beat the bloat.

- ☐ Exercise such as light yoga, walking and swimming can help ease symptoms like cramps and breast soreness.

CYCLE DAY *twenty two*

Date: / /

You're getting sleepy. Today your progesterone levels are at their max, which may equate to an increased tendency to fall asleep in the middle of that super-exciting board meeting.

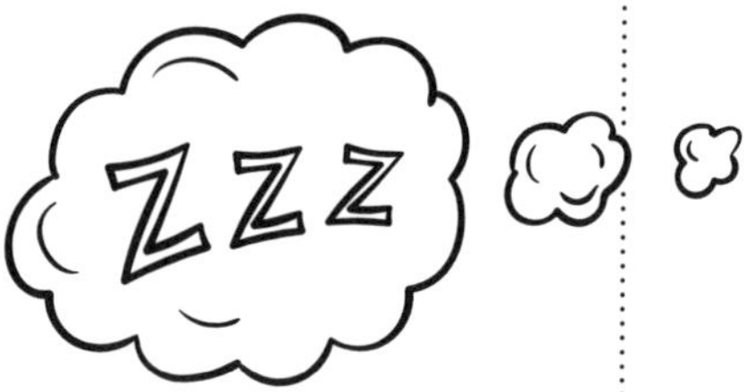

Date: / /

Date: / /

CYCLE DAY *twenty three*

PMS is in full swing. Be gentle with yourself (and others!) today.

Date: / /

Date: / /

Date: / /

CYCLE DAY *twenty four*

Reschedule your waxing appointment. At this time, your body is more susceptible to pain than during other times of the month. Avoid tweezing, waxing or laser hair removal.

Date: / /

Date: / /

Date: / /

CYCLE DAY *twenty five*

Date: / /

This will probably be your worst PMS day. Expect some bloating and don't be surprised if you're feeling extra sensitive or a little weepy.

Date: / /

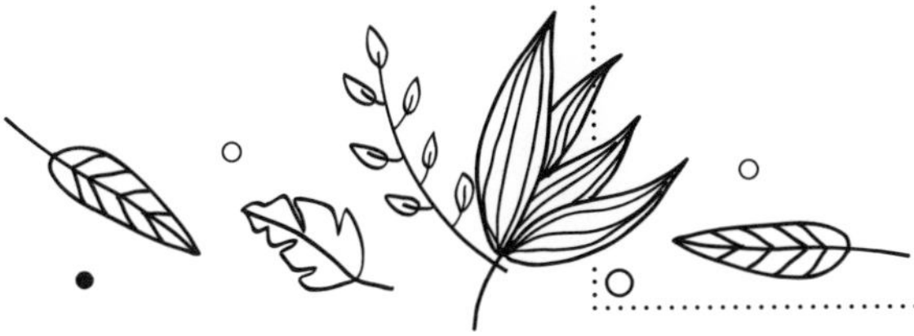

Date: / /

CYCLE DAY *twenty six*

Date: / /

Now is not the time for dieting. Thanks to premenstrual fluid retention, you could see up to 4.5 kgs/10 lbs on the scale today. With all the hormone changes, our bodies tend to hang on to extra water in our system. One of the most ironic cures? Drink more water and go easy on the salt.

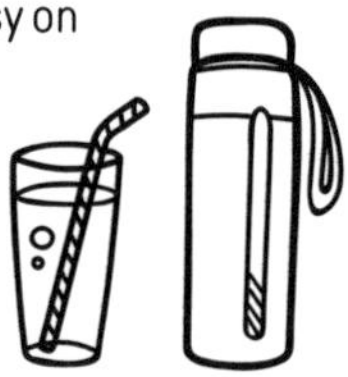

Date: / /

Date: / /

CYCLE DAY *twenty seven*

Got the munchies? At this point in your cycle, your oestrogen (and consequently serotonin) levels are bottoming out. That means you're craving carbohydrates and sugar, which can give you that serotonin hit. Many women experience menstrual cramps a day or two before their period begins. This is because your body has begun producing prostaglandins, which help your uterus contract.

Date: / /

Date: / /

Date: / /

CYCLE DAY *twenty eight*

Date: / /

At this point in your cycle your testosterone levels are higher than oestrogen and progesterone. This causes more stimulation of sebum and a higher chance of cystic acne, oily skin and large pores.

Date: / /

> 'If you notice acne as a precursor to your menstrual cycle, be proactive and up your routine the week before. Reach for an exfoliating mask, a salicylic cleanser or topical retinol to kill bacteria, unclog pores and eliminate excess oils.'
>
> ***– Monica Grohne, Marea Wellness***

Date: / /

CYCLE DAY *twenty nine*

The menstrual cycle is typically described as lasting for 28 days. This means there are 28 days between Day 1 of your period and Day 1 of your next period. Not everyone has this textbook cycle. Your cycle might run for 21–34 days. If your period has started again (bleeding not spotting), go back to the start of this section and begin tracking your next cycle!

Date: / /

Date: / /

Date: / /

CYCLE DAY *thirty*

Date: / /

Try to focus on eating healthily and give any foods that can exacerbate cramps a miss e.g. caffeine. Foods that help to boost serotonin and your libido, and combat fatigue are leafy greens, pumpkin seeds and dark chocolate.

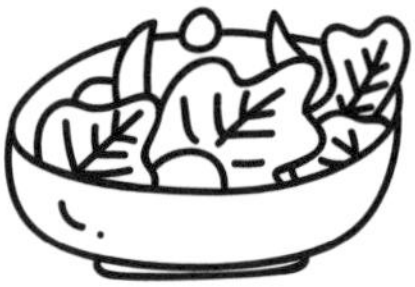

Date: / /

Date: / /

CYCLE DAY *thirty one*

Your energy levels tend to drop at this time as your body prepares for another period cycle. So try to take it easy and opt for lighter exercise such as walking, stretching or gentle yoga.

Date: / /

Date: / /

Date: / /

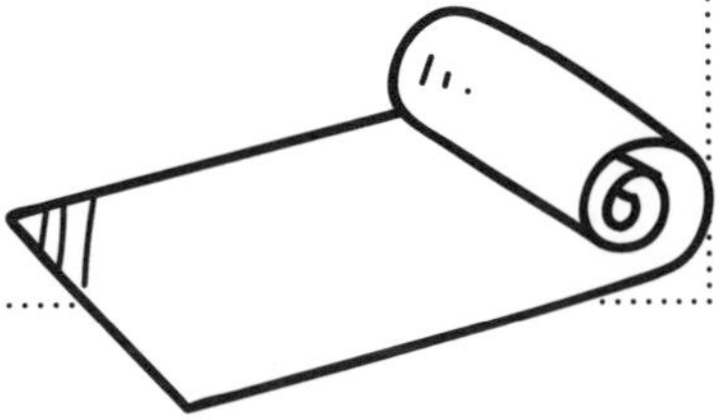

CYCLE DAY *thirty two*

Date: / /

Wondering why you've been dropping things lately? This could be linked to the drop in oestrogen and progesterone experienced in the run up to your period, which can affect coordination. You might feel more clumsy than usual.

Date: / /

Date: / /

CYCLE DAY *thirty three*

Less talked about than cramps and bloating, anxiety is actually another symptom of PMS. This includes nervousness, increased tension and worrying. Experiencing a bit of anxiety 1–2 weeks before your period is fairly common. If you are concerned about the impact of anxiety on your life, don't hesitate to seek support from your doctor.

Date: / /

Date: / /

Date: / /

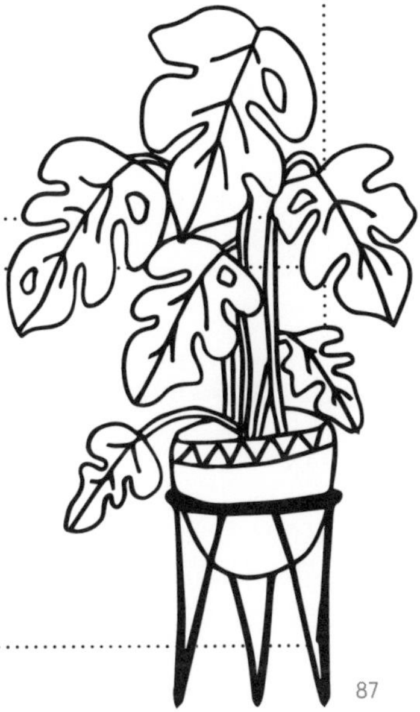

CYCLE DAY *thirty four*

Higher levels of progesterone can have a sedative effect on the body so you may find yourself benefiting from a more refreshing and deeper sleep.

Date: / /

Date: / /

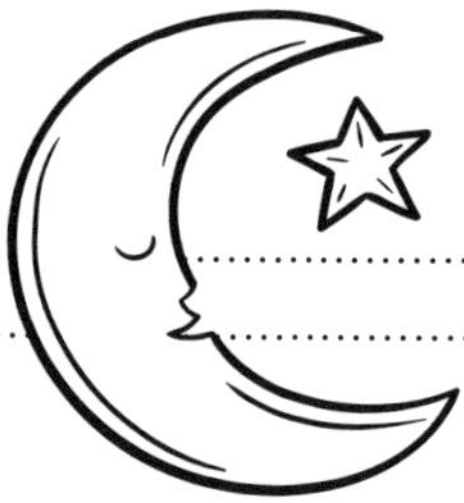

Date: / /

AUTUMN REFLECTION

Look back over each day of your cycle.

What similarities and differences do you notice month to month?

What do you notice about your mood, feelings and energy levels?

What did you struggle with?

What did you enjoy or do you want more of?

DAILY TRACKING

Summary

Now that you have been writing your journal for your last three cycles, you should have built up a pretty consistent picture of the changes you experience and how they make you feel. Below are some questions to help you explore and identify any patterns. There may also be things that you haven't noticed previously, but now make sense as you take the time to reflect.

- Were there any days that seemed to be consistently difficult?
- What days did I regularly feel at 'my best'?
- How were my transition days? (on an average 28-day cycle, transition days usually fall on Day 6, 12, 20 and 28)
- What activities helped me deal with stress?
- Are there any consistent triggers that make me feel down?
- When did I feel most sociable?
- When did I want alone time? What did that look like?

Want to carry on with your daily journal-writing exercise? Head over to wearethehood.com/dailies to download and print out our free templates. Alternatively, you can use the notes section at the back of this journal.

SPACE FOR NOTES

HOW TO

track monthly

Our monthly trackers are designed to support you through your menstrual cycle. You will be able to keep track of your cycle days and period, but we have also left some blank space for you to include whatever you would like to chart. From your daily journal writing, you may have noticed changes at specific times in your cycle. The monthly tracker is a great way to explore further and understand any patterns that may be linked.

Additional things you may like to track could include:

- Exercise
- Sleep – did you get your 8 hours?
- Libido/Sex – When are you having it?
- PMS symptoms – Cramps, spotting, breast tenderness, headaches, etc.
- Skin health – When does hormonal acne show up? Or when is your skin dry/oily/normal?

Take advantage of the larger areas for note taking, colours to reflect your mood or simply one word to summarise how you feel that day.

We recommend you start on Cycle Day 1 (the first day of your period) for a complete view of your cycle on each page. Try to chart at the same time each day; we recommend just before going to bed. Don't worry if you forget or skip a day occasionally.

KEEPING TRACK

Creating your own key for use throughout this journal will make it simple for you to track and compare your periods and symptoms, and how you're feeling from cycle to cycle.

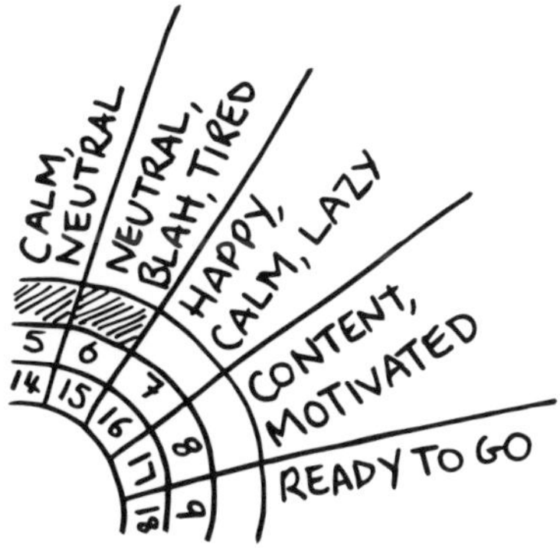

COLOUR CODE

Personalising your journal with colour will make it easier to log your observations, identify patterns and spot changes, and compare trends at a glance.

Period	**Add your own**	
Heavy	○ ______	○ ______
Medium	○ ______	○ ______
Light	○ ______	○ ______
Spotting	○ ______	○ ______

FEELINGS

In addition to tracking your symptoms, you will gain deeper insights into how your mind and body work by noting down how you're feeling from day to day. Here are a few useful prompts to get you started.

yay	*hey*	*meh*	*ugh*	*wah*
Confident	Happy	Neutral	Tired	Stressed
Motivated	Relaxed	Lazy	Irritable	Emotional
Focused	Balanced	Disconnected	Sensitive	Vulnerable
Energetic	Calm	Bored	Discouraged	Anxious
Productive	Present	Distracted	Overwhelmed	Sad
Purposeful	Satisfied	Blah	Insecure	Numb

TIP: Contrasting colours will help you to identify a trend more easily. Stick to a base colour for consistency so it's easier to compare month on month.

Space for observations

Period

Cycle Day

Day

1 2 3 4 5 6 7 8 9 10 11 12 13 14 15 16 17 18 19 20 21 22 23 24 25 26 27 28 29 30 3

Cycle 1

Track your period and habits

Time to reflect

What are the biggest insights I have gained over this cycle?

How have my symptoms, mood, feelings and energy levels evolved throughout?

What did I struggle with most? What am I most concerned about?

What do I want more of? What am I most excited about?

What can I release or let go of?

On a scale of 1–10, how do I feel about this cycle overall?

1 2 3 4 5 6 7 8 9 10

Space for observations

Period

Cycle Day

Day

1 2 3 4 5 6 7 8 9 10 11 12 13 14 15 16 17 18 19 20 21 22 23 24 25 26 27 28 29 30 3

Cycle 2

Track your period and habits

Time to reflect

What are the biggest insights I have gained over this cycle?

How have my symptoms, mood, feelings and energy levels evolved throughout?

What did I struggle with most? What am I most concerned about?

What do I want more of? What am I most excited about?

What can I release or let go of?

On a scale of 1–10, how do I feel about this cycle overall?

1 2 3 4 5 6 7 8 9 10

Space for observations

Period

Cycle Day 1 2 3 4 5 6 7 8 9 10 11 12 13 14 15 16 17 18 19 20 21 22 23 24 25 26 27 28 29 30 31

Day

Cycle 3

Track your period and habits

Time to reflect

What are the biggest insights I have gained over this cycle?

How have my symptoms, mood, feelings and energy levels evolved throughout?

What did I struggle with most? What am I most concerned about?

What do I want more of? What am I most excited about?

What can I release or let go of?

On a scale of 1–10, how do I feel about this cycle overall?

1 2 3 4 5 6 7 8 9 10

Space for observations

Period

Cycle Day

Day

1 2 3 4 5 6 7 8 9 10 11 12 13 14 15 16 17 18 19 20 21 22 23 24 25 26 27 28 29 30 31

Cycle 4

Track your period and habits

Time to reflect

What are the biggest insights
I have gained over this cycle?

How have my symptoms, mood,
feelings and energy levels
evolved throughout?

What did I struggle with most?
What am I most concerned about?

What do I want more of?
What am I most excited about?

What can I release or let go of?

On a scale of 1–10, how do I feel about this cycle overall?

1 2 3 4 5 6 7 8 9 10

Space for observations

Period

Cycle Day 1 2 3 4 5 6 7 8 9 10 11 12 13 14 15 16 17 18 19 20 21 22 23 24 25 26 27 28 29 30 31

Day

Cycle 5

Track your period and habits

Time to reflect

What are the biggest insights I have gained over this cycle?

How have my symptoms, mood, feelings and energy levels evolved throughout?

What did I struggle with most? What am I most concerned about?

What do I want more of? What am I most excited about?

What can I release or let go of?

On a scale of 1–10, how do I feel about this cycle overall?

1 · 2 · 3 · 4 · 5 · 6 · 7 · 8 · 9 · 10

Space for observations

Period

Cycle Day

Day

1 2 3 4 5 6 7 8 9 10 11 12 13 14 15 16 17 18 19 20 21 22 23 24 25 26 27 28 29 30 31

Cycle 6

Track your period and habits

Time to reflect

What are the biggest insights I have gained over this cycle?

How have my symptoms, mood, feelings and energy levels evolved throughout?

What did I struggle with most? What am I most concerned about?

What do I want more of? What am I most excited about?

What can I release or let go of?

On a scale of 1–10, how do I feel about this cycle overall?

1 2 3 4 5 6 7 8 9 10

Space for observations

Period

Cycle Day 1 2 3 4 5 6 7 8 9 10 11 12 13 14 15 16 17 18 19 20 21 22 23 24 25 26 27 28 29 30 31

Day

Cycle 7

Track your period and habits

Time to reflect

What are the biggest insights
I have gained over this cycle?

How have my symptoms, mood,
feelings and energy levels
evolved throughout?

What did I struggle with most?
What am I most concerned about?

What do I want more of?
What am I most excited about?

What can I release or let go of?

On a scale of 1–10, how do I feel about this cycle overall?

1 ····· 2 ····· 3 ····· 4 ····· 5 ····· 6 ····· 7 ····· 8 ····· 9 ····· 10

Space for observations

Period

Cycle Day

Day

1 2 3 4 5 6 7 8 9 10 11 12 13 14 15 16 17 18 19 20 21 22 23 24 25 26 27 28 29 30 31

Cycle 8

Track your period and habits

Time to reflect

What are the biggest insights I have gained over this cycle?

How have my symptoms, mood, feelings and energy levels evolved throughout?

What did I struggle with most? What am I most concerned about?

What do I want more of? What am I most excited about?

What can I release or let go of?

On a scale of 1–10, how do I feel about this cycle overall?

1 · 2 · 3 · 4 · 5 · 6 · 7 · 8 · 9 · 10

Space for observations

Period

Cycle Day

Day

1 2 3 4 5 6 7 8 9 10 11 12 13 14 15 16 17 18 19 20 21 22 23 24 25 26 27 28 29 30 3

Cycle 9

Track your period and habits

Time to reflect

What are the biggest insights I have gained over this cycle?

How have my symptoms, mood, feelings and energy levels evolved throughout?

What did I struggle with most? What am I most concerned about?

What do I want more of? What am I most excited about?

What can I release or let go of?

On a scale of 1–10, how do I feel about this cycle overall?

1 2 3 4 5 6 7 8 9 10

Cycle 10

Track your period and habits

Space for observations

Period

Cycle Day

Day

1 2 3 4 5 6 7 8 9 10 11 12 13 14 15 16 17 18 19 20 21 22 23 24 25 26 27 28 29 30 31

Time to reflect

What are the biggest insights I have gained over this cycle?

How have my symptoms, mood, feelings and energy levels evolved throughout?

What did I struggle with most? What am I most concerned about?

What do I want more of? What am I most excited about?

What can I release or let go of?

On a scale of 1–10, how do I feel about this cycle overall?

1 2 3 4 5 6 7 8 9 10

Space for observations

Period

Cycle Day 1 2 3 4 5 6 7 8 9 10 11 12 13 14 15 16 17 18 19 20 21 22 23 24 25 26 27 28 29 30 31

Day

Cycle 11

Track your period and habits

Time to reflect

What are the biggest insights I have gained over this cycle?

How have my symptoms, mood, feelings and energy levels evolved throughout?

What did I struggle with most? What am I most concerned about?

What do I want more of? What am I most excited about?

What can I release or let go of?

On a scale of 1–10, how do I feel about this cycle overall?

1 2 3 4 5 6 7 8 9 10

Space for observations

Period

Cycle Day

Day

1 2 3 4 5 6 7 8 9 10 11 12 13 14 15 16 17 18 19 20 21 22 23 24 25 26 27 28 29 30 31

Cycle 12

Track your period and habits

Time to reflect

What are the biggest insights I have gained over this cycle?

How have my symptoms, mood, feelings and energy levels evolved throughout?

What did I struggle with most? What am I most concerned about?

What do I want more of? What am I most excited about?

What can I release or let go of?

On a scale of 1–10, how do I feel about this cycle overall?

1 2 3 4 5 6 7 8 9 10

Getting to know you

'I believe true freedom, with regards to our physical health, will only come when we are fully aware of our own bodies – ultimately, we must be responsible for ourselves. For me, this means educating ourselves, connecting with our own body's rhythms and listening to its needs. And I would suggest we start with sex. Not because it is more important than knowing about our gynaecological or reproductive health – but because, I believe, it's where the deepest stigma lies. Only when women, and men, can free ourselves from this acute shame, steeped in historical judgement – will we be truly free to be intimate with others and ourselves. And when I say ourselves – I really do mean 'ourselves'. Starting with self pleasure. If you don't know how to give yourself pleasure, you shouldn't assume someone else will automatically be able to. Learn how to do it yourself so that you can tell your partner exactly what you like and not have to compromise.'

– Mika Simmons, The Happy Vagina

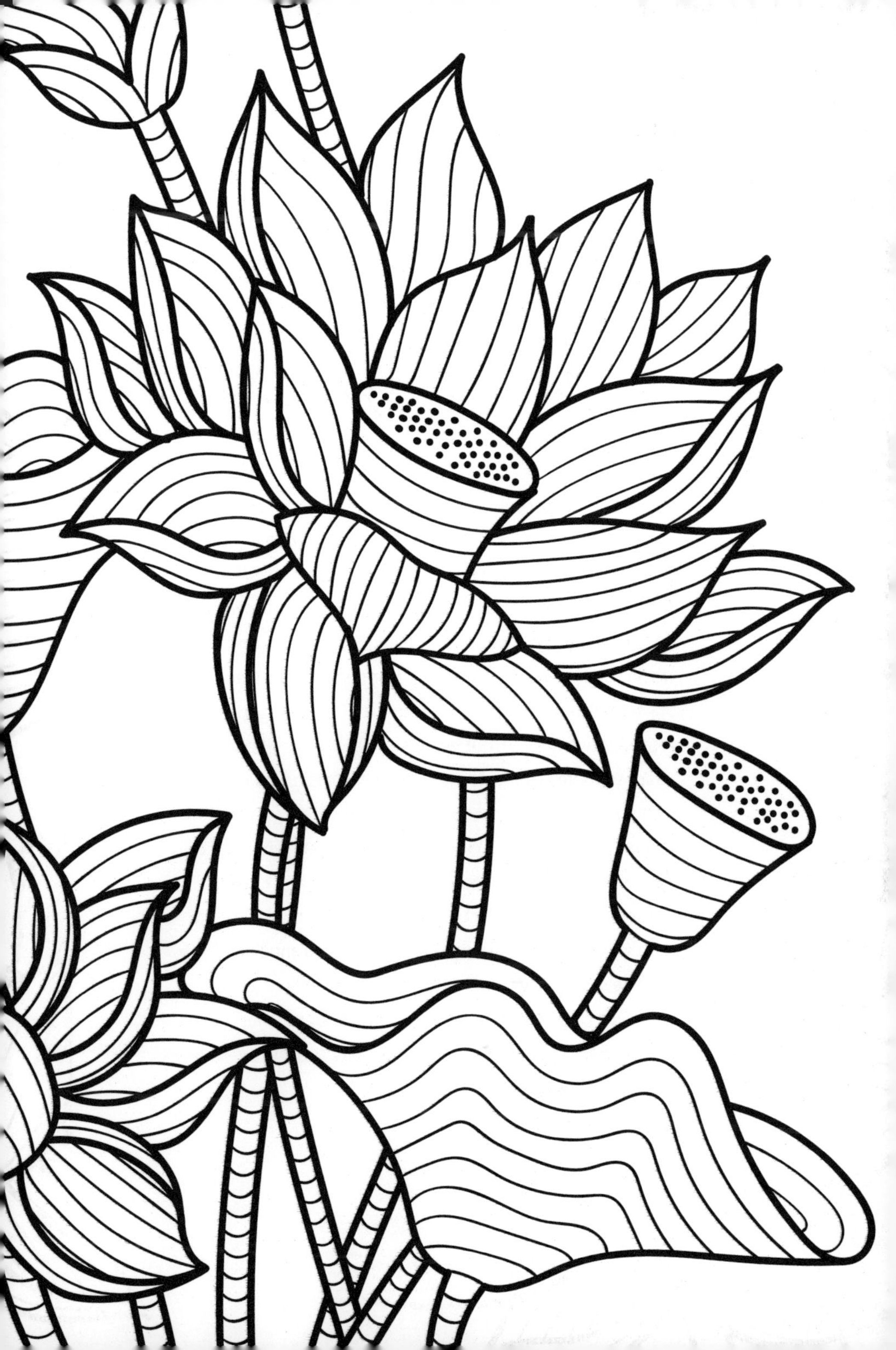

SPACE FOR NOTES

SPACE FOR NOTES

SPACE FOR NOTES

Want to go digital?

If you would prefer to replace or complement your offline period tracking with an online solution, here are a few apps you might like to check out and what they are known for:

Symptom tracking

Clue

MyFlo

Period Tracker Period Calendar

Eve by Glow

Moody Month

Fertility

Glow

Ovia

Perimenopause

mySysters

Athletes

FitrWoman

Teens

MagicGirl

Books we love ♡

Period Power
Maisie Hill

Wild Power
Alexandra Pope and
Sjanie Hugo Wurlitzer

Sweetening the Pill
Holly Grigg-Spall

The Period Repair Manual
Lara Briden ND

50 Things You Need To Know About Periods
Claire Baker

Your Period Handbook
Natasha Richardson

Invisible Women
Caroline Criado Perez

This Is Your Brain On Birth Control
Sarah E Hill

Hormonal
Eleanor Morgan

Code Red
Lisa Lister

The Fifth Vital Sign: Master Your Cycles & Optimize Your Fertility
Lisa Hendrickson-Jack

It's About Bloody Time, Period.
Emma Barnett

Fix your period
Nicole Jardim

The Vagina Book: An Owner's Manual for Taking Care of Your Down There
Thinx

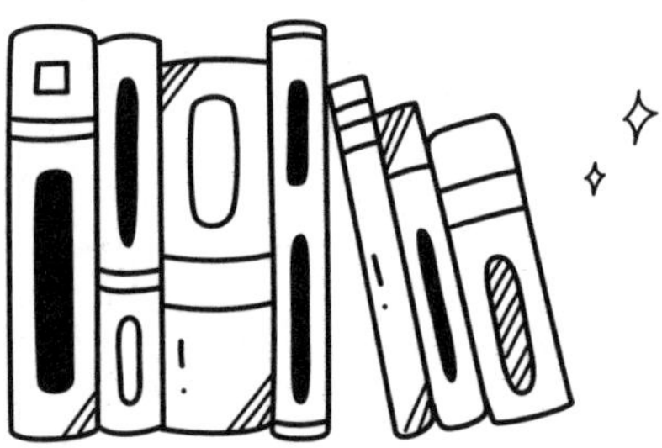

Resources

BLOGS AND WEBSITES

Endometriosis

peacewithendo.com

endometriosis-uk.org

PCOS

pcosdiva.com/category/blog

pcosnutrition.com

verity-pcos.org.uk

PMD/PMDD

iapmd.org/blog

iapmd.org/provider-directory

Menopause

drannacabeca.com/pages/blog

thebms.org.uk

Fibroids

floliving.com/guide-to-fibroids

britishfibroidtrust.org.uk/index.php

Hormones

happyhormonesforlife.com/blog

nicolejardim.com/blog

mareawellness.com/blogs/news

PODCASTS

The Fertility Podcast

thefertilitypodcast.com

Holistic Wellness

holisticwellness.ca/podcast

The Happy Vagina

thehappyvagina.co/podcast-1

Eat Love Move

eatlovemove.com/period-story-podcast

SISTERHOOD

The Journal

First published 2020

Published under licence by Brown Dog Books and
The Self-Publishing Partnership, 7 Green Park Station, Bath BA1 1JB
www.selfpublishingpartnership.co.uk

ISBN printed book: 978-1-83952-241-3
Printed and bound in the UK
This book is printed on FSC certified paper

FSC
www.fsc.org
MIX
Paper from responsible sources
FSC® C114687

Blind Faith

By the World's Worst Treasure Hunter
(Possibly maybe)

NAMBAN TETSU IN
Japanese under water.

THANKS FOR YOUR SUPPORT

SUUNTO UK www.suunto.com

0three custom drysuits www.0three.co.uk

Daniel Surf www.danielsurf.com

Aquascan International www.aquascan.co.uk

The Ginger witch R.I.P

All Plymouth Dive centres and charter boats.

My great family x x x x

Front Cover: Some random passer by.

Disclaimer

First let me state that no fish or marine life was hurt during the making of this book.

Some of the activities in this book are not normal scuba diving practises as taught at your local dive school. You will not find the ways of the adventurer, searcher or treasure hunter in your sports diving manuals. The path we follow and the way we dive is not without risk. A good way to avoid risk and disappointment is to stick to diving known wrecks on a certified charter diving boat. This book is written in a certain style, with a warts and all attitude that may not suit all readers. There will be spelling mistakes, punctuation mistakes and possibly the odd word missing. The book is written in the same tone as the Blair Witch project and Donnie Darko. Be aware it lives on the edge of copy right and slander, to anyone who feels they might have a copy right issue we are happy to offer a discount off your book purchase. If this offends or upsets anyone please accept our apologies, this was not our intention. Treasure hunting in the UK is fantastic! But it does come with a certain wealth warning. Sadly some of the characters in this book our addicts; they are addicted to drinking tea. They have been advised to go to Rehab, but they said No No No. If you find yourself enjoying our story, and you are inspired to take up underwater treasure hunting, we are very sorry but we cannot accept any responsibility for this.

Captain Black.
Take everything, give nothing back.

This is an OCD free product.

Statement of Significance

The Dutch East India Company (VOC, Verenigde Oostindische Compagnie), Founded in 1602 and dissolved in 1795, was a Dutch trading company. It was the largest and most impressive of the early modern European trading Companies having sent almost a million Europeans to work in the Asia trade on 4,785 ships.6 The Company's extensive archives, registered by UNESCO as part of the Memory of the World programme, have allowed for Comprehensive study of VOC operations which have been widely published (See, for example, Prakash 1994 and Blak *et al* 2007).

The basic VOC trading pattern was to export silver and gold to Asia, and with this to purchase and return to Europe valuable spices, silks and porcelain which would then be sold at auctions. Silver was particularly important as it was much more valuable in Asia than in Europe, so it's mere transportation to the East realised a profit (Marsden 1997: 91).

Archives of the Dutch East India Company, Nomination submitted by Netherlands in 2002 forinclusion in the UNESCO Memory of the World International Register.

Although the return voyages to Asia in support of Company activities were long ones, they rarely ended fatally. Out of a total of 8000 voyages (including those under the earlier Voorcompagnieën), less than 8% (*i.e.* 1 in 12½) came to an untimely end (source: www.vocshipwrecks.nl) For a number of reasons (principally associated with the survival of documentary evidence and the reputation of these vessels as treasure ships) the wreck sites of many Dutch East Indiamen have been investigated around the coasts of Europe, Southern Africa and Western Australia. As a group, they indicate graphically the commodities and products involved in this commerce and the extent of VOC operations.

The wrecks of Dutch VOC ships in British waters form an important subcomponent of discovered maritime archaeological sites, and include the designated *Kennemerland*, wrecked on Skerries in 1664 and the *Hollandia*, lost off St. Agnes in 1743. In all, England's National Monuments Record (NMR) records 26 Dutch VOC losses in English waters dated from the *Golden Lion*, lost in 1592, to the loss of the *Zeelilie*, lost in 1795.

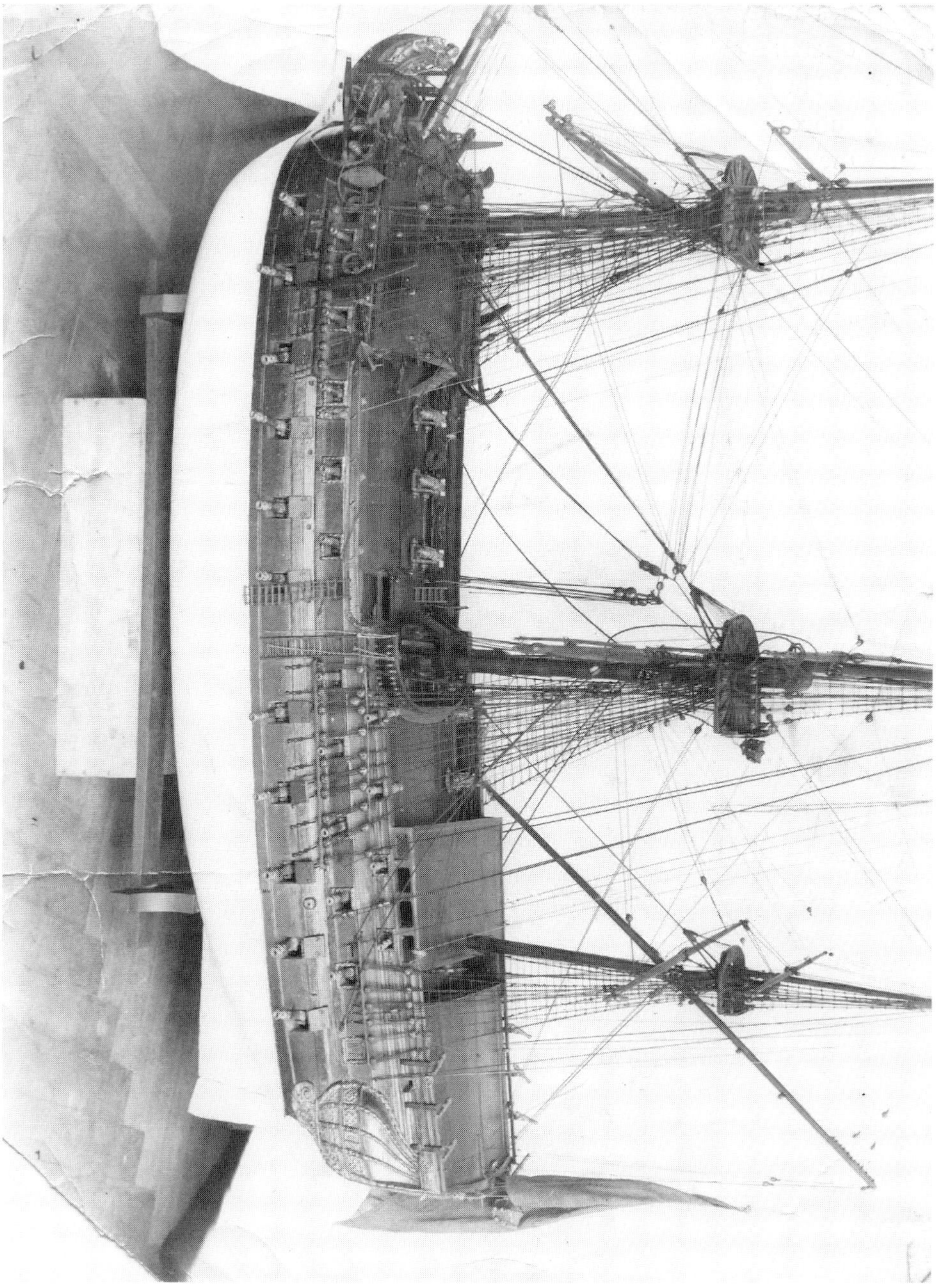

Plymouth Maritime History Timeline

6500 BC	Britain became an island when the channel plains flooded with rising sea levels.
2500 BC	Bronze age settlement at Sutton Pool.
9th century	Plymouth is known as Tamaworth. Vikings raided Britain. Vikings fleet wrecked of Mount Batten Plymouth. King Alfred raised a navy to counter this and the first sea battle against them is thought to have been fought in 875 AD. Vikings sail inland up the river Tamar.
11th century	Plymouth becomes a major fishing port.
1066	Northern Britain was attacked by King Herald of Norway and Tostig Godwinson in 300-500 ships. The Norman conquest of England, in the autumn of 1066, occurred after a seaborne invasion at Hastings.
1147	A fleet of 167 ships sailed from Dartmouth on a crusade to capture Lisbon from the Moors.
1211	Tamarworth becomes known as 'Plym Mouth'
1241	William Maurice was convicted of piracy and is the first person known to have been hanged, drawn and quartered.
1254	Plymouth is granted a charter.
1339	18 French ships attack Plymouth houses burning several down.
1340	During the Hundred Years' War (1337-1453) the French fleet was initially stronger than the English one, but was almost completely destroyed at the Battle of Sluys.
1362	Tarrit is the first shipwreck recorded in Plymouth.
1337	Plymouth is sacked by the French.
14th	Century Edward III's navy had 712 ships.
1408	The post of "Lord Admiral of England" was created.
1453	The Hundred year war ends.

1545	The Admiralty was set up as the King's Council of the Marine.
1509 and 1511	The Mary Rose was built in Portsmouth for Henry VIII. She was the flagship of his navy and one of the first with gun ports. She was rebuilt in 1536. Mary Rose sank on 19 July 1545 off Portsmouth.
1542	Francis Drake was born in Tavistock. He later sailed on the first English slaving voyages, taking Africans to the New World. Drake attacked Spanish ships sailing back from South America laden with silver. He took their treasure for himself and his queen.
1554-1618	Walter Raleigh was a favourite of Queen Elizabeth. He built a warship which he named the "Ark Raleigh" later changed by the queen to the Ark Royal. He is generally credited with introducing tobacco and potatoes to Britain from America.
1578	Sir Francis Drake in the course of his circumnavigation of the world discovered Cape Horn at the tip of South America. The sea between this and Antarctica is now known as Drake Passage.
1588	The Spanish Armada sailed against England and consisted of about 130 warships and converted merchant ships. It was attacked by an English fleet of about 200 vessels. A fire ship attack drove the Spanish ships from their anchorage. The Armada attempted to return to Spain by sailing around Scotland but many ships were wrecked off Ireland.
1596.	Drake died at sea in Nombre de Dios bay, Panama in January. 1578 The first modern underwater boat proposal was made by the Englishman William Bourne who designed a prototype submarine. Unfortunately for him these ideas never got past the planning stage.
1599	The Honourable East India Company was set up, also the Hudson's Bay Company.
	In 1600 Queen Elizabeth had given the Honourable East India Company the right to trade east of the Cape of Good Hope. By 1804 the company's fleet from India was said to be worth £6M.
1620 to 1624	The first modern submersible to be actually built was that of Cornelius Drebbel, a Dutchman. Its exact design is not known but versions were tested in the River Thames.
1620	The Mayflower sailed from Plymouth. The connection between the American colonies and Britain, with shipping as its cornerstone continued to grow unhindered for almost two hundred years.
1652 to 1653	The First Anglo–Dutch War was fought between. Battles were fought at Dungeness, Portland, the Gabbard and Scheveningen.
	William, Prince of Orange lands at Brixham Devon and his fleet is welcomed into Plymouth sound.
1689	HMS Centurion and HMS Henrietta are wrecked on rocks at Mount Batten.
1690	1st day of the fourth month privateer Black Pearl wrecked off shipwreck cove.
1691	HMS Coronation wrecked off Penlee Point.
1699	The first offshore lighthouse was that built on the Eddystone Rocks.

17th century	Trade expanded with. The Royal African Company which had a monopoly of the African trade until 1712 but there was much privateering. Later a major part of this trade was in the "Triangular trade" which involved taking goods from Britain to West Africa, slaves from Africa to the West Indies and America, then sugar to Britain. The main ports involved were London, Bristol and Liverpool and Plymouth.
1721	Dutch East Indian (VOC) ship Aaktekerke is wrecked off Plymouth.

Move forward nearly 300 years

April 2008 Captain Black started to take treasure hunting a bit more serious and devote lots of time plus resources to identifying three good targets.

April 2009 lead a expedition to dive on the VOC wreck site of the "De Liffe" wrecked in 1711 on the Shetland Islands. Found the site of the wreck and had a fantastic weeks diving. He learned a few valuable lessons, the first being research is very important. The second is look for a target closer to home, so if you find your a shipwreck you actually have time and resources to do something about it. Third lesson choose your team wisely, you need a good crew with tight lips. Next lesson, which I must admit was learned quicker by Mr Green than by myself, metal detectors are the absolute weapon of choice.

And last but by no means the least, enjoy yourself, have fun and let your dreams and imagination run wild. Reality is much less exciting place to dive, who cares about the truth live the dream.

May 2009 Start looking for new targets, found two good ones and the chase is on!

June 2009-June 2010 diving the places where our research has led us, but no finds.

July 2010 change to target number two, diving and searching the areas we believe the wreck to be but no joy.

August 2010 hire Starfish side scan sonar, towed the fish for miles and miles, but with no results. Fantastic images a great bit of kit. But alas no cannons or anything resembling a shipwreck.

September 2010 borrowed a Magnetometer from local dive shop, but again no targets.

Winter 2010 to March 2010 back to the library, internet and all the usual research.

April 2010 under pressure and need some results quick, came up with, what I thought was a very good idea.

Just an Idea

Hey Mr Green how's it going, good to see you again mate.

Likewise captain Black, how's all the family, they good?

Yep they are on top form and keeping me really busy, every night I've got something going on, swimming lessons, football club, rugby club I'm like a permanent taxi driver. Can't seem to get ahead of the game and Mrs Black is the same. Money just goes out of the house like water, or should I say milk. I can have four litres of milk in the fridge in the morning and by the time I am on the way home at five o'clock Mrs Black is texting me 'need more milk'. Something has got to change soon Mr Green, I know we have to dive when the weather is good and all things like visibility and tides come together, but I can't keep taking days off to go and find didily scwat!

Even doing it on as low a budget as possible with our tiny rubber boat and the eight horsepower engine it still adds up to a twenty pound day. And I just aint got many more £20's to throw away. The pressure is on and I'm close to calling it a day, I am so broke I am losing my smile. And that's fine for me but not good for my kids, and the long haired Sergeant Major! deserves better. Wow that was a good rant Captain, feeling any better now? Sounds like you are running out of patients, and faith.

All I'm saying is our lives are different and our time scales for striking pay dirt and finding some treasure that we can sell, then go home to significant other and say there's the cash. Because I'm at a place where the only thing that's going to take the pressure off is good hard cash

And I don't mean old artefacts that are really cool and we love them for their history, the story they can tell and the link with our past. I mean treasure found, sold and hard cash on the table.

Well it's only been two years, how long did you think it was going to take to find her, two years is nothing in the big scheme of treasure hunting. If it only took us two years to find a treasure ship, my god every diver who ever looked would say we are the luckiest guys alive.

That's spoken by a man who has little money worries, who has wife earns a really good wedge and isn't getting ass bent over bills and shit.

Come on Captain Black it's not like you to get pissed off and fed up. Like we keep saying once we found the first one and we have our big fat wedge in our back pockets we were will have the time and money to find lots more, we just need a bit of luck I'm sure were really close.

I know and I agree but two years of diving in different locations, two years of our so called good research leading us to some god forsaken shitty old gully full of kelp and sand and nothing else, starts to wear on my confidence and most of all my wallet.

Well what do you suggest? If you know another way of finding the type of money we are dreaming of I am all ears fat boy.

Well I did have one idea which I know you're not going to like much.

Shoot, lets here it.

Every read any conspiracy theory books or watched any documentaries on conspiracy theories?

I've seen some stuff on them but not thought much of it, I reckon most of them are rubbish and the books are just written to make some sad person lots of money.

Do you think the Yanks landed on the moon? Was that footage of "one giant step for mankind" done in a Hollywood studio or was it on the moon. Lots of people say they could see the flag moving in the wind, and yet there is no wind on the moon.

What's your point?

Was the Titanic actually the Titanic or in fact her sister ship swapped or here at the last minute because the Titanic was ready, and are all those people buying an artefact from the Titanic actually not!

No still don't get it!! And the day is moving on as is the tide, so get to the point.

What about JFK was he shot, was he even in Dallas! Ever watch the Blair Witch project?

No I haven't and what is it with this obsession with bloody witches any way.

But you must have heard of the Blair Witch project right?

Of course there was massive hype sounding the film before it came out and everyone was talking about it.

And can you remember what everyone was saying about it?

They were discussing, well arguing whether it was real or not, if there was a Witch or not, or if there was even a wood.

Now you're on it, and it was made with people running around with small cam corders strapped to their heads. Had to be the lowest budget movie ever, just like our budget for treasure hunting.

O no, no you don't I see exactly where you are going with this, and there no way you can do that.

Just here me out that's all I am asking.

You are chuffing nuts if you think you can pull that off. Stark raving nuts!

Just shut up a minute and calm down, don't poo poo it until you've heard what I have to say, just sit down look out to sea and hear. what I have to say. Then if you can honestly look me in the eye and tell me that you and me are not capable of pulling it off I will never mention it again.

So what you're suggesting, if I have got this right is blag the whole finding a wreck thing and make money off the hype?

Yep that's what I'm saying.

Well I can tell your not going to go diving until you've told me your foolish scheme, so go on then you nutter, get it off your chest.

Right the way to think of it is like a crime.

That's because it would be a bloody crime.

No it can't be a crime, it can't be anything illegal, we tell a story and people believe what they want to believe just like Bair Witch or Donny Darko.

But if it was a crime and you where a detective, as in the movies they would say, do we have the motive? Without doubt I do, I am so skint it's scary, I am broke with three kids to feed and clothe. Like I said before I'm under pressure and it's about to pop. That pressures it enough to take a chance, not the kind of chance that might send me to prison as I could not bear to be away from the kids, but a chance none the less.

Your motive is a lot less I agree. But your motive is to help a mate in need and by doing so you have a dive buddy that can spend all day every day treasure hunting with you is a good one. And make some money. Every knows we are looking for a wreck so it's not out of the question that we find one. Second do we have the means, and that is a big fat yes, we have two boats, engines, dive kit, metal detectors the whole shooting match. Plus everyone knows we have been looking for a certain treasure ship for two years. We are ocean men and capable of doing pretty much anything under water. Anyone who knows us would have no doubt that we could salvage a wreck site. Lift cannons; dredge the sea bed, whatever it takes.

Do we have the opportunity, absolutely we do, we could find it today or next week, we are diving every day and could stage the press realises and news articles to suit are time line.

Ok let me get this straight, what your saying is lets pretend we found the wreck we are looking for and just blag it all, everything lock stock and barrel.

Yep that's what I am saying.

So if there's no wreck, then there's no treasure and if there is no treasure there is no bloody money, so what the hell would be the point.

And in Blair witch you never actually saw a witch.

Don't start on stupid witches again your doing my head in with that shit.

So answer me this Mr Green, maybe there was no witch in Blair witch, but did they make shit loads of money?

Yes millions, from the movie and the hype.

Exactly we will make the money from a book and the hype; we will blag everything and then write a book all about our wreck discovery and salvage. Plus as with every worth less artefact we will add a mountain of province. And then as with the Titanic everything that comes off her is worth a small fortune.

So get some old iron cannon ball that no one knows where it came from, worth lest say £20 give it a load of false provenance from a historical shipwreck and hey presto its worth £100.

Isn't that breaking the law?

No I don't think so, more of a bend I would say.

Ok just for one minute I buy it to this crazy idea of yours, where do we get all the stuff we need to fabricate a ship wreck? Can you imagine all the stuff we would need? Cannon, cannon balls, musket shots, bits of old crockery, bits of timber. We would need photographs of everything. We would need to be holding the finds and under water photos of us finding the stuff. Where on earth do you think we are going to get all that stuff..... And you're a bastard because you know that as those worlds are coming out of my mouth, you know that I know where we can get them. I hate it when you do that, you smug git.

"Uncle Orange's museum"

Uncle Orange's museum, he has it all, and you knew that I was going to think of that just as I was saying it, DIDNT YOU?

Yep well it's not rocket science, he has it all, and I mean all. He has cannon balls, musket shots, silver coins, gold coins, old crockery old timbers, loads of crustation everything we would need.

Yeh but what about cannons, there is no way he would lend us his bronze VOC cannon.

I know! we would have to find and bring up a old iron cannon with loads of crud on it and then sex it up a bit, you know like the weapons of mass destruction document. There's a fine example of fabricating evidence to make a good story. So what I am saying if it's good enough for parliament it's good enough for the diving magazines and their readers if it's not illegal for them to say things that aren't true, well I'm happy to live by the same sword.

Do you think the diving magazines and press would buy it?

You were smiling as you said that Mr Green because you know how they love a good story of course they would, there hungry for news stories and they wouldn't even question it, I mean why they would?

Free story, free photographs they would bite our hands off.

You still didn't answer the question on where we would get old cannon?

I know where there is some off Pier cellars, there is some off Drakes Island and the back of the Mewstone we just choose one the right size and age and go and get it.

What if people saw us lifting it and where we got it from?

No one is going to see us, we go mid week, get one ready to lift and then sling it under the Rigid Raider and wait for it to get dark land it ashore.

What after we have it, we lie low for a couple of weeks.

And then we take it back to the slipway and then call the press and pretend we have just found it.

But I don't see how the rest of the story gets people excited.

Well what we do is the same as making a jigsaw puzzle start at the end with a picture, in our case a name of a ship that sunk and then make the pieces of the puzzle to fit.

Wow you certainly have been giving it some thought Captain, and it sounds like a fun idea but times moving on and I have finished my coffee so let's get the boat off your car roof and in the water, today is the day and I'm feeling lucky.

Your right Mr Green all we need is a good positive attitude and good old lady luck.

End of the days diving......................That was bloody hard work; I swear that engine is getting heavier every time I carry back up those bloody steps. Another wasted day, another day when our research lead us to the same place, absolutely no where!

Well at least we know where she isn't

You say that every time Mr Green and it's stating to get on my tits.

You're not still thinking of your hair brained idea are you Captain?

No it was just a thought.

CONTENTS

Chapter One

Choosing a Target

Come in Mr Green! Have a seat; do you want a tea or coffee?

"Tea please Captain Black."

So how's the practice going with that new toy of yours?

"Yeh really good, I have rigged it in a different way and it's much easier to work with."

How small an object can it find underwater?

"I would say smaller than a new five pence piece under about 2 feet of sand with its small search head and under about 3 feet of sand with the larger head."

Cool, keep practising mate - we are going to depend on the metal detector I'm sure of it. Here's your cuppa, an' don't spill it.

"So how's your research going Captain?"

Mind blowing!

"...Mind blowing in a good way I hope."

Yep. Just hard to make sense of it all. Here you go, I want you to read this new article on the Aagtekerke.

"Who wrote it?"

I'm not saying, and it's not important, just read...

Much mystery surrounds the ill-fated voyage of the Aagtekerke and her final resting place beneath the waves...

One of three Zeeland Chamber, Dutch East India Company (*Vereenigde Oost-Indische Compagnie*, VOC) ships that set sail from the Netherlands in December 1721, headed for the Indian Ocean, the Aagtekerke would have been carrying many large chests of gold and silver bars and coins, ready for trade in the East.

The VOC official site lists the ship as 145 feet, weighing 800 tons, and setting sail from Rammekens on 17th December 1721, with 250 crew under the captainship of Nicolaas Rabodus.

Whilst the final destinies of her two companion ships (The Samaritaan and The Steenhoven - both making it to Batavia, meeting their respective ends on subsequent voyages in years later) are well known, records regarding the Aagtekerke appear muddled and have led several authors to write-up very disparate accounts of her journey.

Official documentation of the Aagtekerke's maiden voyage, including reports made by Nicolaas Rabodus are in existence, held in a private archive of the Rademacher family (lawyers to the VOC for many years) and have been reviewed by maritime historians and shipwreck enthusiasts alike. Eighteenth century Dutch is notoriously difficult to clearly translate, perhaps accounting for such wild discrepancies in their conclusions.

It is known that all three ships fell subject to severe storms as they journeyed south, skirting the waters of the English coast during December 1721, but it seems that while her companion vessels made it out those stormy seas, the Aagtekerke fell foul to the brutal winds and waves...

Somewhere in the waters around Cornwall and the Scilly Isles, things began to go wrong for the Aagtekerke and her crew. In a storm at the beginning of the dog watch one evening, the ship was thrown about and began to take on water.

Accounts differ so dramatically from here on in, that even a most careful comparison of the two most prominent analyses does little to uncover the truth of what happened beyond this juncture.

One interpretation talks of the mainsail and floating anchors failing before three tempestuous weeks were spent in the stormy seas, tirelessly pumping out water, ditching whatever ballast possible – including guns, cannons and even some of the riches (unbeknownst to the Captain!) - and building to an ultimate revolt against Nicolaas Rabodus by an exhausted, desperate and rebellious crew: forcing the captain along with the rest of the crew to board 3 England bound vessels to save themselves, finally watching the Aagtekerke sink into the night somewhere in the English Channel on the 17th of March 1722, taking with her up to 8 chests of the gold and silver bars and coins which had been stored below deck.

Another account, based on analysis of document No.247 from the Radermacher collection, tells of the strong gales and stormy seas on December 23rd throwing the vessel about and pushing water in through gun and scupper holes, forcing the Aagtekerke to aim for shelter around Rame Head, in Cawsand Bay (on the west side of Plymouth Sound). On the morning of the 24th, the researchers claim, even fiercer winds whipped up the sea, snapping the anchor rope and driving the ship towards the rocks. Panicked, and thinking the rocks were closer than was reality, many tried to jump for their lives, and drowned. In the days that followed the ship was pillaged by locals, and, tired of fighting they eventually watched the Aagtekerke and her stowed treasure chests sink...

The one consistency of details in both versions, with regards to the final watching of the vessel sinking taking some, or all of the treasure chests with her, is of little help given the discrepancy of dates and locations. However, a further piece of the puzzle may indicate that there is somewhat more accuracy to the grounding in the second account – letters sent between local lords and the Collector of Customs living and serving in Plymouth at that time refer to a Batavia bound ship, named Aagtekerke, captained by Nicolaas Rabodus, running aground near Bovisand and being subjected to riotous locals who fought the crew and made off with goods such as wine and brandy. The letters beg for additional officers and law enforcement to prevent further looting by the violent local 'mob', and, most interestingly refer to a Mr Calmady the local MP, living near the point of wreckage.

Critically, the Calmady family owned and lived at Landon Court, a manor house on the headland encompassing Wembury, Heybrook Bay, Bovisand, Jenny Cliff and Ramscliff Point on the opposite side of Plymouth Sound to Rame Head and Cawsand.

So what do you make of that Mr Green?

"Well, very interesting captain, but it didn't tell us anything more than we already knew, did it? ...or am I missing something?"

Yep you are, and it's the author's personality.

I will tell you what I think: because I know the person who wrote that new summary, and because I know their personality and the way they think, I can now make more sense of the article by Patric Jongen and the article by Richard Larn. The person who wrote the new article only likes to deal in absolutes - they only like facts and science. They've a Masters Degree in a science subject and would find it hard to write make believe or just waffle on about something!

"And how does that help us?"

Well now I can understand the personalities of the other authors and it helps me make sense of why their articles of the Aaktekerke's wrecking are so very different.

I want you to read Patrick Jongen's article again, but this time read it with his personality in mind: A man who would prefer if possible to deal in fact and has gone to great lengths to translate the events correctly.

...But a man who will also will insert a bit of his interpretation where he is not 100% sure of things. He says it himself *"Translation into modern day English was also quite a challenge! Trying to stick faithfully to the original document has unfortunately made some of the text quite stilted"*. In other words, never let the truth spoil a good story. Try your best and fill in the gaps where necessary. Also I can see that Patricks has more experiece in researching ship wreck articles and treasure hunting research than he has actually diving and searching.

You can see he loves VOC history, but I doubt he has ever found a VOC treasure wreck or any other old virgin wreck site.

Bear that in mind Mr Green and have another read of Patricks article written in spring 2005.

SPELT WRONG, SHOULD BE AAGTEKERK

VOC Ship Aegtekerken

Written by Patrick Jongen

The following article about the VOC ship *Aegtekerken* (also referred to as *Aechtekerk* in some documents) is based upon research undertaken by Mr Patrick Jongen in The Netherlands. Mr Jongen gained access to the private archive of the Rademacher family in The Hague – this family were lawyers to the massive VOC company for many years.

VOC ship *Aegtekerken* set sail from Texel bound for Goa, India, in the company of the ship *Samaritaan* in late December 1721. Both ships perished off the south-west of England in 1722 taking with them over 50,000 lbs of gold and silver bars and coins. Only 25 of the 38 chests were salvaged or otherwise accounted for – leaving 13 chests still to be discovered.

The one and only document held in this private collection concerning the abandoning and lost of the ship *Aegtekerken* is written in an old fashioned Dutch language and was, at times, hard to decipher. Translation into modern day English was also quite a challenge! Trying to stick faithfully to the original document, has unfortunately made some of the following text quite stilted but it is hoped the reader will still be able to make sense of it.

FOLIO 1

Aegtekerken shipmaster Koole and the merchant Fraichereau signed the following report:

February 22nd :
– Sorlinghen (believed to be in the vicinity of the Scilly Isles) 30 to 33 miles West; wind East-South-East; wind increasing.
We took in reefs in the sails and in the afternoon a second reef Followed by the foresail and shortly after that the top main sail. At sunset the foresail bowed and floated on the mainsail. During the second watch the mainsail fell down and soon afterwards the topmast hit the deck. We weren't able to clear the deck.

February 24th :
Two days later we lost the mizzenmast and dropped out the floating anchor. Due to the increasing bad weather we had to chop the anchor rope.

February 26th :
– High and bowed sea; the ship yawed extremely. Everything moved and rolled from one end to the other. We had difficulties keeping the two water pumps working. We tried to fix the mizzenmast behind the stump of the main mast. However all in vain, it broke into two pieces. We tried again by putting the foresail in its place and were successful. As we threw all excess weight overboard, the chests (holding the gold and silver bars and coins) started to move alarmingly. The steersman and the officers wanted to throw the chests overboard, however the shipmaster and the merchant refused. They ordered them to be made fast, as good as possible, and if that were not possible the chests were to be brought up to the shipmaster's cabin and made secure. Some chests were brought up to the cabin under loud protests from the uppersteersman.

February 27th:
– The storm increased, coming from the SE. The chests started to move again. The steersman and the officers once more pleaded that the chests were thrown overboard. The shipmaster refused and forbade this action. Nevertheless the First Officer prised open 4 chests in the shipmaster's cabin and disposed of the contents. Hesitating however, he didn't know what to do with the rest, due to impossibility of storing loose coins and silver bars. He spared the other 8 boxes and took them back down below where they remained.

FOLIO 2

February 28th:
– We had a hard time trying to put the foresail behind the stump of the mainmast. We continued to pump and tried to balance the ship as well as we could. However, *Aegtekerken* yawed more and more.

<u>March 1st</u>
– The storm continued. We couldn't do anything else but pump out water and try to maintain balance. We headed in a south-westerly direction and estimated our position to be approximately 78 miles from Sorlinghen.

<u>March 2nd</u>
– Still stormy weather. We pumped and balanced. We sighted a hooker, heading for Bordeaux but quickly lost sight of her. We tried to bring the foremast behind the mizzenmast.

<u>March 4th</u>
– A little ship, outbound from Lisbon heading to London, approached us and we gave her a letter to forward for us. The crew, having pumped day and night, were exhausted and wanted to stop pumping and abandon *Aegtekerken*, and board the visiting ship. The First Officer even suggested capturing the new arrival. The shipmaster forbade it.
Sorlinghen estimated to be SSE at a distance of 69 miles.

<u>March 5th</u>
– The shipmaster summoned the whole crew who believed that in order to stay alive they had to abandon ship. The shipmaster stood alone, as even the officers were of the opinion of the general crew. He commanded the crew to remain at their posts and to have faith. Reassuring all onboard that they would shelter in the first available harbour. He promised double ransom and double wages upon arrival. The shipmaster shouted that if everything turned out not to be as he said, than they were allowed to throw him overboard! The reluctant crew eventually obeyed orders under protest and returned to work.
At last the pumps were back in action.
Wind ESE. Heading: East.

<u>March 6th</u>
– Wind East veering ESE. Sorlinghen estimated to be 49 miles away. Hard time balancing the ship.

<u>March 7th</u>
– Wind ESE backing ENE. *Aegtekerken* was pushed in a north-westerly direction for 2 days.

<u>March 8th</u>
– Sorlinghen: SSE 47 miles. The officers wanted to discuss heading south. We examined the possibility of heading to the Azores or the Canary Islands, even Lisbon.

<u>March 9th</u>
The wind NE and ENE. We sailed SSW and tracked 16½ miles. The crew continued pumping and balancing the ship.

<u>March 10th</u>
– Wind: Easterly. We sailed 9½ miles in a SSW direction and estimated Sorlinghen to be at a distance of 65½ miles. In the morning we saw two ships SSW. The crew, still wanting to abandon ship if possible, became excited and prepared to fire shots and capture the vessels if they approached. However, they kept their distance then turned away.

<u>March 11th</u>
– Wind: East. The sea was high and the ship yawed extensively making pumping almost impossible. It was decided that the two upper canons should be thrown overboard. We reckoned that we had sailed 14 miles in a SSW direction. Sorlinghen: 74 miles NNE.

<u>March 12th</u>
– Wind SSE. Extreme yawing. It was calculated that we had sailed 6 miles in a WNW direction leaving Sorlinghen 78 miles away to the NNE. Changed direction and headed East.

<u>March 13th</u>
– Wind SSW and we continued to track eastwards covering 8 miles. Sorlinghen 70 miles NE. In the afternoon we saw a sail on the horizon. The crew and the officers forced the shipmaster to signal. The ship approached. It was a ship from Jamaica headed for London and the First Officer onboard spoke very good English. The new ship stayed nearby all night long.

March 14th:
~ Wind South, changing to SSW. We continued to sail eastwards, 9 miles. Sorlinghen 69 miles NNE. The crew forced the shipmaster to prepare the boats in order to go onboard the England-bound ship during the third watch regardless of limited food supplies.

March 15th:
~ Wind East and ENE. Fair weather. The ship yawed. In the afternoon we saw two more ships. The ship from Jamaica approached them and reported to *Aegtekerken* that the two new ships would approach the next day.

March 16th:
~ The three English speaking captains of the visiting ships came onboard and spoke with *Aegtekerken*'s officers (the shipmaster was not invited. Sick and humiliated he retired in his cabin). The uppersteersman informed the shipmaster that they intended to abandon the ship. The shipmaster asked for a meeting with the board of the ship and asked them to re-evaluate whether the ship could be saved. However, all voted to abandon the vessel, except for the merchant. The shipmaster stated that if everybody did their utmost to save the ship he was sure they would all survive, and he begged the board to reconsider their decision but all his efforts were in vain. They wanted to carry out the agreed resolution.

March 17th:
~ The uppersteersman let the boats out and sailed back and forth under protest of the shipmaster who summoned the uppersteersman to explain his actions. On hearing that goods were being transferred to the England-bound ship, the shipmaster fainted, whilst the steersman laughed and continued to supervise three boats to ferry supplies. Mr Gerlach (Navy Commander) and his wife were the first to board the nearby England-bound ship. In the afternoon the First Officer asked the shipmaster (who was still in his sickbed) to pack his goods in order to abandon the ship. The shipmaster refused, whereupon the First Officer said remaining onboard would mean certain death. Eventually the shipmaster agreed to abandon ship too, as alone he would be in no situation to save *Aegtekerken*. He ordered that the money chests had to accompany him but the officer wanted at least half of the chests to go onboard one of the other ships bound for Beddefort (thought to be near Plymouth). Being in a weak state, the shipmaster agreed on the condition that the merchant travelled with the chests. The officer thought this was not a good idea and that he, himself, should be in charge of the valuables. The loose coins and silver bars were put into sacks and went on board of the ship from Jamaica. The Consul signed a paper and sealed the sacks. In the late afternoon the shipmaster wanted to inspect the new storage arrangements of these sacks of precious cargo. Although too tired to carry out the task himself he believed the merchant to be onboard the ship from Jamaica and he could carry out the inspection. However, the merchant was in fact on the same vessel as the shipmaster and so no inspection took place! Meanwhile, the officers attempted to gain access to *Aegtekerken's* lower deck where the sealed chests were stored but rising water forced them back. Fearing the ship would roll over and capsize at any moment and they quickly retreated to the ship bound for Beddefort.

With the *Aegtekerken* pumps now abandoned she filled with water and the ship's crew, now safely all aboard their rescue vessels, remained nearby throughout the night until they watched her and the treasure chests finally sink.

Supplementary information:

March 12th:
~ The uppersteersman held a secret meeting without the shipmaster's knowledge but with the authorisation of the Navy Commander Mr Gerlach.

March 13th:
The shipmaster was forced to send at least one officer to the ship from Jamaica.

March 14th:
~ The crew was rebellious. Exhausted from maintaining the pumps someone shouted "overboard with the shipmaster". The shipmaster was furious and asked who had shouted this but no one answered, not

even the officers volunteered any information. Thereupon the shipmaster grabbed one of the crew and beat him saying "You'll have to kill me before I surrender. The one who tries, I'll cleave his head!"

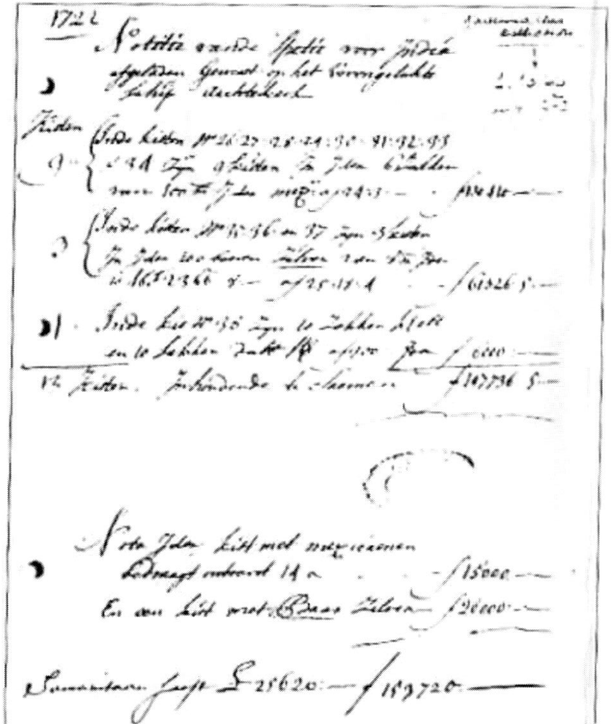

Document listing Aegtekerken's lost cargo
Source: Rademacher Collection, Algemeen Rijksarchief Den Haag.
Ref: 1.10.69 inventory no. 247

March 15th
– The two ships came over.

March 16th
– The crew was wild and wanted to go onboard of the other ships immediately. The ships offered to share the rescued crew and food supplies between them. The board came together again in order to consider everything and voted to abandon the ship. The shipmaster and the merchant were the only ones who wanted to stay on board *Aegtekerken*. The First Officer muttered that they better be careful otherwise the crew would throw them overboard! The officers agreed that it was possible to sail to a repairing harbour as long as the weather remained fair but any storm or change of weather would be disastrous. The shipmaster replied: "and if the weather stays this way, what next?". The First Officer laughed and answered : "we will take care of that !". The shipmaster assumed that they would scuttle the ship but the steersman protested because of his pride and honour. Next the First Officer declared that he and the Commander Gerlach with three steersmen would board of the ship to Beddefort. Then it's believed the First Officer gave 115 bars of silver to the Beddefort bound ship for the help they were offering. The shipmaster wanted to stay with the rest of the valuables. The steersman, however, wanted to divide the remainder into 3 parts but the First Officer commanded a 4-way split. The shipmaster ensured everybody had plenty to drink and succeeded in getting his way.

Many thanks to Patrick Jongen
for submitting his research to ***Shipwrecks*** magazine.

"OK so I kind of get where you're coming from Capt'n Black - so what do we take as fact and what is fiction? ...or is it all fiction and so it's all just a wild goose chase?"

I think we have to take about half of it as fact and take the rest as being 'sexed up'.

"So how does the second article by Richard Larns square up?"

Well this sent me into a tail spin, his so called 'facts' are so far adrift it's like it was done on purpose...

Richard and the rest of those guys he mentions are well respected, experienced treasure hunters, who have searched for and found many old wrecks. They are very passionate about what they do and very good at it. The way Richard's article has a pop at Patrick's and insinuates it's not accurate or somewhat fabricated beggars belief when you take into account he says he *"literally mowed the lawn for days inside Plymouth breakwater... looking for the wreck of the Steenhoven"*. I believe therefore, the article was written by a very passionate man who for some reason was very angry with Patrick's article and was trying to throw readers off the scent.

Because why was he searching for the "Steenhoven" when she didn't actually sink!

The VOC website and archives state. The "Steenhoven left Holland on the 17-12-1721 and arrived at the cape on 19-04-1722. She then Departed from the cape on the 20-05-22 and arrived at her destination "Batavia" now known as Jakarter Indonisia on the 02-07-22.

Here you are Mr Green, have another read and try to separate the facts from all the errors. We now know that since he was on his high horse, his article could have gaps in it as wide as the Atlantic. The question is, did he put all the errors in his article on purpose? And if so, was it because Patrick's article was too close to the bone, such that he panicked and tried to throw in a curve ball to throw any would be treasure hunters off on a fools errand. Read on MacDuff!

(17)

Dutch East Indiamen *Aagtekerke*, *Samaritaan* and *Steenhoven* – 1721

By Richard Larn

Patrick Jongen's interesting article concerning the VOC. ship ***Aagtekerke*** was of particular interest to me, since in the early 1980's I spent a considerable amount of time and effort, in company with Rex Cowan, Peter McBride, Anthony Lonsdale and Simon Keeble, attempting to find the wreck of the ***Steenhoven*** which had accompanied the ***Aagtekerke***. Using Decca as our position finding equipment, we literally 'mowed the lawn' for days inside Plymouth Breakwater, towing a specially adapted proton magnetometer.

By inference, Patrick Jongen implies that he was priveledged to have sight of VOC documents in the possession of the Rademacher family. These had already been indexed and transcribed in the 1970's, and with help of the late Bas Kist, of the Rijksmuseum, Amsterdam, and Rex Cowan, who had a contractural agreement with the Dutch Government to search for VOC. wrecks, we had copies of the relevant research documents, including details of the treasure carried on board the ships.

Three Zeeland Chamber VOC. ships sailed from Rammekens on 17 December 1721, bound direct for Batavia. The largest was the 850-ton ***Steenhoven***, Captain Jakob Lijnsen, which had been built in 1718 and carried a complement of 225. The ***Aagtekerke***, Captain Nikolaas Rabodus, was the second largest at 800-tons, built in 1720, with 250 crew, passengers and soldiers. At only 600-tons, the fluit ***Samaritaan*** was the smallest, having been built in 1718 and carried only 94 people.

Details of what happened to the ***Steenhoven*** are contained in the Radermacher Collection, document No.247, and it is worth reproducing this in full, in order to get the full flavour of events in the English Channel, between 17th and 24th December.

'Report made by Nikolaas Rabodus, Isaac Labilien, Jan Coetres and Peter Sorgeloos. With three ships to East India, signed on 16th December with ***Steenhoven***, skipper Maarten Crijnsen as commander or bearer of the pennant; ***Samaritaan***, skipper Jan Credo, and ***Aagtekerke***, skipper Nikolaas Rabodus. Sailed the 17th from the Roads of Rannelties, with easterly winds.' There follows a description of their passage until the 23rd, which is of little interest, then '– 23rd. the daywatch turned round to look for the ***Samaritaan***. Saw their signals and steered to the wind, again NW, to the shore. In the afternoon guessed Hoek van Doodmans Hooft (the Deadman's or Dodman Head) NW 2 miles from us. Let her run NE at a quarter mile from the shore but being afraid that we could not pull through before nightfall (we had agreed to put into Plymouth), we signalled the skipper Credo to put out to sea knowing it to be dangerous to ride with these winter nights in the Vioers (the outer roads of Pleijmout(Plymouth). Steered for the shore, SSE sailing with the jib, foretop sail, knij sail and mizzen.

By evening we guessed Hoek van Doodmans Hooft to be 6 miles from us, and Hoek van Lesard(Lizard) WNW five and a half miles , the Vioers of Pleijmout NE 8 miles. Thinking we were far enough out to sea we made the signal for floating, wind being SW with topgallant breeze, good weather, overcast sky, which skipper Credo answered. Steered SSE, guessed to have floated a mile ENE in the first dogwatch in the first night also 2 miles. We had decided to steer down at the beginning of the day watch and to steer NE, but at the beginning of the dog-watch we got a heavy gale with

3

rain, thunder and lightning, which pushed the ship so much over that the lee holes(gun-ports) made water, but in 5 glasses we got the topsails to at last. We could not have any sails; sometimes the ship heeled so much over that we had water in the scupper holes. With the squalls we got very much borne down upon the lee shore but hoped to have enough drift till day.

Being 6 glasses into the dog-watch I was being told as skipper that someone standing on the quarterdeck near the night-light had sighted land abreast, and staying there for a while, I knew it immediately as the Vioers or outer roads of Pleijmout.With the steersman and further officers we decided to have the anchors ready because on neither tack could we keep off 20 to 30 fathom deep. Got the heavy ropes on deck, that being coiled we measured 20 fathoms, let go the daily anchor for approximately 2 ropes we got her still and rode steady. Got the jib close and took in the mizzen, fired for pilots and hoped to pull through till daylight. Were busy to look after the rope with a piece of leather in the hawse hole, secured the jib and braced the yard to port so that we could put to starboard in case the rope snapped and put into Costenbaay (Cawsand) near a fishing village and good sandy ground, this was our last hope. Took bearings of Ramshooft(Rame Head) at W and the E corner of the Vioers NE. Found ourselves nearer to the shore than we had guessed which was the most important cause of our accident.

24th. In the morning at the beginning of the day-watch, fierce S wind. By way of precaution we slipped our anchor a bit. Even more wind S to SW with gusts of rain, the ship slipped to port and the anchor rope snapped (by some mysterious cause with all sorts of rope). Not knowing that the rope had snapped I ordered the aft-anchor out hoping that the anchor would catch again, but what ever trouble we took, no use. After this we quickly neared the shore. We cut down the trailing ropes and ordered to take in the flying jib and put the helm to windward, to put into a little sand bay which I knew to be there or an inlet, before the wind, so that the hurling sea could not beat so much. Thinking to be better off there than any other place, but because of the strong wind the jib went high up and we could not pull it in, and the ship jolted and turned round immediately with the bow before the wind. To get the wind from port and the jib flapping to pieces on the mast we drifted with our starboard side against the shore in the mentioned inlet. No orders anymore and much moaning – great panic – and more when they touched ground. Perceiving that we were on a flat ascending rocky ground I shouted that their lives were saved because I hoped that (because of the rising water(tide) we would jolt so far that we could reach a steep rock and they should stop crying and behave like men. Some went on the boat and thought they could jump on shore, thinking the shore to be nearer because of the going down of the sea and the darkness, and this way a lot of people drowned.

In a short time the mast fell to starboard and shortly afterwards the mizzen followed, from which I had the tackle cut to let it fall on a rock, but it broke too high so that it was of no use. They fired(cannon) for help as long as they had dry powder and in the meantime daylight came and a lot of people were on the shore. They showed their flag to show us what nation they were from, but the flag blew to pieces immediately. At last got a rope to the shore and got two people there to ask for help from the authorities. After a few days fighting against the robbers and being robbed of a lot of stuff, we returned home.'

(5

The ***Aagtekerke*** as we know became a total wreck, the Rademacher archives stating that 'they remained nearby throughout the night until they watched her and the treasure chests finally sink', whereas Dutch-Asiatic Shipping in the 17th & 18th Centuries, Vol.II (outward bound voyages 1595-1794), page 362-3 states 'the ship ran ashore near Plymouth in December 1721'. The ***Steenhoven*** was also a total wreck, but tthe ***Samaritaan*** survived, remaining at anchor in Plymouth from 24th December until 14th January 1722,(where 6 sailors and 2 soldiers deserted), the ship eventually reaching Batavia on 24th November 1722. Of the 94 seamen and officers on board when she sailed, only 65 survived the voyage, and of the original 61 soldiers, 34 reached Batavia; a total loss of 56 men on the outward voyage alone. She then left the Far East on 21st January 1723 and was back at Rammekens four months later.'

There appear to be a number of inconsistencies between Patrick's Rademacher account and other VOC. sources, in that the ships were bound direct for Batavia, not Goa, and that the ***Samaritaan*** did not perish off the south-west of England, since we know she reached Batavia, and later returned to the Texel. There also appears to be something wrong regarding dates, since it would be most unlikely that a VOC. ship leaving the Texel in December 1721 would still only be off the Sorlinghen (Isles of Scilly), the following March. After almost three months at sea she would be short of both food and water, and unable to proceed for the Far East. Patrick's log entry for the ***Aagtekerke*** for the 14th March, the last indication of her position, shows 'Sorlinghen 69 miles NNE', which places the ship at the mouth of the English Channel, in 360ft(110m) of water, at roughly 49N, 07.30W. The log states she sank on 17th March, three days later, and if previous daily distances covered were as little as 9, 8 and 6 miles respectively, when she was obviously only drifting, did she actually sink in the middle of the English Channel, miles from anywhere, or did she then make 50 miles a day east, for three successive days against the wind, to become stranded and lost near Plymouth? We may never know.

So what do you make of that Mr Green? Now that you've read it taking into account the person, and mood in which it was written rather than what it actually says?

"Well, I'll tell you what; I don't know what to believe and what not to anymore! I'm going to be like the mystery author of that first article and only deal in absolutes."

"I know that's not your way but you're the dreamer amongst us not me. And the only thing I'll say I know for sure now is that; 1, a Duch East Indian ship called Aaktekerke was wrecked somewhere - when and where I have no idea!; 2, She was 800 tonnes and had 250 men on board; and 3, she had lots of treasure and some of it went down with her."

"And that's it. That's all I safely believe at this moment."

Ok, I can see why you are saying that. So now take a look at the copies of the two letters written at the time by the local customs officer and the local land owner and resident landlord of Langdon Court which is near Wembury.

Read these letters writen at the time the first is from the local customs officer asking for help, the second is from the local MP/land owner at Langdon Court (on this stick)

Aagtekercke

7 Jan 1722 Plymouth Copy
a letter written 17 Dec 1721
I beg have to inform you,
that on the 13th instant a
violent storm happened on our
coast, which drove on shoar,
at a place called Bovey Sand
within this harbour a
merchantman of Middleburg
bound to Batavia, called the
Aagtekercke, Nicolas Rabodus,
commander. Her cargo consisted
of 13 chests of silver money,
which is salv'd; a large
quantity of wine, brandy &
some bale goods, which have
been rifled & carried away by
the country, notwithstanding
the endeavours of Mr Calmady

6

who is a member of Parliament,
& lives near the place where
the ship was drove on shoar.
Mr Whaddon our landsurveyor
& as many other officers as
could be spared to assist him,
& a lieut with 50 soldiers spared
us, upon application made
to the governor of our citadel.
Also Sir John Rogers
appeared & read to the rude
assembly the proclamation
against riots, but to
little purpose, until a
greater reinforcement of
soldiers came, with a
resolution to disperse them
by force, at which they
seem daunted until several
of their comrades were killed
which caused them to

9

Aagtekerke.

remove for that time
at a greater distance; but
as the ship remains whole
as yet, & has a considerable
quantity of iron and other
valuable goods on board,
we are apprehensive they will
make a further attempt
upon their endeavours, against
which we have made the best
provision we can to oppose
them, & heartily wish some
legal course might be taken
to inflict exemplary punish-
ment on men of substance
that shall be discovered to
have carried off any of the
effects, or any ways encouraged
such inhuman practices in
a christian country.

D. Morris PTO
(collector of custom)

Mr Calmady's place
was Langdon Court

4 miles S E Plymouth
please check with
Plymouth Lib

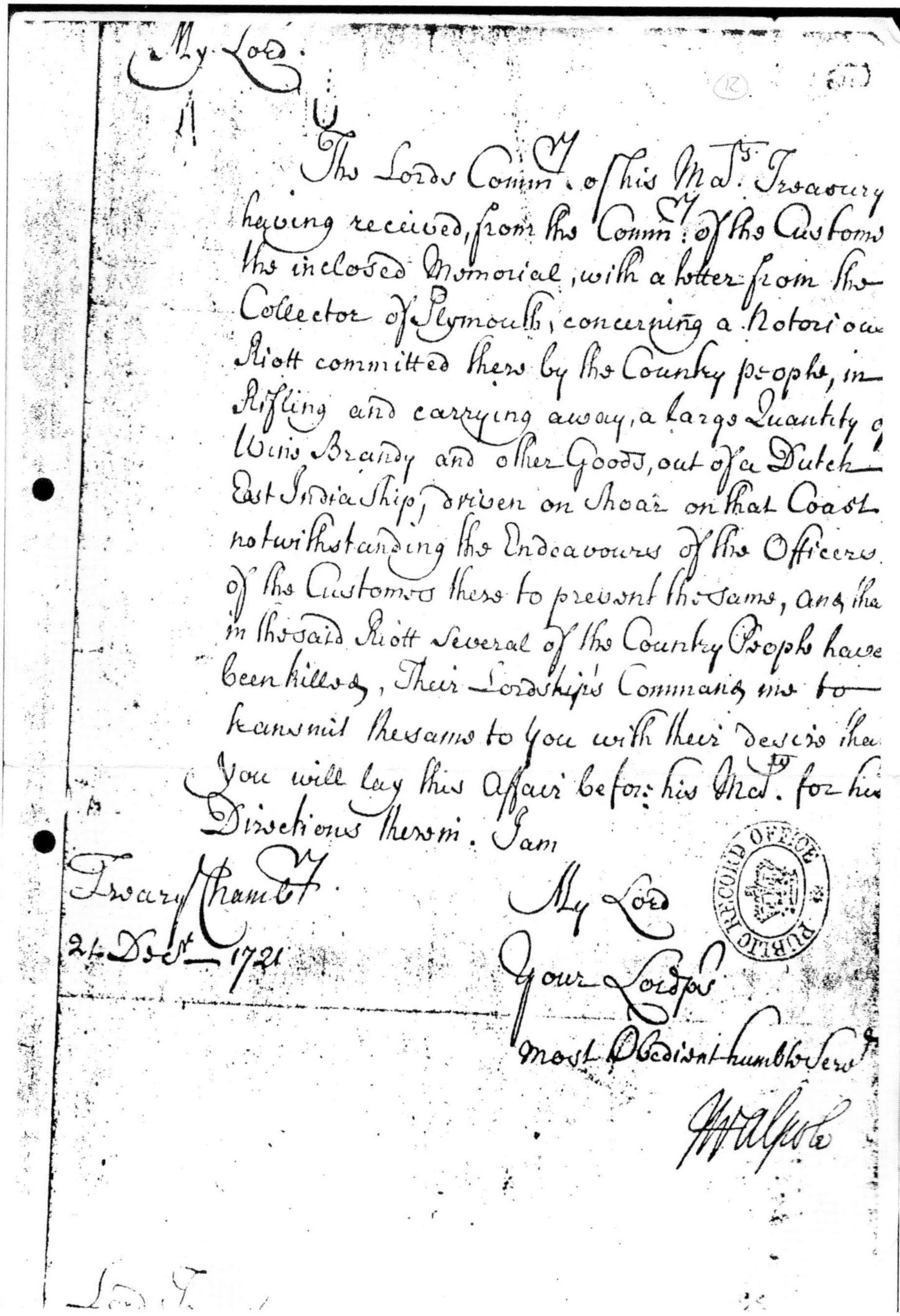
My Lord

The Lords Commrs. of his Matys. Treasury having received, from the Commrs. of the Customs the inclosed Memorial, with a letter from the Collector of Plymouth, concerning a Notorious Riott committed there by the Country people, in Rifling and carrying away, a large Quantity of Wine Brandy and other Goods, out of a Dutch East India Ship, driven on Shoar on that Coast notwithstanding the Endeavours of the Officers of the Customs there to prevent the same, and tha in the said Riott Several of the Country People have been killed, Their Lordships Command me to transmit the same to you with their desire tha You will lay this Affair before his Maty. for his Directions therein. I am

Treary Chambrs.
24 Decr 1721

My Lord
Your Lordps
most Obedient humble Servt
R Walpole

PUBLIC RECORD OFFICE

What do you make of them then Mr Green?

No different at all, all you done is proved to me is that it's just like the age old saying "you can't believe everything you read" And those letters would have been easy to make, I have a friend who is fantastic at old English writing. He could have made those letters easily.

Ok I accept that, but what you have to ask your self is why? Why would any one fordge them? What the hell purpose would do they serve?

They serve the exact same purpose that you are showing them to me for, to add credibility to the story.

Ok here's your fresh cup of tea, and don't let *this* one go cold without taking a sip.

An' come on the Captain Sensible, what do you think now that you've read those letters again?

"I now believe she did hit a cliff near Bovisands Bay, and that her crew were murdered and robbed by the people of Plymouth. I can believe the local authorities did try to stop the murderous crowd."

"And, I can see that none of the dates on the letters tie up with either Patricks article or Richard's article, so I'm still sticking with the mystery author."

"I can see you're not going to move from that position and I hope your head is now as messed up as mine is! I've been going round the twist try to make it all tie up."

"So what's the plan of attack now then Captain Black?"

Well all we can do its keep going...

You practise with that metal detector and I will keep on with the research.

And when the time comes, I'll drop you right on top of the wreck and you better find me some good shit with that detector or it's no more cups of tea for you.

Now take your cup out. ...I've got to get on with some real work.

Chapter Two

Been Here Before

Hi I'm the captain, actually I'm not a real captain,(or maybe I am) but I'm guessing some of you might have figured that out. Especially if your interest in this book is that you're like me a want to be treasure hunter with a big imagination and even bigger dreams. I mean have you spent the money already a hundred times in your head. Have you bought that new boat, that new top of the range Aqua pulse metal detector, that magnatoeter. Have you see in your semi conscious as you try to get to sleep the vision of you coming home to your wife, partner, kids and just saying those worlds we all dare to dream one day get to say, the words it took Mel Fisher 17 years to say. As you place your booty on the table with a loud thud "for us the search over, today was the day"!

Have you mentally prepared your press statement, you know your story, your tale of endeavours off by heart, where you will be when you tell it and here the gasps from the response from the listeners. Have you seen it and felt it so bad that you grow ten feet tall and you almost cry the tears of the man who proved to the world and all the sceptics in it, that you are indeed a treasure finder.

What is it you have pictured in your hand? Is it gold coins, is it silver bars, diamonds, gold bars what is it in your vision that you have found that will change your life forever. I bet it's the same in every dream, I bet you that no matter how much you think you are in control of that vision you can't change the object the find that's in your hand, the booty. I bet it's the same every time.

I read a great book once written by Napoleon Hill called "Think and grow rich" it sold millions on millions of copies and to me it kind of sums up treasure hunting and treasure hunters.

Think and grow rich, the whole ethos of the book was that if you can think it hard enough you can have it, and if you can't think yourself ever having it, then you never will. Now why does that have anything to do with treasure hunting. Well there are those who buy books like that, you know self empowerment books, self development books and those that don't. The ones that don't believe and will tell you in very strong terms that anyone who buys those books is mad, and the only reasons the people who write them have any money is because stupid idiots like me buy them. And then there are people like me who buy them and never will the two agree.

So there are people like me who believe there is an enormous wealth of sunken treasure still be found and that one day I will find some, and are those who think I am nuts and I completely wasting my time and living in cuckoo land. And I buy the how to find books and they don't.

But it's the think and grow rich process that gets you out on bed on those shitty rainy days, the thing that drags you to the library to do yet more boring old research that leads nowhere. Gets you into that wet wetsuits when it's blowing a cold easterly wind, and drives you to carry that heavy gear up and down the beach. It's the thought that you will find something that no was has ever found before, the thought of hitting pay dirt. And for be the best reward of all, proving to yourself that you can do it, you can research a target, maybe a 300 year old Pirate ship. You can find every clue, turn every page and listen to every story. Then take all the parts of the jig saw put it together and then dive where the research leads, and hey by the grace of god go I ....a ship wreck!

Can I and Mr Green do that? Well the answer you will know by now is Yes! We think we can 100% we think we can. We see it in our dreams, we see it when we are driving, we see it when we are doing the washing up in fact it's always in our minds eye.

So where does one start? I would start taking a few silent honest moments and looking at your skills and strengths. Are you the Diver/researcher? Are you a diver/worker or maybe just a bloody good researcher? I guess where you live and the oceans that surround you have a massive influence on your answer. Let me explain, I'm guessing most of you reading this are scuba divers or have done some of diving or snorkelling and would call yourselves divers. And there are lots of places in the world where it is easier to dive then others. Crystal clear waters, no currents, warm waters etc and if you live and dive in those oceans then I am very jealous (not really) and the percentage of people who would consider themselves worker/divers would be very high. Bring the figure down massively if we return home to good old blighty where is cold, green and quiet often miserable with strong currents.

Here is kind of a test, if you go diving out of Plymouth UK where I live, there are many large steel wrecks to dive on all well documented and all have been dive thousands upon thousands of times the James Egan Lane, the Persia the Main and blow me down if they didn't even sink a war ship the HMS Scylla on purpose to make a artificial wreck/reef. All the dive charter boats will take you there every day you wish, or you can join a club dive on a large rigid inflatable boat that will put you on the well known wrecks. Now your thought process should be either yes that is what I happy doing, and that's in my confidence zone. Or no I am not happy with just doing that and I am confident I can dive un supervised and unorganised. With me so far? Good.

Now how if I told you that myself and Mr Green have lived in Plymouth for over 40 years and have been diving for ever and have never dived on any of these wrecks or any other known tourist wreck you might see where we are coming from.

So have a think to yourself, see there's that word "think "again. Now think would I be happy launching a small rubber boat, with a small out board engine your own fuel and paddles and all the rest of the kit you would need to dive on the mark your research has taken you too, and dive one up one down?

So with us Mr Green dives first and I paddle the boat behind his bubbles, and when he is done we switch over and it's my turn to dive.

And you know all the very expensive dive gear you've bought, well we share a weight belt, share regs, we share and stab jacket and we share the fins. We don't share mask and snorkels or knives. The reason we dive this is so that the diver can follow his nose, his instincts or a signal from the metal detector and he knows that where ever he comes up the boat is right next to him. And as for the lack of kit, well we like to travel as light as possible because lots of times we have to launch the boat from some god dam awful places. Across beaches, down cliffs up rivers etc very rarely on a nice concrete slipway. We know the sea, we know the tides, we know the hazards, we would consider ourselves to be ocean men. Respectful of the sea, but not afraid of it. We show the ocean immense respect and know when to call it and when to go for it. When it's doable, and when it's one of those days when after all the hard work of launching the boat and kitting up, there is a change in the air and today is not the day, today is over without even getting wet.

Also we never look for wrecks deeper than 15m and we never dive into decompression stops. Its old school diving stepping back 30 years, there isn't any diver lifts and there isn't any one to dress you, or make a you a cup of tea. No one to tell you it's safe to dive and no one to tell you when the tides are slack. No one to check you're dressed correctly and no one to check you know what the hell your doing. No buddy to follow or to make stupid hand signs at you, no one to get you out of the shit. No one to lend you their knife because you forgot yours. No one to trust but yourself.

And this is why we dive shallow, as shallow as possible, when everyone is heading straight out full speed on their hard boats to dive some -30m old tug; we are the guys you are laughing out. You know you could you have seen us before, the two guys in the little rubber boat with the tiny put put engine. The ones who are turning left and heading straight for the cliffs. The two guys who look like they should be selling the big issue or in the soup kitchens, you know the ocean men!!

We don't just dive shallow because it's safer, it's because we know that nearly all ships the sank hit the cliffs, very few sank out to sea. Before the 19th century about 90% of all ships that sank hit the cliffs.

So hopefully that helps you kind of know which camp you're in, the researcher camp or diver camp, or if you have time maybe both. But not all divers are good at research and not all great researchers can dive. So now if one is ready to start, the first thing is to find a target, you do this by either research, snorkelling along the cliffs or talking to old divers and old fishermen. Local knowledge and stories are the best form of information, you just need to work out the true bits from the sexed up bits, or fisherman's yarns as they are effectionally known.

And that's it! You just start. Just like taking your first sip of cold Guinness you are hooked, and nothing is the same ever again You think about finding treasure every day and you get started on your quest and your quest won't be the same as any one else's that has gone before yours, or will come after yours, it's your search, yours alone your holy grail.

So here we are again, Mr Green and I on the small rubber boat about to dive, once again playing the highly emotional game called "treasure hunting snakes and ladders. What happens is your find a new piece of information, a new piece of the jigsaw and it's like rolling a six on the dice. Six places forward on the board and you land on a ladder. Wow nearly half way up the board and at the top its pay dirt, riches beyond your wildest dreams. Having studied both Richard Larns article and Patricks article and picked it to its bare bones, we are convinced we know where the wreck of the Aaktekerka lies.

It's another roll of the dice on that good old snakes and ladders board. Six places forward and beautiful, I landed on another tall ladder, found another clue.. So close I can taste it, spending the money already and then when you think you have all the answers and nothing can stop you this time, you dive to the bottom of the big green ocean and all your troubles are as good as over.

Make sure you've got a big strong bag I tell Mr Green you're going to need it for all the gold coins. Mr Green leaves surface with a rye smile, his ever faithful Aqua Pulse metal detector in hand. I paddle behind his bubbles all the time thinking of the things he might be finding. His bubbles are still, he's not moving, could be a target thinks I, 5 minutes pass and he hasn't moved, must be to something good thinks I. His bubbles start to move again paddle I paddle behind him, near one hour passed so he will be coming up soon, bag full of swagger. First I see his hand break the surface, then his head and I look for his eyes they will tell me what I need to know. And bollocks its bad news I can tell, I can see it in his eyes it's not today. We have just thrown a one on the dice and landed on a big fat slippery snake back half way down the board.

Not too worried, it's not over yet as it's my turn to dive, I know she is here somewhere and I am just going to dive a bit shallower and more to the North she is bound to be up those deep Northern gullies.

I get to the sea bed and sort myself out, check my weight and get out my knife, always like to dive with my razor sharp green river knife in my hand.

Mr Green likes to use his Aqua pulse I like to follow my nose and see where it leads me, not very scientific I know. But lots of wrecks and artefacts have been found by people you have a sixth sense or a gut feeling on which way to fin. I look everywhere, every gully and every crevasse, between every stalk of kelp and under every ledge and what do I find a big fat zero, not a sausage, diddly squat. Didn't even get to stab a nice plaice for my supper, seems I have even lost my touch as a good hunter gatherer amongst other things.

The only thing I have achieved is landing on the head of another big fat horrible windy snake and here I go weeeeeeeeeeeeeee all the back to "start" back to the bottom back to the beginning. Another day I didn't work, another twenty pounds down the swanny and even worse another day my little five year old will run down the drive when he sees my car and with the same undying enthusiasm shout out "did you find the treasure Daddy ? And I think to myself, maybe I should give up, maybe I already have the treasure right here in my arms, someone with unconditional love for me whether I have the treasure or whether I am the "world's worst treasure hunter". To him as with my other beautiful kids the fact that I made it home safe and I am as they say not like other Dads, I am a fun loving Pirate" and its enough for them, more than enough.

Do I give up this treasure hunting dream or do I try even harder, it's got to be one or the other. Something has to give, maybe I'm not thinking straight, and maybe I'm not looking in the right place for clues. Richard Larns, Rex Cowan and Pater McBride couldn't find the Aakterker so maybe there's no point in following their research, I mean why am I following the research of three guys who failed surely that's a bit mad, I've all ways been told the first sign of madness is to keep doing what you're doing and expect things to change. And what about Patrick ...... does he dive! Has he ever even been to Plymouth?

At least I know the three old timers have found wrecks before and in their time they where three great divers and treasure hunters. That's more than I know about Patrick. But if I am brutally honest, all of them failed, with the information they had which seems pretty sound they still failed to find the Aaktekerke.

So maybe it's time to forget there research and do my own, one last stab at it and then if I can't find some treasure this year it's get a normal nine to five job for me, I will quit. I will have to admit to all those so called friends that they were right, and I was just chasing rainbows, and life doesn't work like that.

So where do I start. What is it that's not quite right come on Captain think, think?

Well one thing has always bothered me, and has always seemed a little strange. How did three guys with such strong personalities and who usually keep everything to themselves team up together?

What was the common denominator that brought them all together? Yeh! That seems like a good place to start around, I'm going to do my own research, but before I start on the sinking of the Aaktekerke I'm going to have a bit of a dig around those good old boys and see want turns, see if there is any skeletons in there deep blue closet,

Chapter Three

Seeing Things That Aren't There or are They

SIX WEEKS AFTER THE LAST DIVE

Ring Ring..Hello! Ah Mr Green how goes it? Its Captain Black here.

It goes fine mate what's happening with you?

Well my brain is in melt down again and I can't switch it off at night, need to empty my thoughts on to you so I can get some bloody sleep. After all the months of research and digging around I have been doing I think I have finally nailed it. I think I know where the Aagtekerke sank.

Can you get your ass down here tomorrow and I will tell you my theory?

Yep can get there at 10am if that works for you?

Yep see you then

Mr Green in his mid late thirties about 5'7" and of heavy build, he is married with one little boy. He is Captain Blacks freediving buddy, diving buddy and treasure hunting buddy, he is the sensible one, the one that slows everything down and made sure things were safe. Caution and safety where his middle names and whilst together they would do extreme and unorthodox things he would always keep Captain Black in check. Mr Green also like toys, and would always invest in the best quality and maintain it to the highest standard d. He had very little time for fools and incompetence. Having recently becoming a father he was now a house husband as his wife had a very well paid job.

Captain Black is a total contrast to Mr Green and that's why there partnership worked so well. The captain to put it nicely was the ideas man, and to put it truthfully he was a dreamer that somehow managed to pull things off that no one thought possible. He was in his late forties, of strong build and caricature and was the type of guy that made things happen and went with his dreams and impulses. The captain is married with three kids and lived in Plymouth.

"Come in Mr Green..T or coffee"? "T please Captain Black"

Ok let's look at the facts or what we believe to be the fact, we know the Dutch and especially the VOC were meticulous about records and log keeping. So we have no reason to doubt their accounts we have previously read, and those we have based our research for the Aaktekerke on.

I'm not so sure we can trust them 100%, they have been translated from Old Dutch, and who knows who had stuff to hide or stuff away. It happens now and you can be sure it happened then.

Ok point taken but I think we have to accept what we have got or we will never move forward. It's going to take a lot time and hard graft and we have to believe in something. Or else we will be like the rest of the sceptics out there who tell us there no treasure left under the sea, and if there was anything there someone would have found it by now.

Your right just thought I would chuck in my usual bucket of caution

So I will start again, we know the Aatekerkre ran aground on the rocks and sank near Plymouth near Bovisand bay.

Correct..

We know this happened in 1721 and she was a Dutch VOC ship..

Correct.

We know she carried about 40 cannons, 240 men and weighed 800 tonnes and was 145 feet long. We also know she sank with about half her treasure still on board which we believe is about ten to fifteen chest of silver bars and coins.. We also know that she dumped a few cannons and her anchors in the madness of the storms...

Correct.

And you know that I also thought she sank off Noah's cove.

Yep and not without good reason Captain Black.

Well after digging up so many very old copper and iron nails which date to roughly the same age as the Aatekerkre I was pretty certain she must be off that cove.

Well you convinced me so what's changed your mind?

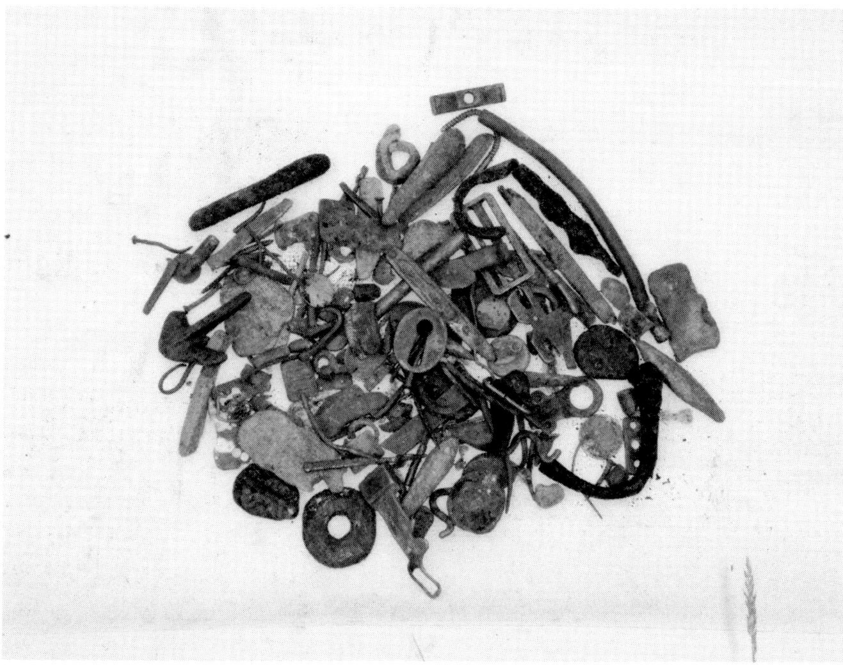

Well here's the thing as the weather has been so shit and work so scarce that I have had some time on my hands I have done lots more digging around. Plus I had a great big dollop of good luck. I tell you for all the wonders of the internet and Google the best information comes from people and their stories and knowledge. The only thing is, that one person only has one part of the jigsaw, and sometimes they don't even know they are holding a piece or even that there is a jigsaw.

So you have to kiss a lot of frogs to find a prince.

Exactly Mr Green and I notice it's me doing all the frog kissing. The other day I was talking to Uncle Orange about cannon balls, and asked him where he got all his stuff from, and did he know where I could go and dive for one. Because a mate of mine keeps bugging me for an old cannon ball, wants it for a door stop or something.. You know the score ha ha never for me always for a mate. Any way Uncle Orange told me that some times after a day's training at Fort Bovisands where he worked for years teaching commercial diving, the commercial diving students would ask him to take them somewhere where they could find old cannon balls. He would take some of the lads to a certain gully where there were cannon balls wedged in between the rocks and they would dig them out.

'That sounds interesting, as there certainly would of been hundreds of cannon balls on board the Aatekerkre and you would expect them to be everywhere around the area where she ran aground and sank.

Yeh that's what I thought and loads of cannons as well..

'Yeh I agree not the 40 cannons as we know she dump some but at least I would say 20 or so.

How much effort do you think the locals or the Navy at the time would have put into salvaging the cannons?

'Depends on how easy it was to lift them and transport them, they were very ingenious and Iron cannons would have fetched good money. But if it was a very steep inaccessible cliff a long way from a good track. Or if it was deep and strong tides they would of found it very hard, but in shallow water and not much tide and weather they would have made a big effort. I have seen old drawings of them salvaging wrecks back in the seventieth century. They would blow the shipwrecks apart with black powder barrels and then grapple for the big stuff, cannons etc Sometime s they would do this for a couple of years such where the value of large iron cannons.

And don't forget they had been murdering the crew and were wanted men.

It wouldn't have been the mob on the cliff that salvaged her it would have been the Navy from Devonport Naval base. They would have had the barges and man power to do it. Not some crazed mob.

Ok point taken Mr Green, What about the bronze cannons?.

Well we know all VOC ships carried two bronze cannons and they were a lot more valuable, so I think if they could have salvaged them if they could have, hey but the same for the chest of treasure..If they could of they would of. But they could only grapple and get large stuff, they had no way of seeing things and small stuff would still be there I am sure.

Does Uncle Orange still have any cannon balls?

Yeh he's got loads, the problem is he's in his seventies now and his memory is a bit clouded and can tell me which of his cannon balls came from the gully.

That's a shame, stupid old codger I will give him some shit next time I see him, don't think it would have told us much anyway. One cannon ball is much the same as the other.

Yeh but! If it had been let's say a 32 pounder, and we know the Aatekerkre was not carrying 32 pound cannons then we would be barking up the wrong tree, or swimming in the wrong gully. I will ask him if he can remember what size the balls where as I am sure he will know if they were huge 32 ponders or small 6 pounders. Do we know exactly what size cannons she was carrying? no but a good guess would be 6 pounders, 9 pounders, 24 pounders and some small swivel guns as well as the two bronze cannons.

How about muskets and swords?

Yeh shit loads.

Let's try and find out off the VOC in Holland a complete inventory of her cargo and size of her cannons?

I can certainly try Mr Green but you will have to put your short arms in those deep pockets as they will charge us.

More T vicar?

Yeh lovely.

Write num nuts here's you. What we need to do now is name the area we are talking about and then we can refer to it as said area. Sounds good to me how about treasure area?

You're such a knobber Mr Green no wonder I'm the ideas man you stick to the technical stuff. I will give you three choices

1 Plunder cliff
2 Phionix bay
3 Monkeys Graveyard

You're off your head Captain Black ...but if you are making me chose a name; it's got to be Monkey's Graveyard.

Write that's its then we shall only ever refer that area as Monkey's Graveyard. Now let me carry on with the bits of the Jigsaw.

A few weeks ago I went down to check on the vis and the rubber boat at Discovery Divers, and I bumped into Pinkie and Perky. They kindly made me a cup of coffee and we started to chat. Perky was in his usual happy and chatty mood so I did what I do what I do best. Yeh I know you ask question without asking a question. You got it in one.

So there we were shooting the shit, putting the worlds to rights...and then I drop the old favourite buy telling him where I been diving and some semi interesting things I had found. Then adding the old ditty "keep it quiet though mate it's a bit of a secret. Then as old sailors always do, the old black cat comes right back at me. He told me that about 10 years ago he was on a training dive and he swam past two cannons facing each other and a pile of ballast stones.

Was it close to here I asked as we where sat on the wall at Bovisands, and he said yep and pointed to a small area off a point where the cannons where. Now as we know from all our studying, a couple of cannons doesn't make a wreck site.

Yep ships would use old cannons as ballast, or dump them over board when they were in trouble.

I'm glad you've been taking it all in Mr Green.

But cannons with ballast stones, well that's a different story.

Yep too right it is!.

Have you ever found or seen any old ballast stones Captain. No never have but would I would love to. How obvious do you think they would look? I mean do you think they would just jump out of the sea bed at you?

Not sure Mr Green, I kind of think they would just look wrong. As we know they were taken from fresh water rivers and very round so they didn't damage the wooded ships. They would just be different than the surrounding rocks and formations. I reckon they would look very fragile, not sure why that's just how I imagine them. In Dr Robert Max treasure hunting books he always says the first part of any wreck site to search is under the ballast stones, as lots of heavy stuff like silver and unworked precious metals was kept in the lower decks or in with the ballast.

Yeh I remember reading that, but I also remember reading that lifting and searching under the ballast stones is always the most dangerous part of wreck salvage.

Hm, I must have missed that bit, never mind how dangerous can it be. Couple of stones! Piece of cake.

How deep the cannons captain?

-8meters about 2 hours after low water. Let's say the Aatekerker had a draft of 4m, and that spot at low water would be about 6m ten she could have passed that point and run aground on the cliff.

Yeh and then after being battered on the cliff for a few days, holed and flooded she slipped back and sunk at -10m high water.

Also Mr Green she could have easy been on her side by then as the documents tell us she was close to capsizing.

Yeh plus with hours of being on the cliff she would of been filling up with sand and being holed every where and when she finally sank she wouldn't of gone very far at all.

Ah well! I have more information that tells us she very quickly filled with sand.

Hold that tale Captain I'm dying for a piss.

Cool I'll get the kettle on and the biscuits out.

As luck would have it, I came across some information that reported that in 1968 a dive club from London fond a neck of a jar sticking out of the sand. They dug it out and it was a complete very old olive jar.

One of the only ones ever found complete anywhere ever. And guess what?

what?

It was sent to the London museum and dated.. And you guessed it; it was dated to probably the 18 century.

Wow that is cool!.

No no no Mr Green the cool bit is, they said it probably came from Holland.

Double wow!! Double cool!

No shit double wow Mr Green

So for the Jar to have remained intact for nearly 300 hundred years it must have got buried in sand very quickly, and stayed covered most of those 300years.

Yeh I would agree with that, and a jug like that is quite a buoyant item even if it was full of stuff. So imagine how quick a bar of silver or bronze cannon would have sunk. And how deep it would have sunk.

I told you that underwater metal detector you bought would come in handy some time. I reckon when Perky saw those cannons and ballast stones it was just one of those days when a storm had shifted all the sand.

So my good plan would be, if I do all the detecting and Captain you lucky lucky man you get to all the dredging and digging.

And where do you think the Jar was found?

Monkey's graveyard?

Yep you should have been a brain surgeon.

And now you've got to keep switch on as I have got more hot info. Check this out if you've got the brain space.

Yeh give it to me Captain I'm so excited now just want to grab my kit and get in amongst it.

Ok so next part of the jigsaw is just as good so go for piss now if you need to?

Good idea and I will have another brew if there's one going.

In 1972 as scuba club, let's call them scuba club R sent a letter to the owner of Fort Bovisand under water centre, who name was Commander Silver, who was a ex Royal Naval commander. In the letter they asked the commander if they could come to Bovisands and do an archaeology course.

To cut a long story short they set dates to come down and do their sea bed surveys and archaeology reports. They asked the commander if he had an area he could suggest they could survey. As the commander was going to get the results of the survey which area do you think he suggested they might like to survey?

Monkey Graveyard?

Well yes and no, a small area clipped Monkey Graveyard, but mostly the area was right next to it, on the northern side.

And you don't think that is just coincidence captain?

Hmm coincidence once maybe.

Did you get to see the results of that survey?

No, Mr Green I couldn't find the results only their method statement. Not even sure if they actually did the course or survey. Help yourself to some biscuits and open those ears wide cause here comes the next bit of the puzzle.

In 1978 guess what?

Don't tell me the same thing happened?

A different dive club wrote to commander Silver and asked if they could do an underwater armature archaeology course at Bovisands. He wrote back telling them it would happy for it to be to be done over several weekends and they set some plans and dates. As we know you have to dive the sea when it's good, and not set a date and dive even if its shit, this was their first mistake.

Did they ask the commander if he could suggest an area?

Yes they did.

Did he give them the same area as before?

As near as damm it, he gave them an area that overlapped the last area and came South East.

And did they find anything this time?

They certainly did Ollie! They found a object sticking out of the sea bed which they have called a swivel gun, they found a cannon ball, a unidentified piece of metal sticking out of the sea bed, and some bits of old wood.

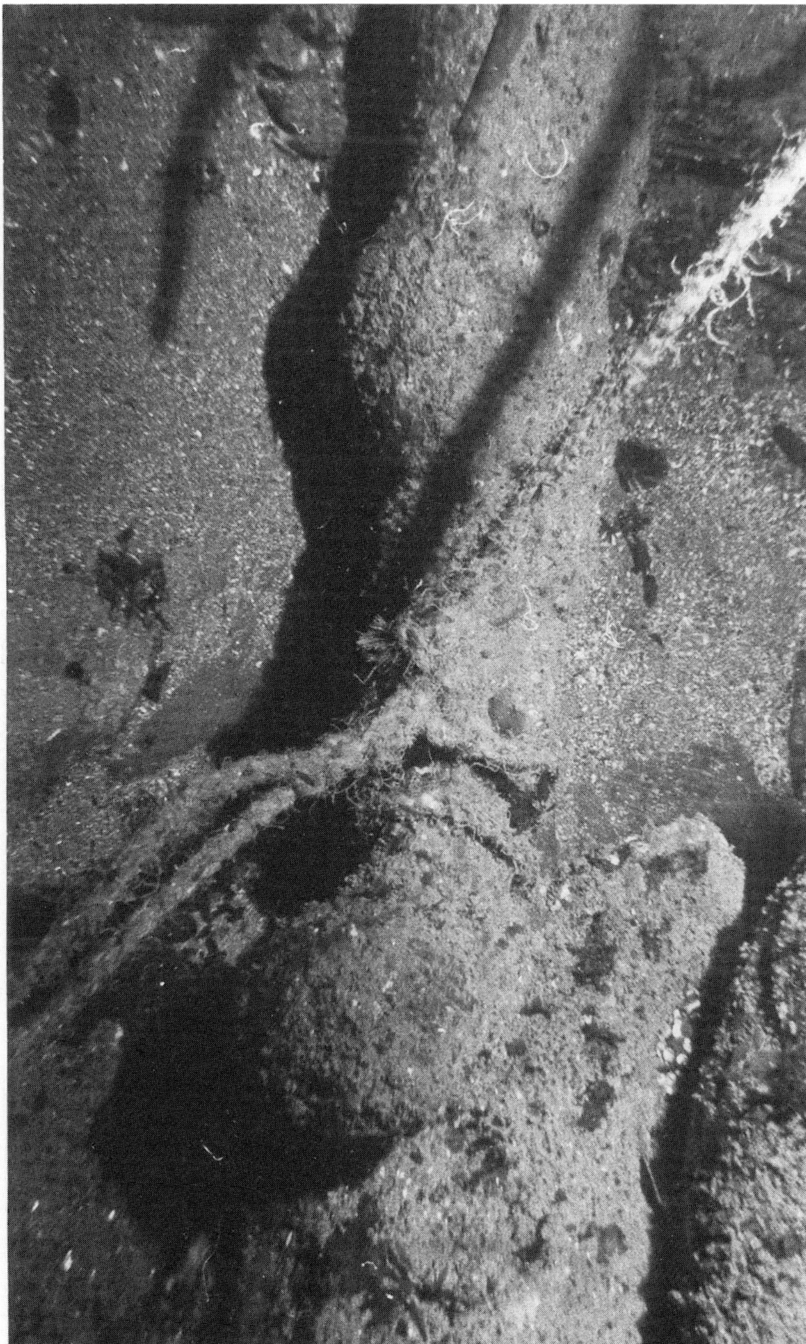

Swivel gun

Have you got or seen a drawing of the objects and where they found them. Yes to both even have a black and white photo of the object they our calling a swivel gun.

Excellent! You are definitely the man Captain.

Let have a look at the photo then.

There you go mate what do you make of that?

Not sure, can't see how they think it's a swivel gun can you ?

No I have no idea what the hell it is, but somebody must of as it's not a name you just call something.

I agree, why didn't they dig it up? I think by the time they done all there surveys they ran out of time, or did not have the right equipment to dig it up.

I'm surprised they did not find the cannons and ballast stones aren't you Captain Black?

No I'm not and I will tell you why. The mistake they made which I mentioned earlier is that they planned their weekend diving several weeks in advance and we have done the same. When they turned up to dive the visibility was pants, maybe only 2meters and the sea was not flat and the sky over cast. You tell me what the visibility was like around here a couple of weeks ago? 8-10meters vis, flat calm sea and sunny as you like.

Yes sir it was.

So the lesson learnt is you have to go dive when the conditions are fab and not when its shit just because you have planed it.

So do you think they would have found cannons and other stuff if they had better vis?

I'm not saying that, but they would have had a lot better chance and definitely found more than they did. To be sure of finding the cannons and ballast stones I think you would need the perfect day. Good vis, sunny sky, flat sea and lots of sand having been shifted by a storm.

Oh you don't want much then, how about we chuck in some big chested mermaid as well.

Yes please and Ill chuck in a merman for you, you knobber.

Stay there I need another leak. Then I have question for Mr Green. How deep will your metal detector find and object?

Depends.

I knew there was going to be a depends answer and not just a simple depth.

Well it depends on the size of the object and the sea bed material. Also what size search head I have on.

Ok well we are looking for a six foot cannon, in fine sand and silt with your biggest bests search head. How deep?

I m guessing about 4-5 feet.

Hmm that's not bad, not bad at all.

Yeh it's a good bit of kit in the right hand in the right place, and the thing is if something is only buried a couple of inches and you haven't got a metal detector you will swim right over it. You might come close but you might just as well be diving on the moon. You know the saying Captain "miss it by an itch, miss it by a mile"

I'm hearing you Mr Green loud and clear, and kind of makes up the plan for the search. A fab day with good vis and your metal detector.

What we going to dig with?

A trowel to start with then I will make an air lift and hire a road compressor if needed. Or you can make one of those water lifts you are always going on about.

And lifting a heavy object?

Not sure yet because I think the first thing we need to do it protect our interest and hard work on this site, and try and positively identify the wreck. Before anyone see us actually working over the site.

So what the plan man? Your always the man with the plan no matter how shit your plans are I take my hat off to you, you have always got a plan.

Ah yes the plan! First we need to try and get as many dives in as possible on the site without arising suspicion.

That's is bloody hard to do with all the pirates that live round here, if they see us diving there a few days in a row on the same site, they will wonder what we are up to and take a look when we are gone.

Yeh I know so we have to be careful, when we are certain we have found a site that is of interest to us, and we are going to work the site. Then we want to able to establish a "Salvor in possession" right.

How does that work?

Well when I went to the shipwreck conference last year I had the good fortune of meeting Professor Blue. He is a top maritime lawyer and has helped people like ourselves get salvage in possession orders before. I spent some time talking to him and he roughly explained to me how to go about it. He also said he was coming to live in Plymouth and would help me if needed, and he gave me all he contact details.

So what do we have to do?

Well basically we need to prove that we have spent time and money on looking and investigating this site. By keeping records and receipts of everything we do, and maintain a dive log.

Which we have done.

And we need to lift something off the bottom to prove we are in possession.

Something like a signal gun.

Ding dong the penny drops for Mr Green.

Cool

Coooolish I would say, because professor blue said that if the wreck gets identified or dated the whole thing changes.ie if…, lets paid 250 years old, English Heritage and a whole load of over pencil pushers will get involved. If it is a VOC wreck then we will have to do a deal with the Dutch Government as all VOC wrecks are still owned by them.

Would we be able to date the wreck from cannon?

We would be able to date the cannon, but cannons can come from anywhere. I think we would need more than that, maybe some timber of crockery or a ships bell would be nice.

What about a positive id? Would we need something with the VOC mark on it?

Yeh or something that was unusual and logged in its cargo manifesto when it left Holland.

I'm quite into the preservation bit and it would be good to try and preserve a cannon or other historical artefacts.

Sounds good to me, you have just volunteered yourself for that job then Mr Green. Not sure why we are talking so much about cannons, I mean it's not like we have found one and the only cannon we could conserve and lift would be quite a small one.

I agree but what I don't want to do is lift something and then start thinking about how we are going to conserve it. We need to have some conservation plans in place first, before we lift anything.

God you are so practical and caring, I will leave all that stuff to you. But the "Receiver of Wrecks" will come into play at some stage.

How about receiver of wrecks, where does she fit in? And where does she fit in with professor Blue?

Well I guess we still have to follow the letter of the law which states "that anything found in the ocean must be reported to the receiver of wrecks within 30 days" Then she has 1 year to find an owner for the item. Once the owner is found, they are asked if they wish to have the item. If they do they then need to pay the finder a fair salvage reward for the finder's services. This is determined by valuation collected by the Receiver of wrecks. If after one year no owner is found or comes forward, the object then belongs to the crown. The receiver then contacts museums etc to find a buyer or a home for the item. If no one wants its then it becomes our property.

How long could that whole process take?

Well like most government departments they have lost staff and our undermanned, so I would say about 18-20 months.

Seems to me that once we commit we've got to commit, and then the big change is when or if we can date or identify the wreck. I mean how sure are you that's where the Aartikerka lies, it could be any wreck with cannon balls and a swivel gun, hundreds of ships must have sunk around these parts hitting the cliff. What makes you think the silver commander had any idea that there was a wreck there or that it might be carrying treasure? He could have just chosen that area because it was nice to dive. It's protected by the weather, close to Bovisands and a safe area for divers at the right depth. An maybe that live jar just got washed in from where ever the Aakteferfer or any other Dutch ship or even a British ship could use them for storage.

See that why we make such a good team, as you are always there to bring me back down to earth and get out of my dream world. But what's the most important quality a treasure hunter?

Yeh, I know they must be dreamers!

Without being a dreamer you would never be a treasure hunter, it's the dream that is the buzz the passion and the energy. I don't actually think the actual treasure when we find it is going to be the best bit. I think it's the chase, putting together the 300 year old puzzle and maybe inspiring others to have ago.

Glad you feel that way about it Captain Black. Does that mean I can keep all the treasure for myself?

I never said that, you know it's all going to be mine and I'm going to be richer than my wildest dreams. And it will be time to do the dance…

Now then let me tell you a story, in the 1960; s Commander Silver led an expedition whilst in the Navy to the Shetland Islands North of Scotland. The task was to find the wreck of a ship called DeLife which hit a cliff in 1711 and guess where the ship came from? Holland?

Yep it was a VOC ship carrying Silver coins, Gold coins and some bullion. The Commander went back a couple of times and was successful in finding about 4000 silver coins and a hundred gold coins all dated 1711. They also found lots of artefacts like spoons, knifes sword handles and about of other stuff. You and I know in order to do that he must of done lots of research, and not like easy research on the World Wide Web I'm talking 1965. Wet suits, primitive gear and primitive research.

So what you're saying is that at some stage he must have had access to some VOC files and archives.

Exactly and during that research he must have came across the files on the Aaktekerker especially as it was wrecked in Plymouth on his back door step. And if you where him where would you send people who would want to do some archaeological research?

You went to the area where you thought she sank.

Yep and he would have absolutely known of that live jar and where it was found. It wouldn't surprise me if there was other stuff that was found there, that he became aware of during his 30years running at Bovisands dive centre.

You know it has always puzzled me that Richard Larns, Rex Cowern and Peter Mc Bride teamed up to search for the Aaktekeker and I couldn't figure what was the common denominator. Well it wasn't what the common denominator was; it was who the common denominator was.

And guess who was in the Royal Navy with Commander Silver in Scotland on that expedition?

No idea

Peter Mcbride

And guess who had a deal with the Dutch Government to salvage VOC wrecks, and also knew Commander Silver?

Rex Cowan

Correct

And who else was in the Royal Navy under Commander Silvers watch?

Richard Larn

Yep your right again, now you tell me it was just a coincidence the Commander sent everyone to survey the same area where a Dutch 300 year old Jar was found. And who was Uncle Orange working for when he took the students to find cannon balls, you know the answer and you know I'm right, he bloody well knew where she was.

All right Captain you have convinced me it's worth a look, I mean after the last two years we've had we couldn't do any worse, I'm in, when the weather turns good let's go look.

Cool now, Pass me your cup and I will tidy up a bit before the long haired sergeant major gets home.

So the plan is I will contact the Professor and see if I can meet him for coffee. And you get practising with your metal detector. And the next day of good vis and flat seas we need to dive the site and get to work.

That sound good, keep an eye on the weather and give me as much notice as possible.

No problem, I will do that, I have seen the long range forecast and it's really bad, so lots of time for more research. I'm hoping the next time we go it's a really flat day because we also need to detect on the foreshore at low water.

Whys that?

Oh didn't I tell you, I heard the painted man saying something about some iron cannons in a kind of rock pool cave type of thing that is cut off at low water right in the middle of Monkeys Graveyard.

So another mystery how did heavy iron cannons get into a rock pool which is cut off from the sea at low water, the storms would roll them. But it won't lift them into rock pools.

What are your thoughts?

Fell off a ship that hit the cliff and the capsized. Now get the hell out of here. And keep your lips sealed dude.

Off course I will, it's best if it's just me and you that know what we know.

The only person I will have to tell some info to is the Professor… And of course the Ginger Witch will have to know.

Of course she will! Im not that brave or stupid to think we can keep anything from her.

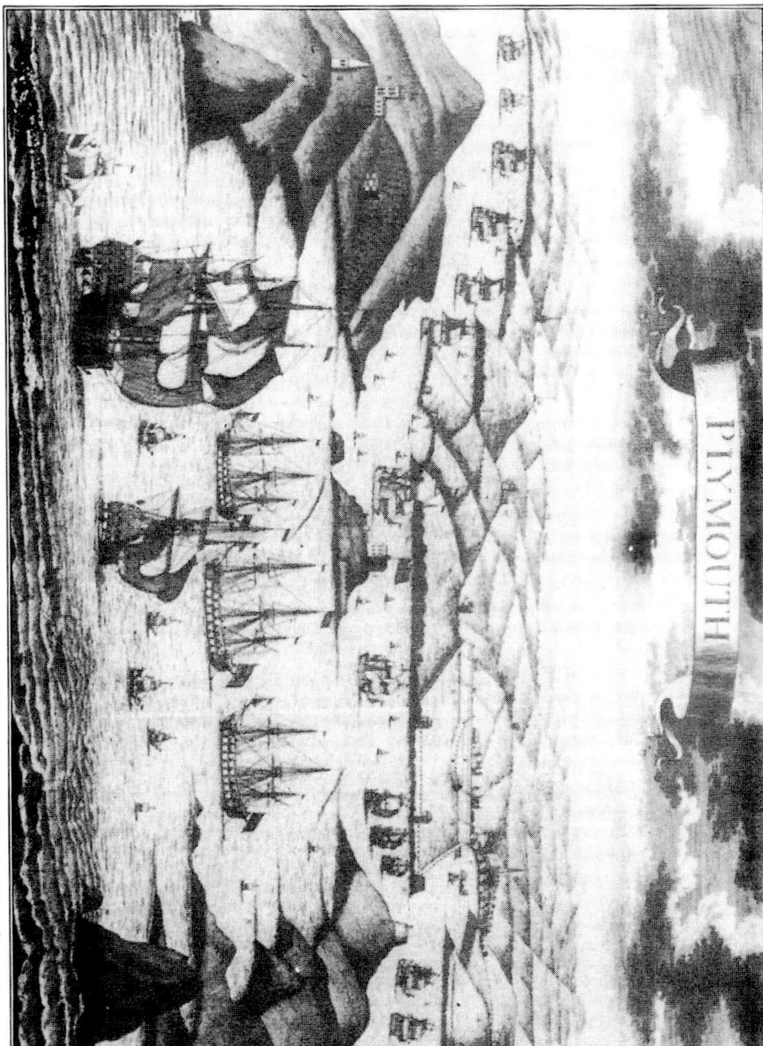

This print dated 1724 of Plymouth Sound shows big ships anchored off Bovisand while waiting for water.

Chapter Four

The Penny Drops

Oh my god! I am so stupid that is incredible, I must be so bloody stupid; I can believe how the hell I haven't noticed that before. Oh my god! Oh my god! That is unbelievable! Call myself a treasure hunter and a captain I am such a plonker. I need to sit down and watch the de vinci code all over again about a hundred times. How could I miss a clue like that?

How the hell could anyone, how all those people who have looked for the place where the Aaktekerker ran a ground have missed it. What about all the previous expeditions I have read about, how could they have missed it? And that Jar is actually called the xxxxxxxxx Jar.

I must phone Mr Green, wait to he finds out how stupid he is.

Hi Mr Green it's the greatest treasure of modern times here.

Yeh well let me know when you're a treasure finder and not a treasure hunter.

How about if I told you that we are in fact the possible "the world's worst treasure hunters" and we couldn't spot a big fat clue if it bit us in the ass.

Go on then give it to me Captain.

Ok well we both know nearly all marks on a admiralty chart, bays, headlands, reefs etc are named for some good reason. Even Rocks and have a name.

Yep

And we know that those names are not just made up or plucked out of thin air. They nuts of got their names from somewhere or someone. Even surf breaks that have well know names, that some time in the past someone named.

Go on.

Well I had a absolute eureka moment and my whole body was shaking and I was screaming out loud at myself for being so stupid. Anyway, when I calmed down which took a while? I did a bit more research just to convince myself that I finally hadn't gone mad. We both know that day is not far off, in fact my wife and her mates think that day is long gone.

Get to the point will you.

This is what I found out Bovisands bay a s we know it today used to be the place where for hundreds of years ships would come in to collect fresh water. Either at the start of their voyage or during their voyage when there supplies where running low. It was one of the only safe places to anchor to send their small boats in for water. And the stream still runs there even now, all the way onto the beach. And it even states in the article I was reading that is was the best fresh water in the whole of Devonshire. What they used to have was a big buoy with old barrows tied together, and then anchored to the sea bed so ships could come in and tie up alongside.

And on the 1690 sea chart is marked as "Buoy sands". And later on Benjamin Donns chart is was marked as "Bovey sands".

And now it's marked as "Bovi sands" and now no body knows why that bay is called Bovisands, and if you even asked people who live there where did it gets its name from they would have no idea.

It's amazing is it?

Yeh that is incredible, and very interesting, but how does that help us?

Ok so you and I both see how names get changed slightly over hundreds of years, but in the beginning when they were named, is was some good reason.

Got it, Like Plymouth being the at the mouth of the river Plym.

Now look at the area we are calling Monkeys Graveyard is called on today's admiralty chart

Yeh "Ramscliff point" I have read it a thousand times before. So What?

I know so have I, and so have thousands of people. And so did all those guys who surveyed the area before us for Commander Silver. And so must of Richard Larns, Peter Mc Bride and Rex Cowan. Maybe even Patric ..... I mean for god sake it was even called the “Ramscliff Jar”

No don’t get it Captain. Don’t get it at all; I think you have lost the plot.

OK let’s try this a different way, when a car hits another car what do you call it?

A crash?

Keep guessing

A smash up? Umm a collision? aah a bang ?

Ok that’s not working; try this one, what if a car runs into a stationary car hard?

No sorry not getting anything.

What about if you where attacking an old fort and you had to break the wooded doors down? Or in more modern times smash a car into a shop window to steel things.

Smash the doors?

Nearly

Ram the doors?

Bingo Mr Green! Now split the name of the place into two

“Rams Cliff”

Yep on the chart it’s called “ Rams Cliff Point”.

Hello you still there Mr Green Hello any one there Hello Mr Green.

Yeh yeh I’m still here.

Well have I gone nuts or what?

No you’re a bloody genius; I can’t believe I am so damm stupid. I must be the thickest man on the planet.

I know it’s just incredible isn’t it, and to think everyone else has missed it as well.

So what we are saying is that some big even i.e. a huge ship smashed into the cliff right there at that point.

Yep and is was a big enough event to be remembered, and to be referred to as the place the or a ship “Ramed the Cliff” for many years. So much so that it became known as “Rams Cliff Point” And then as with all these names it makes it on to the Sea Charts. Then just as with the Bovisand story the name gets changed. In this case it gets changed to one word.

So if that is true we should be able to look at the old charts, se when that place was first named "Ramscliiff" and also find out when it became two words.

That's exactly what we need to do.

And if it was called "Ramscliff" before 1721 then whichever ship hit that cliff point, it was not the Aaktekerker. So maybe there is still a shipwreck there Captain but! It's not the one we've been looking for.

So what you going to do now, you seem to be on a roll mate, you're on fire? But hold on a minuete what about your Noah's cove theory. Remember at one stage you had me convicted the Aagtekerke ran aground there.

Yeh well now I'm thinking when she finally smashed up that maybe a larger piece of wood with all the nails in drifted off to near Noah's cove. And don't forget we already know that Noah's cove is an accretion point. And that if you took a modern day ten pence piece and threw it in the sea say a mile out to sea that it would always wash up in Noah's cove. That's why throughout history people have found and referred to accretion points.

One of the strangest TV programmes I ever watched was about this beach comber who lived in Porth Towan in Cornwall. What he did was explain accretion points and how things of the same weight and density would always wash up on the same beach right next to each other.

Surely that depended on how far away from the beach they were when they went into the ocean. No not at all, as long as they went in the sea at the same time they could cross the Atlantic Ocean and wash up next to each other.

What thousands s of miles?

Yep once this guy fond two shotgun cartridges next to each other on the beach, he traced the shop that sold them, and then the guy who bought them. And where do you think they entered the water?

Go on surprise me.

The guy was shooting geese waste deep in water in Canada.

So the two shell casings crossed thousands of miles or storms and, the whole Atlantic and landed next to each other on the same beach. I have got to see that video some day!!

Yep because they had the same weight and density that's what they do. And you also know that when I dig up those copper nails I also dig up old sixpences and thrupences as well as new coins. Anyway stop side tracking me I dread to think of the size of my phone bill. The time of research has passed and it's time to dive and have a look.

Those documents from the Dutch National Archives have been ordered I will let you know how much they cost and when they arrive.

See you Friday, Big Balls.

Chapter Five

The First Glimmer of Hope

The forecast is good light south westerly's force 3-4, suns out and the sky is blue and beautiful day. Having done some more research and climbed a few ladders and we are near the top of the snakes and ladders board. Our peckers up and we have got a good swagger about us. Same rubber boat with the old but trustee Yamaha 8hp on the back. Dive bottles are charged and we are ready to drop the anchor right down on top of the mother load, on the exact mark has lead us to. No GPS, now SAT NAV and no depth finder, just a good old fashioned admiralty chart and a compass.

Left a bit Mr Green and ten meters ahead, ok a bit further and stop there.

How does that look to you Captain Black?

Yes nearly but not quite I don't think she could have come in this close as she had a five meter draft. Let's go out just a tickle, ok that's it throw the hook over there, that's the money shot Mr Green I'm telling you where on it.

Don't give me that look Mr Green I know I have said those words a hundred times before, but this time we are on it I can feel it in my water.

No that's all that tea you've been drinking, and now you're going to move me old the way so you can take a piss off the back aren't you?

You know me so well, and you also know that some of it will go over the out board engine the same as it always does.

Your bloody disgusting, your worse than any dog.

Shut up and get dressed in and find me something good with that useless metal detactor your always raving about, I can't face another day of slippery slimy snakes.

Ok see you in about an hour Captain and just keep an eye on the tide dropping if we are going to stay anchoured up today.

Yeah yeh get down there and don't come up to you find something I don't care if you have any air left or not, I don't want to see your ugly mug again until you have something in your hand, now get lost and leave me to have a coffee in piece.....

Bloody hell!! What are you playing at! You've only been down a couple of minutes what the hell have you forgot now.

I haven't forgotten anything; I just can't find a sausage.

What?

I can't find a sausage Captain, but! It's a good job because I'm not looking for sausages so you better help me with this chuffing heavy cannon ball.

Old my god! You sly old fox you slimy old dog, wow that is a beautiful cannon ball one of the best I have ever seen.

Yep and I'm off again got some more signals on the good old Aqua pulse, see yu later!

Pass it to me, what is it this time.

Here you go, be careful it's some musket shots.

Fantastic, I've got them now get your ass back down there and find some more stuff.

What you got this time, open your hand.

Nothing in my hand this time I'm afraid; just want to tell you I have found cannon.

UN believable!

Yeh and that's not all, it's still got its tampion in the end which means it's still loaded and primed. There are signals everywhere Captain, we have only gone and done it, we found ourselves a ship wreck. Maybe not the one we are looking for, but a bloody old ship wreck.

And so Mr Green the adventure begins no slippery snakes for us. Well not today any way. And when the little speedster runs out to greet me tonight he is going to get the shock of his life, his popsy is no longer a shipwreck hunter, but a shipwreck finder.

So what next then Captain? Well what we need to do next is lift that cannon and see what is under neath it. We need to bring it up as intact as possible and keep all the crud attached to it. Last two weeks ago in

FRIDAY 31ST JULY 2010

Vessel	Tomb Raider (mrk 1 Royal marine Rigid Raider)
Weather	Poor
Vis	4m
Dives	3 dives
Depth	-8m
Seabed	Rocks, kelp and sandy gullies
Items found	one Large Cannon Ball, two musket shots. Small cannon heavily crustated.
Items recovered	Cannon ball, musket shots.

**Divers Captain Black, Mr Green, coxswain Son of Captain Black*

SUNDAY 1ST AUGUST 2010

Vessel	Tomb Raider
Weather	Fair
Vis	3m
Dives	2
Depth	-8m
Seabed	Rocks, kelp and sandy gullies
Items Found	Lots target signals on the metal detector
Items Removed	0 (working on small cannon, getting ready for recovery. Photos taken of cannon)

**Divers Captain Black, Mr Green.*

Florida divers recovered a small swivel gun and inside the gun and the crud were loads of gold and silver coins.

Yeh like we're going to be that lucky. Well that's not all it turn out the gun was bronze.

I thought bronze cannons didn't get curded up? Yeh me to but I have seen the photos on the net and its very heavily cruded. How long would you say the cannon are Mr Green?

It's about 86cm

And do you think its iron or bronze?

I would say Iron, but because it's so small it could be bronze?

And was the Aaktekerke carrying any small Iron or Bronze cannons?

We know all VOC ships carried two bronze cannons but they would have been about 2m long not tiny like this thing.

Well we need to get it up and then I plan to get it x-rayed before we nock any of the crud off.

How you going to do that, well I am going to ask Babcock's in Devon port Dockyard to do it for me.

Think you can blag that favour?

Yep you leave that to me, let's get the lifting bags and tools ready and plan the next day's diving, We will need a 3rd man. Wink wink He is already loaded and primed; Uncle Orange is good to go.

"Let me tell you a little something about Uncle Orange. First of all he is not my real Uncle, when he was young dumb and full of cum he was a young Royal Marine serving his Queen and country. But he did not bold well to discipline and was danger of being kicked out of the cor. My dad was colour sergeant PTI down the gym, and he said send that scaly wag down to me, I will teach him how to box and turn him around. To cut a long story short, they became lifelong friends. I have known Uncle Orange all my life; in fact he was one of my inspirations for getting into diving. After leaving the marines he became a hard hat diver, then a off shore saturation diver. Now at the grand old age of 76 he is still going well, as skinny as a rake, weighs about 3 stone soaking wet. He cycles everywhere and never rides past a skip full of someone's disregarded crap without having rummage through it. In his prime Uncle Orange was one of the world's best and most sort after North Sea divers for sure. Now days he has slowed down a bit on land but still does a good working dive, the hard bit is getting him dressed and in the water. The old goat can't get his own fins or gloves on any more, and his neck is so skinny every suit he wears leaks like a sieve. He needs so much weight to get under the water, the only way is to stamp on his head and push him under. Uncle Orange like the Chiseller has the nose for finding things, and never throws anything away, and I mean any thing"

"He has a forty feet container full of every diving thing you can imagine and lots of things you could not imagine. He has Cannon balls, swords, riffles, muskets, standard diving sets, VOC bronze cannon, just thousands upon thousands of artefacts. He is quite a wealthy man, but if you passed him in the streets you would expect him to be shouting out "BIG ISSUE" or asking you for tupence for a cup of soup. I give him a hard time sometimes and shout at the deaf old bastard, but he is a one off and I love the old git. He would do anything for me and my kids, in fact he would do anything to help anyone."

Chapter Six

Recovering The Cannon

The day's diary

Loaded the Tomb Raider with all the kit we thought we would need to separate the cannon from the rocks and lift it. Lump hammers, crow bars, pink bars, chisels, lifting strops, shackles, lifting bags and lots of rope.5 dive bottles and all our dive kit with 5mm wetsuits.

Launched the Raider and travelled to the Monkeys Graveyard, as always the 70hp engine was not working properly and could only chug along at 3 knots.

Mr Green dive first, once on the cannon and we could hear him working, Uncle Orange went in to join him. Good progress made on first two dives, excavation going well and every care is taken not to take off more crud than is needed and not to damage the cannon.

Captain Black next in and carries on excavation, cannon nearly free. Quick cup of coffee and sandwich and back in for Captain Black and Mr Green. Cannon free and starting to attach lifting bags and plastic 25 litter drums. Captain out of air. Mr Green fills lift bags and the cannon is raised and secured about 1.5m under the boat with ropes and strops. All divers out of water and discuss what to do next. Do we wet store the cannon and pick it up another day as the tide is way out and its spring tides? Or do we go for it and tow it back to the mount batten centre where we launched from?

Decision made and we set of very slowly, making about 1knot which should take us about 1 hour.

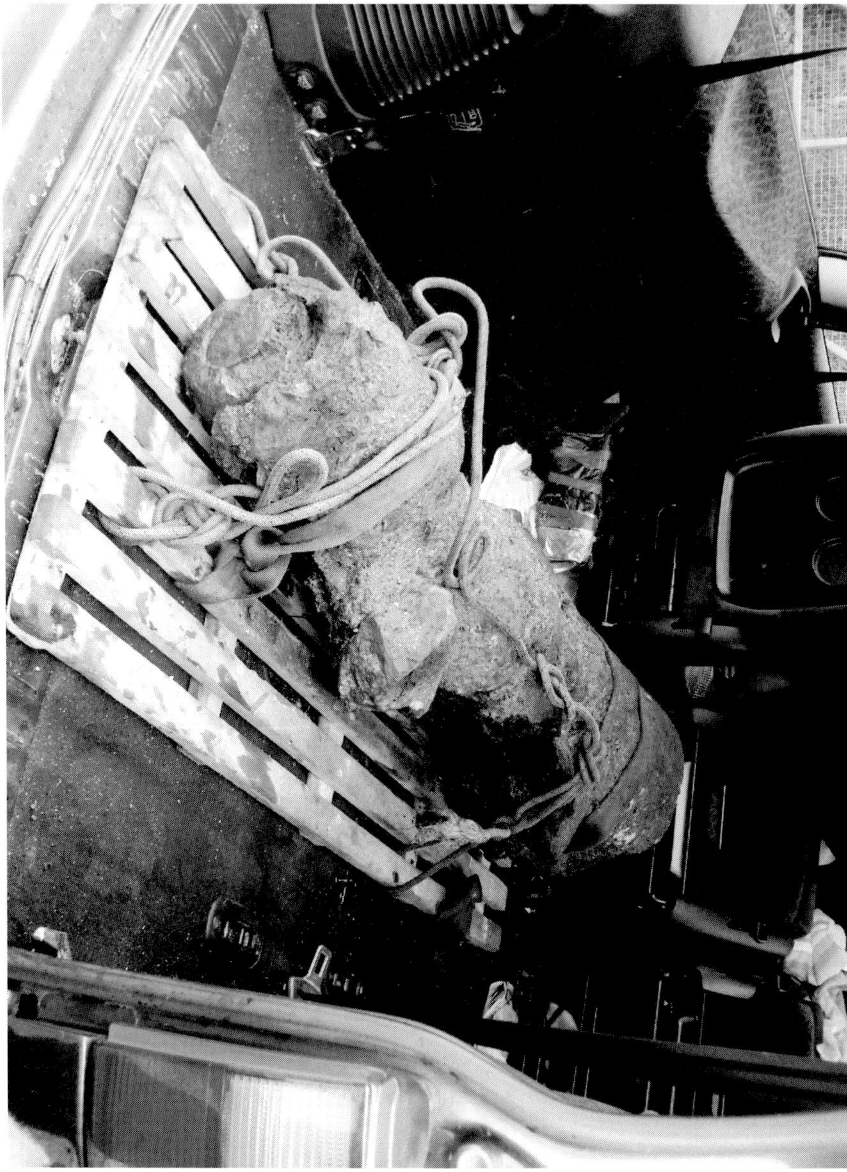

Arrive at Mountbatten centre to find the tide is too low to get the boat with the cannon slug underneath on the pontoon or slip way. Tie up to a buoy in the middle of the river and way 2 hours. Uncle Orange has a well earned nap, he did well for an old codger.

We make a plan to lower the boat trailer down the slip with a 30 feet rope tied to the car tow hook and lower the trailer far enough under the water to lower the cannon on the back of it. Then lash it to the trailer.

Dive Log 12,08,2001

Weather	Fair/overcast
Vis	2m
Depth	-6m
Seabed	Rocks, kelp
Items Found	None
Items recovered	Small cannon (now know as the Monkey cannon)

**Divers Captain Black, Mr Green, Uncle Orange*

Tied high enough to make an attempt. Worried that other people or divers might see what where up to or worse the cannon.

Uncle Orange stays in the boat and Captain Black and Mr Orange put on mask and snorkels and stand on the back of the trailer. Cannon positioned over the end of the trailer then lowered and tied to the trailer. Trailer towed up the slipway with cannon safely secured on it. Now the problem of how to get it in the back of the people carrier. Lucky enough we were able to back the car up to the side of the slipway where the boot of the car was level with the wall. And then move the trailer around to the top of the wall, so now the trailer and the boot where the same height. Went for a scranny and came back with a really good wooden pallet that bridged the gap perfectly and we heaved and pushed and got the cannon on the pallet in the back of the car...7pm long day!! But not over yet. It was important to now work fast to get the cannon home and in a tank of water as quickly as possible so it could be stabilised. Captain Black phoned his wife so she could bring all the kids down to see the cannon. The 5 year old was so excited he was tap dancing.

> "Suits off, boat unloaded and we set off for the Captains house where the tank was all ready, how we were going to get the cannon the tank was another challenge. Uncle Orange getting tired after such a long hard day so we dropped him home, in fact we were all knackered now..8pm"

> "Again another stroke of luck as the garden ran up at slope next to the drive and we were able to get the neighbour to move their car and we back the cannon in to the wall at the same height as the boot just like before, cannon now on the pallet on the grass. We moved the car and put the tank in place. Our problem was we planned for the cannon to weigh about 100kg which would of be man handle able and it was closer to 250kg which was not. Man-

aged to get the man across the road and the neighbour to give us a lift. The cannon was safely in its tank which was quickly filled with fresh water and it was time to take stock and have a wee smile."

What are the next plan then Captain?

Nothing at the moment, go home and chill out I will change the water every day and hose the cannon down and we will just lay low for a while.

Let's plan the next dive for about the 20th if that's good with you?

Yep sounds good,we need to pick up all those lumps of crud that came off and have a dig around in the sand where the cannon was.

Yeh I agree, and I'll tell you what it was a good job you brought uncle Orange with us he was fabulous unnder water, really got stuck in.

Yeh well that's not surprising when you think that he has been diving for living nearly all his life. But just to give you a tip, if you're ever the person on the boat dressing him in. Well he is not good at leaving the surface so what you have to do if put your foot over the side and stamp on his head.

You're joking?

No! Straight up you need to stamp on his head and keep pushing to until he is underwater. Then as you say he is as good as any diver you have ever met.

Don't you worry that something might happen to him, I mean at 74 anything could happen.

Nope don't worry at all, diving is his life and he knows the risk and well if he doesn't come up. Hey ho he has had a good innings and he has promised me I can have his watch if he doesn't come back. Now get your ass back to the gorgeous heavily pregnant wife of yours or she will cut your balls off, and probably mine to.

Still can't believe we got the cannon safely back here, do you think any of the local divers or skippers saw us?

Can never be sure but it was good for us that it was such an overcast cold wet day, let's sit tight and see what comes out of the woodwork.

Ok I'm, off see you on the 20th.

Bye mate and well done today, top effort and another best day ever!

Now where's that large glass of wine!

Chapter Seven

Time To Go Public

Don't get out of your car Mr Green we need to go and pick up Uncle Orange he is waiting for us and I can tell you the plan on the way in your car.

So the plan is to lift the cannon out of its tank with that lifting frame you bought on e-bay and the 5 tonne chain hoist I have. Once its up in the air we will move empty the tank and move it out of the way and then put the trailer I have borrowed under neath the cannon and lower it slowly down.

And then what's the plan and timings after we get it in the trailer?

Well we then take it to Mountbatten slip way and place it in the water.

How do we get it out of the trailer and then back in the trailer?

I have borrowed an engine lift from my brother in law you know old scruffy beard.

Sounds like a good plan, how much time we got?

Lots of time the Plymouth Herald and Western Morning News plus BBC South West will be on the slipway at 11am.

Are we going for the full dress up, suits dive tanks the works?

Yep! Not sure how we are going to get Uncle Orange to put his suit on and pretend we have just been diving. But he will have to tow the line and stick with the script.

I think he will be OK as long as we don't let him do any of the talking.

No problem, you keep him busy and I will do all the talking, and when we have finish the media stuff we will take it back to my house and put the cannon back in that larger tank I have acquired fill it with the old water and then wait and see what comes out of the shadows.

THX-E01-S2

The Herald, Saturday August

Divers haul up primed cannon

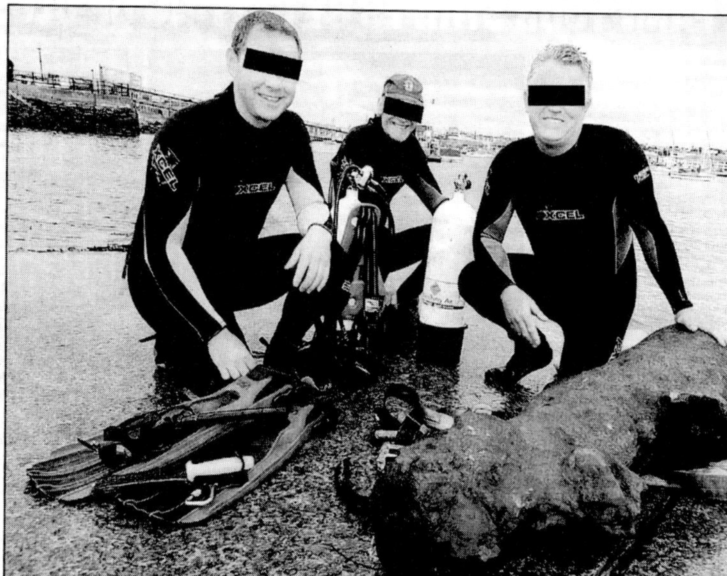

AARRRRRGH me hearties! If you see Captain Jack Sparrow, tell him: the Black Pearl may be lying on the seabed of the Sound.

And she's fully primed and ready for battle.

A team of divers has hauled a small cannon out of the waters off Plymouth. They are refusing to say which ship they believe the cannon came from, nor where exactly it was lying.

But the weapon appears to be ready for a spot of close quarters combat.

[redacted] a commercial diver and amateur marine archaeologist, found the 200kg cannon after researching local shipwrecks.

When [redacted] and his colleagues Chris Bird and Ray Ives hauled the heavily encrusted weapon ashore at Mount Batten yesterday, it was found to have a wooden plug, or tampion, in the end of the barrel.

"If they were in danger or under threat, they would put the ball and charge in and then tap in the tampion to keep the powder dry," [redacted] said.

The men immediately took the cannon to Mr Jones's house, where they immersed it in tanks of fresh water.

"It wouldn't last more than a few hours in the air," [redacted] said.

He is now appealing for experts from the University of Plymouth and any local archaeological groups to come forward to help with an estimated three-year conservation exercise.

Babcock Marine has offered to X-ray the cannon to see what secrets the tampion is concealing.

Meanwhile, [redacted] is putting together a bigger team

where they found the cannon, but he hoped a search of the sand would reveal more finds.

[redacted] said they believed the cannon came from a ship that sank "some time during the 18th century" — a time when the most notorious pirate captains still terrorised the Caribbean and the 'Spanish Main'.

He said there were many other larger cannons on the seabed in the Sound, but it was exciting to discover a new one.

[redacted] said that at just 4ft 6in long and with a barrel estimated at 3in diameter, this was probably a top deck cannon, used for close-quarter fighting.

"But I'm not an expert," he said. "That's why I'd like some experts to come forward and help us to work on this find."

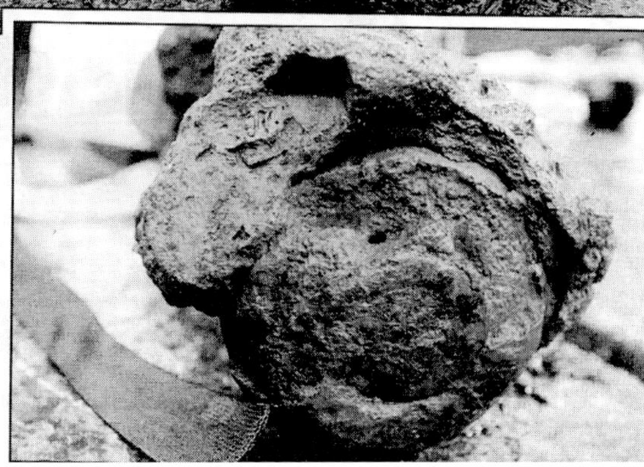

Divers find artefacts from mystery vessel

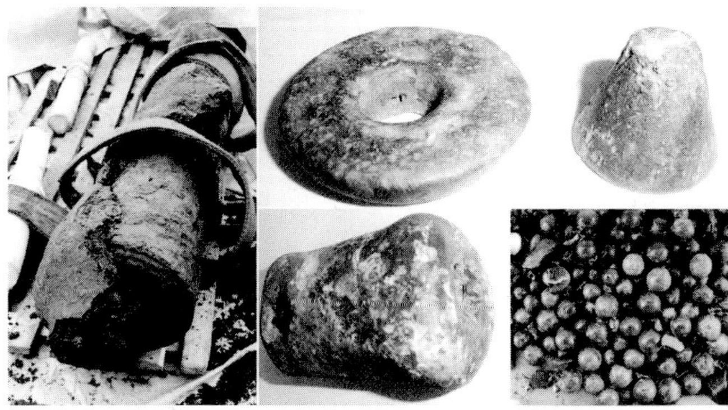
HOWARD JONES

Clockwise from above: Cannon with concretion partly removed; lead disc and small weight; cannonballs of varied size; sounding lead.

FIVE SOUTH DEVON DIVERS have found and raised cannon and other items from a wreck site near Plymouth Sound.

[redacted] Chris Bird, Ray Ives, Dan Bolt and Mike Pellet raised the finds from a 12m-deep area just 30m from the shore.

First up was a 1.5m-long cast iron cannon, heavily concreted. Placed in a conservation tank at one of the diver's homes, it was de-crudded to reveal that a tampion, or wooden end bung, was still in place. This would have been fitted once the cannon was loaded, to keep its powder dry.

"The fact that the cannon was loaded suggests that the ship may have been under threat or in some other sort of hostile environment," team-leader Jones told **DIVER**.

Returning to the site, the divers spotted three more cannon, which were left in place. They then used an Aquascan metal detector to locate and dig out and raise different-sized cast-iron cannonballs and musket balls, and a range of other items, all made of lead.

These include a sounding lead, with hollowed base into which grease would have been put to help crewmen to determine whether a seabed was rocky or sandy; a scupper lining; and items apparently connected with armoury production.

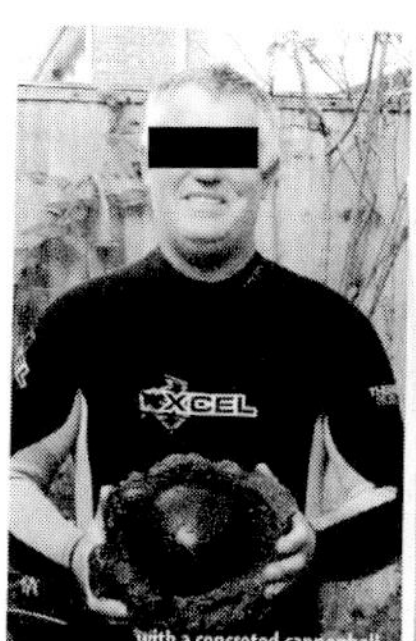

With a concreted cannonball.

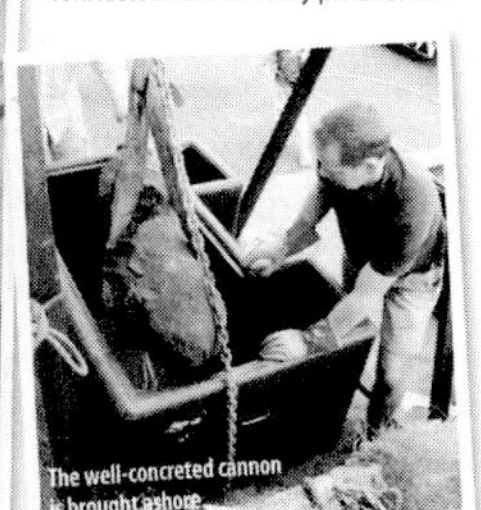
The well-concreted cannon is brought ashore.

A thick lead disc with cannonball-sized hole may have been used in cannonball manufacture, to help cool the balls.

And a 2cm-high pyramid-shaped weight of "exactly two and a quarter ounces" is thought to have been for weighing out musket powder.

Some lead forms could have been used for shaping shoes, while broken crockery, glass and "small bits of leather" were also brought up.

"We think that what we've found is probably a cargo vessel," [redacted] told **DIVER**.

"The finds have been declared to the Receiver of Wreck, who is now using historical records to research what the ship might have been."

He hopes to tour local schools with some of the finds.

[redacted] freely describes the group as "treasure-hunters", with little archaeological experience. They started diving in the area of the wreck site during the summer, after research indicated that a wreck containing valuable materials might lie there. The discovery they made was not what they had intended, but they remained "delighted" with their discoveries.

"We found the site to be covered in about three feet of transient sand and lots of thick kelp, which made searching very hard," said [redacted]

"There was so much sand that it was actually lying on top of the kelp leaves. Once we started excavating a target the visibility went down to near zero, and took a long time to return."

The site was mapped using a rudimentary underwater grid about 50m square, plus small, coloured buoys placed at known locations.

To help mark the positions of finds, GPS positions were taken of an SMB sent up from the appropriate spot on the seabed.

"The water was shallow enough for this to be pretty accurate," said Jones.

The team plans to investigate the site further next spring.

Britons locate French cave-diver's body

TWO LEADING BRITISH DIVERS have located the body of a cave-diver in France, after being called in by the French Cave Rescue service.

Rick Stanton and John Volanthen, who are members of the South & Mid Wales Cave Rescue team, were asked by the Spéléo Secours Français to help search for Eric Establie in mid-October.

The Frenchman, a highly experienced cave-diver who ran an underwater engineering business, was lost in the Ardeche area's Dragonnière Gaud cave, near Labastide de Virac.

It was hoped that he would be found alive in a dry section, after being trapped by a rock fall in the cave passage.

According to a BBC report, Stanton and Volanthen were flown to the area by RAF helicopter as a French team dug through to a dry cave bypassing the rock-fall, which was thought to have occurred about 780m into the system.

Stanton and Volanthen, called in for their cave-diving experience and search and rescue skills, dived to find Establie's remains a reported 900m in from the main cave entrance, eight days after he had entered.

They recovered Establie's dive computer, but the French cave rescue authorities decided against trying to recover his body and putting divers in further danger.

Stanton and Volanthen were recently part of the four-man team that set a remarkable world record penetration of 8.8km (5.5 miles) into Spain's largely unexplored Pozo Azul cave system (*Diving Everest in Pozo Azul*, November).

Any word from Dr Evil Pork Chop?

No not yet...right ssssh Uncle Orange is there waiting on the pavement.

Chapter Eight

Professor Blue Vists

Come in Mr Green but keep really quiet the wife and kids are asleep up stairs. I will get the kettle on.

So what's the plan Captain? Our we still going for a dip in this weather?

Well I'm going call it off and suggest we use the day to do the stuff we keep putting off, the forecast is force 5 SW and the fog is due to stay in all day. Let's have a cup of T and catch up I have lots to tell you.

Sounds good what's new then?

Well I called Professor Blue yesterday and he came over to see the cannon.

And what did he think?

Well first of all we had a cup of T here in the kitchen and something weird happened, he didn't know the name we gave him was professor blue and as we were talking I called him professor Blue and what happened next freaked me out. He turned and said" that's funny how did you know?" I said know what? And he said "well I only got my letter of appointment to professor last week and I didn't think any one new yet, and it came as a surprise to me"

Wow I know what you're thinking, your thinking this is the work of the Ginger Witch aren't you?

Yep! Without a doubt this is the work of the Witch. Mark my word and tread carefully dude

Yeh I will, and I am sooooo glad she is on our side.

Any way moving on, I was a bit worried that the professor would drive all the way over here from the other side of town and then not find the cannon and other stuff very interesting and be a bit disappointed. After all he is part of the team that found the Salcombe wreck with those gold coins on and Bronze Age swords.

Was he disappointed?

No! Quite the opposite it was the blown away he stayed about two hours and he was great to talk too and pick his very large brain. I started talking to him about Richard Larns article and some of the fact that it had some confusing bits in it and guess what he called Richard Larn.

A Pirate?

No he called him Tricky Dickey and said that is what he is referred to by other divers that know him, and he said don't take too much notice of what he writes because he would never write anything in an article that could possibly help anybody find anything he didn't what them to find.

So what the pro was saying is that the mistakes could be on purpose, and that my first guess was right he is a Pirate.

Yep that was kind of the gist of it. Any way we went out to look at the cannon and I drained all the water away so he could see it. And he thought it was fab and even asks if he could take over hosing it down with water. And when was looking out the kitchen window I saw him change the hose from jet to spray so it was nice and gentle ha ha. Just like bathing a baby. And to think I have been doing the same thing some times and I was staring to question whether I was going nuts or not.

Did he have any idea of date or nationality?

No the only thing he thought was that it looked like a kind of mortar cannon because its barrel was so short, but like he said until we get all the crud off its any bodies guess what lies under neath.

Is he going to help us with the legal side of things?

Of course he is, especially after just becoming a professor; he is in good spirits and keen to help.

She is a good old Witch.

Right finish your T and let's get into the pluming centre and buy all the bits we need to make that water dredge you have been keeping on about. Have you finished your design yet?

Ok I have all the drawings with me so let's go.

Cool and then we can go into Plymouth central library and check out the old charts.

Sound good because I want to check for any old paper cutting from that DEC 1721-MARCH 1722

Shortly if there was anything in the local news papers and we can find it then Tricky Dicky would have printed them in his article to prove he was right and Patrick was wrong.

You think?

Ok point taken lets go check it out.

PLYMOUTH CITY MAIN LIBARY LOCAL SECTION.

Right Mr Green I'm going to start over here on the charts and see what I can find and you go to the Micro film section and I'll come over to join you when I have finished.

Where is the Micro film section and where do I get some help?

Over there Mr Green 9 o'clock..In the tight fitting suit, he's your target.

What do you mean my target?

Come off it Mr Green you can see he works here and he's batting for the other side, he will be very pleased to assist you.

Bugger off he's not going to want to help me for any other reason than it's his job.

Look we all no you have a gentle camp side now open the top button, pull you shorts up and be nice to the smart young man.

Cheers some mate you are.

Stop winging and get over there..Oh be sure to comment on his nice goatee.

How are you getting on Mr Green?

Yes good how about you Captain?

Yeh I have finished.

Find out anything?

Yep I found the 1693 chart of Plymouth which is the earliest one I can find, it was produced by Captain G Collins and RAMSCLIFF POINT was not marked on it, and then I found a 1770 chart and it was marked on it.

So only 27 years before the Aaktekerke rammed a cliff there is no RAMS CLIFF POINT, and then in 50 years after there is.

Yeh but the best bit is on the 1770 chart it was written on in two words RAMS CLIFF POINT. Here have a look for yourself.

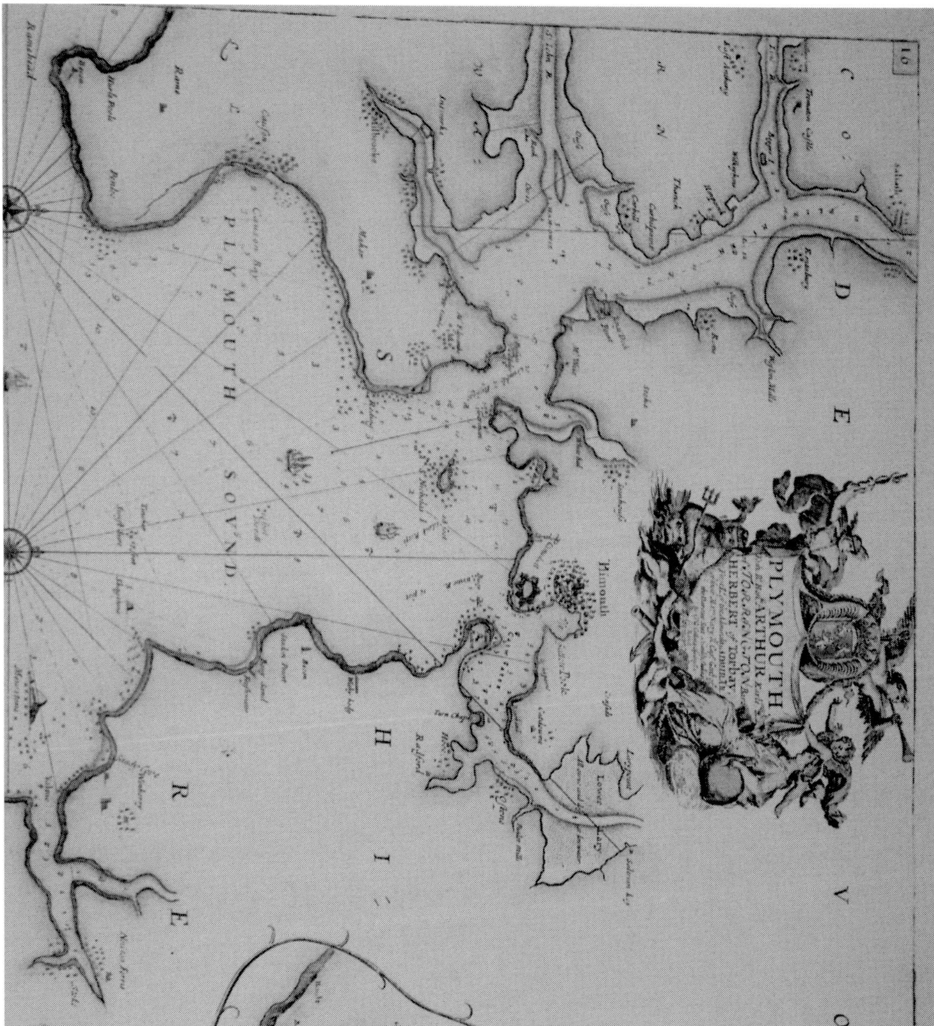

No rams cliff point

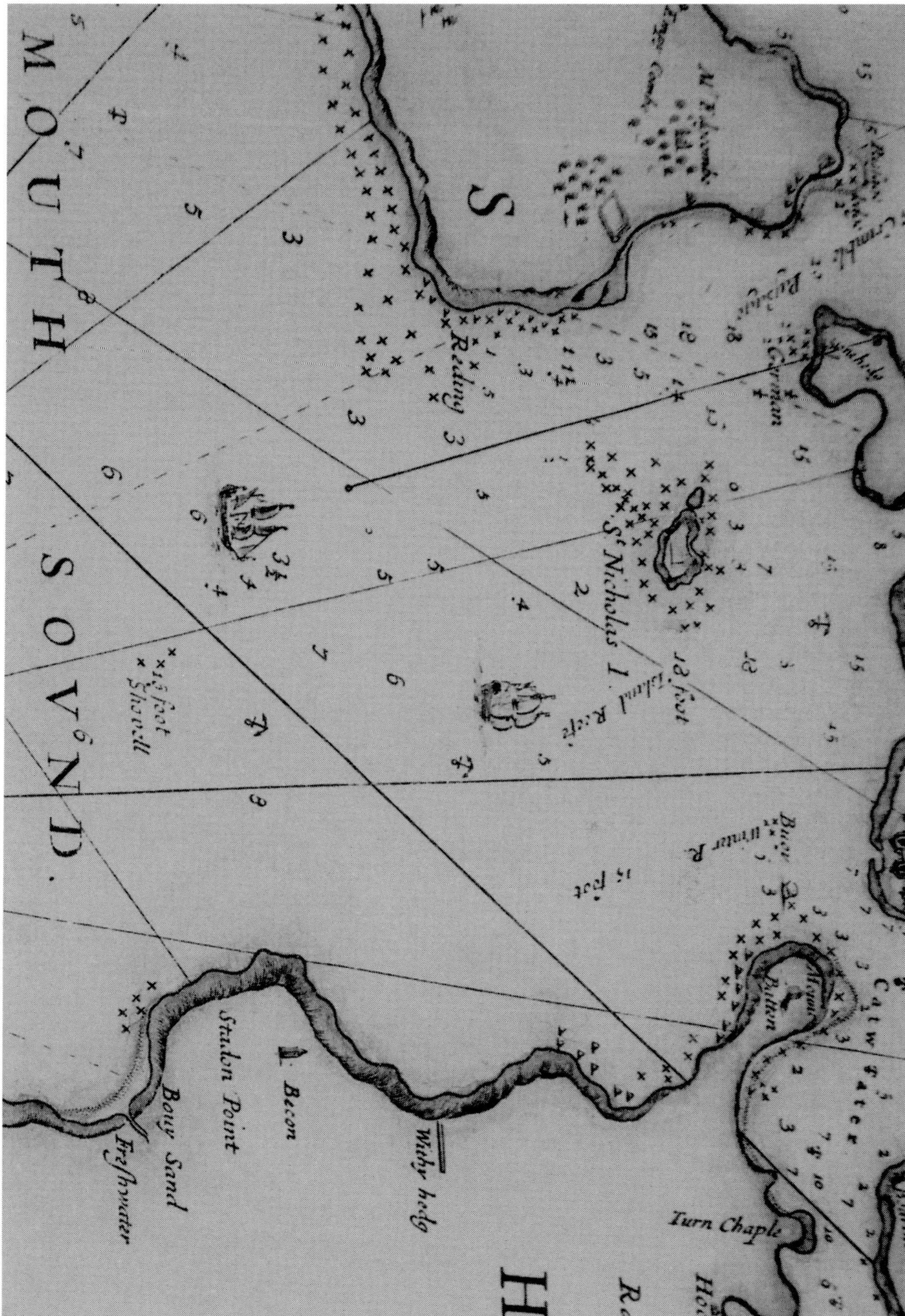

No rams cliff point

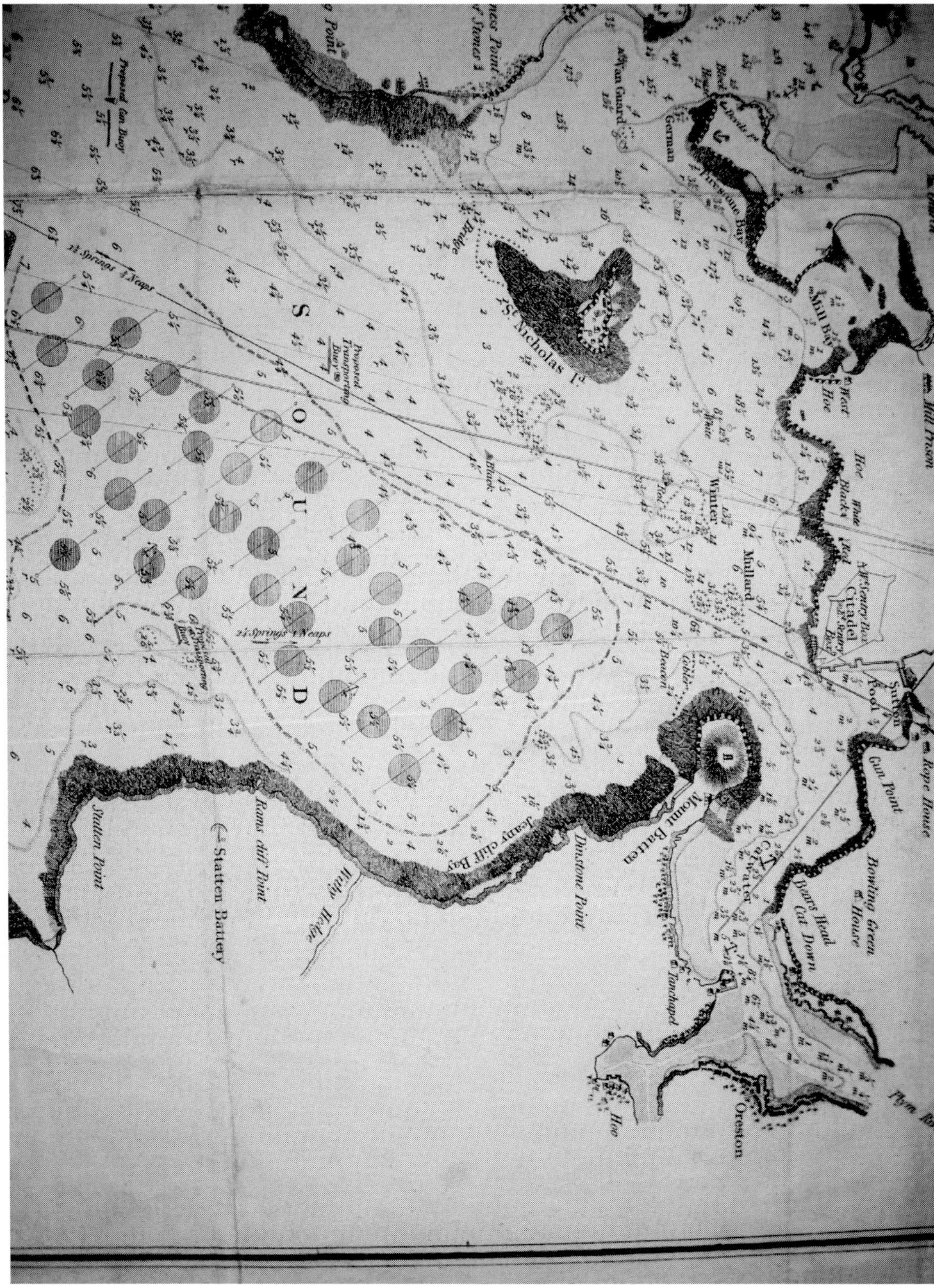

Rams cliff two words

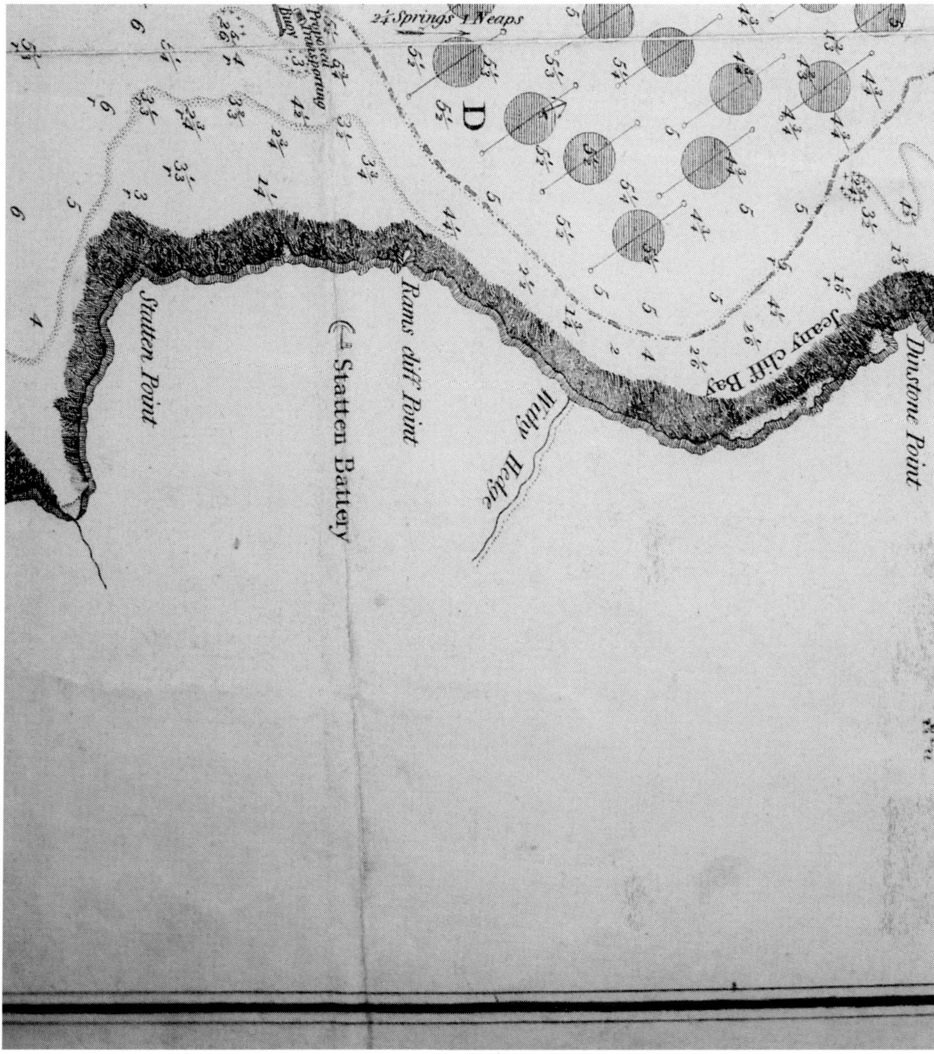

Rams cliff two words

Wow that is good news because it takes many many years for a local's only name to get adopted on to a map or chart.

I know just like surf breaks today, locals have their own name for some reason and years later they are just call and that name and no one can remember why.

It's just like we said before how a Buoy in the bay became on the charts Bouy Sands became Bovey Sands became Bovisands. You can see on the 1660 chart it's marked already as Bovey sands.

Yep big boat rams cliff become locals only "Rams cliff point" then on charts as Rams cliff point then many years becomes "Ramscliff point." And to everyone who reads it and speaks it, it's just another name. And here is the first chart I can find where it's all one word RAMSCLIIFF

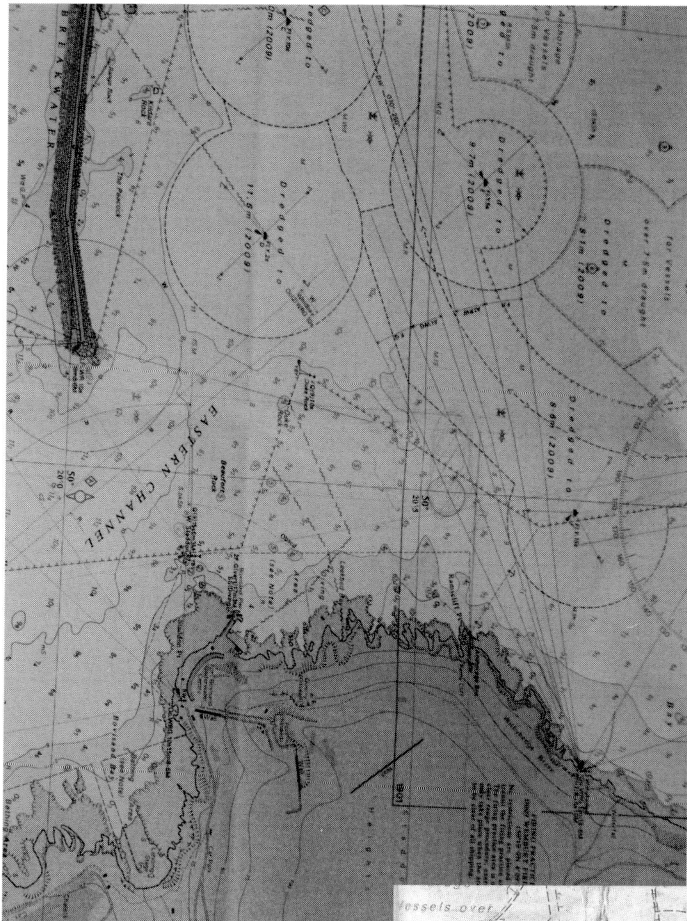

Ramscliff all one word

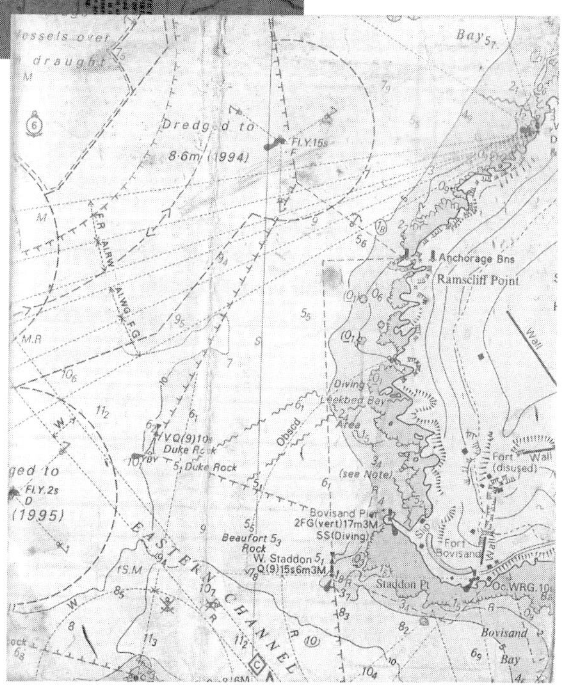

How about you Mr Green how are you and your new best buddy getting on?

Get lost Captain Black he is actually and very helpful guy.

Yeh I be he is bet.

Give me two seconds to put this stuff way and then you can show me what you got.

Ok while you do that, I'm just going to quickly drain the one eyed trouser snake and then I'll show you my findings

Right site down here Captain and read this, it's from an article dated the 19th Dec 1721 and covers between the 15 Dec to the 22 Dec 1721.

Good work Mr Green how difficult was it to find?

Very very simple, once Jason showed me where the micro film was and how to operate the machine it took me only 3 or 4 minutes.

So something Tricky Dickey could have done very simply?

Without a doubt.

The sly old fox he sure is a wise old Pirate.

But even if he had printed this paper cutting what would it of told us that we didn't already know? I mean the dates on this don't match up with either article and I am a confused as ever.

Not sure but there must be something there that he didn't want anyone else to know so we got to just keep reading it and maybe look for what isn't there rather than what is there.

I got some copies of it, here you have a couple.

How much did they cost?

Well there suppose to be 30p a sheet but Jason gave me six copies for nothing.

I bet he did, and if you check the back your find his mobile phone number

Give over will you, and lets go it's my turn to take a leak now and then let's get the hell out of dodge.

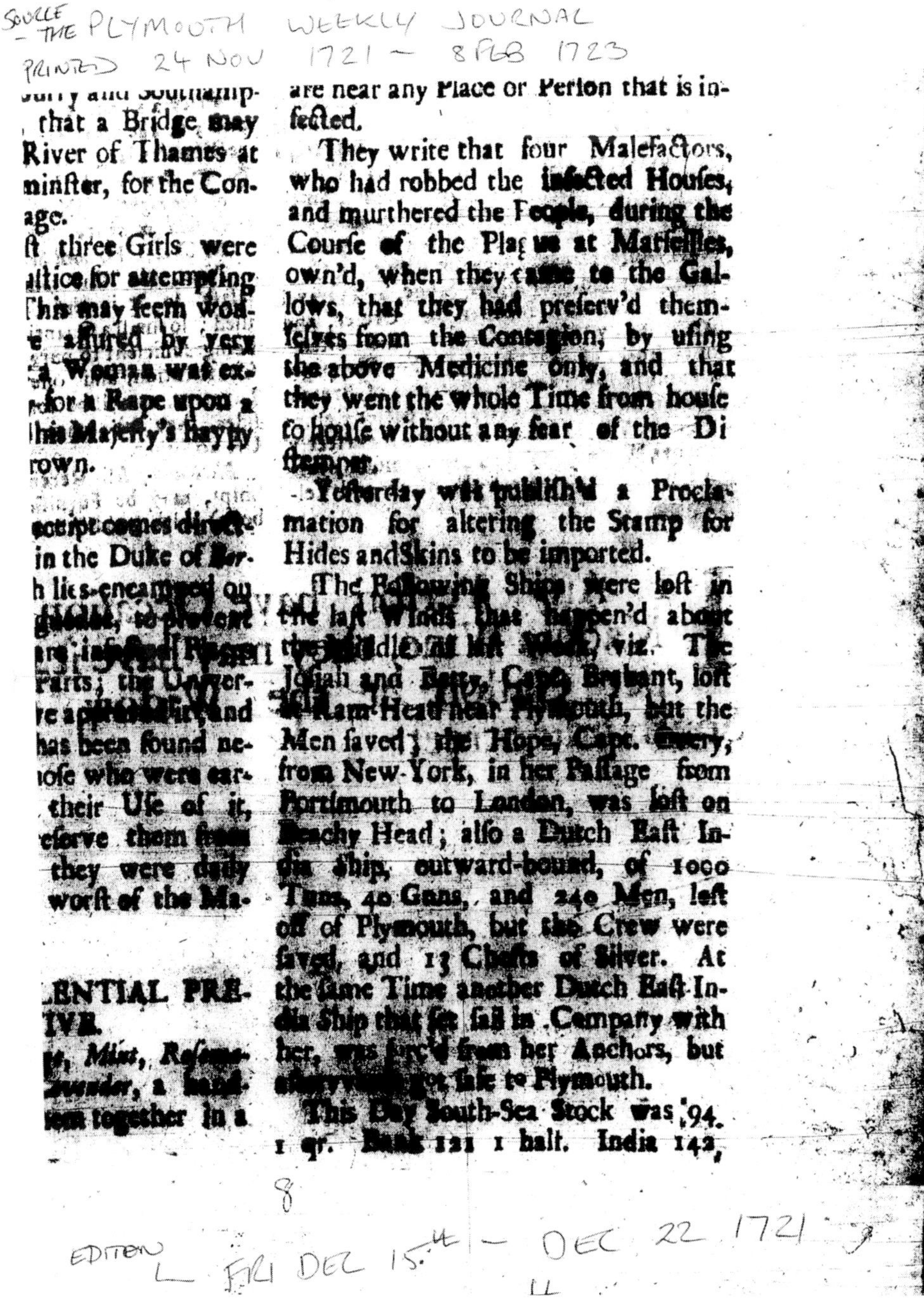

SOURCE – THE PLYMOUTH WEEKLY JOURNAL
PRINTED 24 NOV 1721 – 8 FEB 1723

...rry and Southamp-
, that a Bridge may
River of Thames at
minster, for the Con-
age.
...t three Girls were
...stice for attempting
This may seem won-
...e assured by very
...a Woman was ex-
...for a Rape upon a
...his Majesty's happy
...rown.

...script comes direct-
in the Duke of Ber-
...h lies encamped on
..., to prevent
...re infected Places
...arts; the Univer-
...e apprehensive, and
has been found ne-
...ose who were ear-
...their Use of it,
...eserve them from
...they were daily
...worst of the Ma-

...ENTIAL PRE-
...IVE.
...t, Mint, Rosema-
...ender, a hand-
...em together in a

are near any Place or Person that is infected.

They write that four Malefactors, who had robbed the infected Houses, and murthered the People, during the Course of the Plague at Marseilles, own'd, when they came to the Gallows, that they had preserv'd themselves from the Contagion, by using the above Medicine only, and that they went the whole Time from house to house without any fear of the Distemper.

Yesterday was publish'd a Proclamation for altering the Stamp for Hides and Skins to be imported.

The Following Ships were lost in the last Winds that happen'd about the Middle of last Week, viz. The Josiah and Betty, Capt. Brabant, lost at Ram-Head near Plymouth, but the Men saved; the Hope, Capt. ..., from New-York, in her Passage from Portsmouth to London, was lost on Beachy Head; also a Dutch East India Ship, outward-bound, of 1000 Tuns, 40 Guns, and 240 Men, lost off of Plymouth, but the Crew were saved, and 13 Chests of Silver. At the same Time another Dutch East-India Ship that set sail in Company with her, was forc'd from her Anchors, but ... got safe to Plymouth.

This Day South-Sea Stock was 94 1 qr. Bank 121 1 half. India 142,

8

EDITION L FRI DEC 15th – DEC 22 1721
LL

Chapter Nine

Dates and Calendars

Come in Mr Green, did you see the paper cutting?

No! Where is it, let's have a look.

Here you go and check out your face you don't get any prettier.

Look at Uncle Orange, he looks like Steptoe

But it was a Good Job we had him in the team

That's for sure, what did he say about the paper cutting, was he OK with it?

Yeh he says he's too old to worry and we should never let the truth spoil a good story. Which is kind of what I've been telling you these last few months I can't believe he is 76 years old sometimes, when you work with him it's just like working with someone our own age.

I do feel a bit mean sometimes roping him in on all my mad ideas, that quickly passes and I think that without me keeping him active he would get board and die. And let's face it he survived as a North Sea diver for over thirty years, and you don't do that without enjoying the buzz that comes with taking a risk. And the words "never let the truth spoil a good story" came from his lips not mine. Right a quick cup of T to tell you some other stuff I have found out and also the next plan.

Here you are a nice cup of hot T.

Well where shall I start, right let me tell you that I been thinking a lot about why all the dates of all the information we obtained don't add up. The strangest being that last bit of info we got.

What the news paper article said was, the Aaktekerke was lost of Plymouth about a week before she actually sailed from Holland?

Corectomondo Mr Green, and I have found out what could been the explanation for that. In Patrick's article he states the Aaktekerke finally sank on the 14th of March 1722.

And in Richard Larns article or Tricky Dickeys as we affectionately now refer to him, he writes in order to correct Patrick facts, or as we now suspect to throw people off the trail "the aketerkerke finally sank on the 24th December 1721".

And the local news paper writes on the 19th Dec That's about the middle of last week a Dutch East Indianman Aaktekerke was lost off Plymouth and 13 chest of silver where saved" Which could kind of put the date on about the 14th Dec.

We can also see the date on the letter the customer's office wrote to the Land owner at Langdon court which asked for help against the murders and robbers which was the 13th Dec. And that makes sense as she would still be afloat then.

I agree with everything your stating Captain but I am keen to see how you are going to square the circle.

Check this out, hold on where's that book I had it a second ago, Ah here it is. I'm going to read this to you very slow as I know you're not very quick.

Ha ha Ha very funny get on with it.

Ok here is what it said in a treasure hunting book I was reading....

The World riches wreck By Robert F Marx and Jenifer Marx

"1721 The Dutch East Indiaman Aagtekerke (800 tons/813tonnes) Commanded by Captain Nikolaas Rabodus, sailed for Batavia with 340,000 guilders in gold and silver specie and was lost near Plymouth England. About half of the treasure was saved."

Another important factor to keep in mind when doing research on primary source material is that there was no standardized calendar system followed by all countries. In 1582 Pope Greaogory X111

Ordered that 10days of the year be omitted to bring the calendar and the sun once again into correspondence, thus creating the Gregorian calendar which we use today. For many years afterwards however, all of the protestant countries in Europe continued to use the old calendar.

Until England adopted the Gregorian calendar in 1752, the new year began on March 25th The date of Feb 11th 1733 to the English there, was Feb23 1734 to Catholic Nations.

So hear how my strange mind works, The Dutch say it set sail on the 17th December 1721, which if they were on the Gregorian calendar would of been Dec 7th 1721 here.

That allows it 15 Days at sea being tossed and turned, battered and bruised by high storms before it was wrecked on the cliffs at Plymouth.

Yes I could swallow that, because we know she was almost down by the Lizard at one stage according to Tricky Dickeys report and we have read how bad the seas where and she was unable to make any headway. So 15 days to get from Holland down the English Channel as far as the Lizard off Cornwall then smashed back to Plymouth doesn't seem so long.

I agree, so now we can see that she didn't sink before she set sail but actually 17 days afterwards on the 24th Dec on the English calendar. And the customer's officer's letter was written.

On the 13 Dec English time!

Bingo Mr Green see you're not as slow as people say you are.

But Captain Black that still leaves Patricks dates way off the clock.

Well the only way I can have a stab at explaining that is that his translation was incorrect. I can only guess that as he has already said translating Old Dutch to English was very difficult and where he has put the 14th March it must have said 14 Dec.

Not that a convincing argument as that last explanation Captain.

I know it's pretty week but it's the only way I can square the circle. It's the only way they all end up with the 14 Dec 1721.

I tell you what would be funny.

What?

If when the research from the Dutch archives you have paid for throws up a completely different date for her sinking.

I don't think that would very funny at all Mr Green and if you keep throwing spanners in the works like that then I am going to dick your next cup of tea.

Yuck, so do we have any news on the long awaited research from Holland?

Not yet but I don't really expect it, to after the 15 Sept, I might email them and see if they can dig up specifics on the cannons the Aak-tekerka was carrying at the same time there doing the other research, you know size and numbers etc.

Sounds like a good idea that would be very useful info to have. So what happens next Captain? What's the plan?

Well Babcock Marine have agreed to X-ray the cannon on Wednesday so we need to get there for 11am to pick up our security passes from DML.

Cool how long do they need it for?

Well let's say a hand X-ray has about a 3 second exposure to radiation, how long do you think they need to expose the cannon to radiation for?

I guess 2 hours.

No 12 to 14 hours.

Wow that is a long time; I guess they will shoot it over night.

I think that is the plan, so we need to take a blow up kid's swimming pool for them to put the cannon in when they have finished with it and while they are waiting for us to pick it up.

When will they be able to show us the results?

Straight away when we pick it up. The plan is they will take one shot of the thickest part which is of course the back end where we hope we will see a cannon ball inside. And depending on the results, if we can actually see anything then they will take more shots of the middle and front of the cannon.

And what are the plans after Wednesday?

Next day out for the world's worst treasure hunters is the Friday after, the 10th. On Friday there is a massive tide I think it's about 6.01m and 0.31m.

Yikes that is a big tide for Plymouth, so are we going on the foreshore as we discussed?

Yes we will go on foot and walk down the cliff and use that metal detect in the rock pools and on the beaches. So bring your detector, hammer chisel you know all the tools we will need.

What are you going to wear?

Hey easy Mr Green it's not a date you know, I am not dressing up for you again. You know what happened last time I did that.

You are such a dick head sometimes Captain Black, but you did look nice in that dress ha ha.

Probably going to wear my Shorty wet suit with some shorts over the top, you know like the chaves do when they are tomb stoning off the rocks. And some on training shoes as I think the rocks will be rough and quite sharp. Might also slip a snorkel and mask into my back pack but not sure yet.

Cool I will do the same but also bring my camera.

Good idea Mr Green, in fact best idea you have had all year. And it goes without mention that I will have a flask with lots of hot T.

Ok see you bright and early Wednesday.

Bye, Oh! and don't forget your passport!! You will need it to get in the dockyard.

Chapter Ten

Cannon Collection

Is anyone meeting us at the main dockyard gate Captain?

They said we had to ring them when we get there, and they would send a man up meet us.

Did they say how long it would take to shoot the x-ray?

Well you know I told you when you get your arm or leg x-rayed it has about a thirty second exposure to the source, well how long do you think the cannon is going to exposed to the source i.e. the shot ?

I'm guessing an hour or so?

No over twenty hours, and they still don't know if the results will tell us anything.

So how long do they need the cannon for?

About two days and then they will call us to collect it.

Don't get out of car Mr Green we have to go and collect the engine lift and Uncle Orange, there has been a change of plan and the cannon is ready to collect.

How did they get on? Any results?

They found the cannon to be too thick to get any good results, but they are able to tell us that there is nothing in the crustation. Which means we can now start to clean the cannon and nock off the crustation?

So they can't tell us if the cannon is primed and loaded?

No

Are we able to see the x-rays they took?

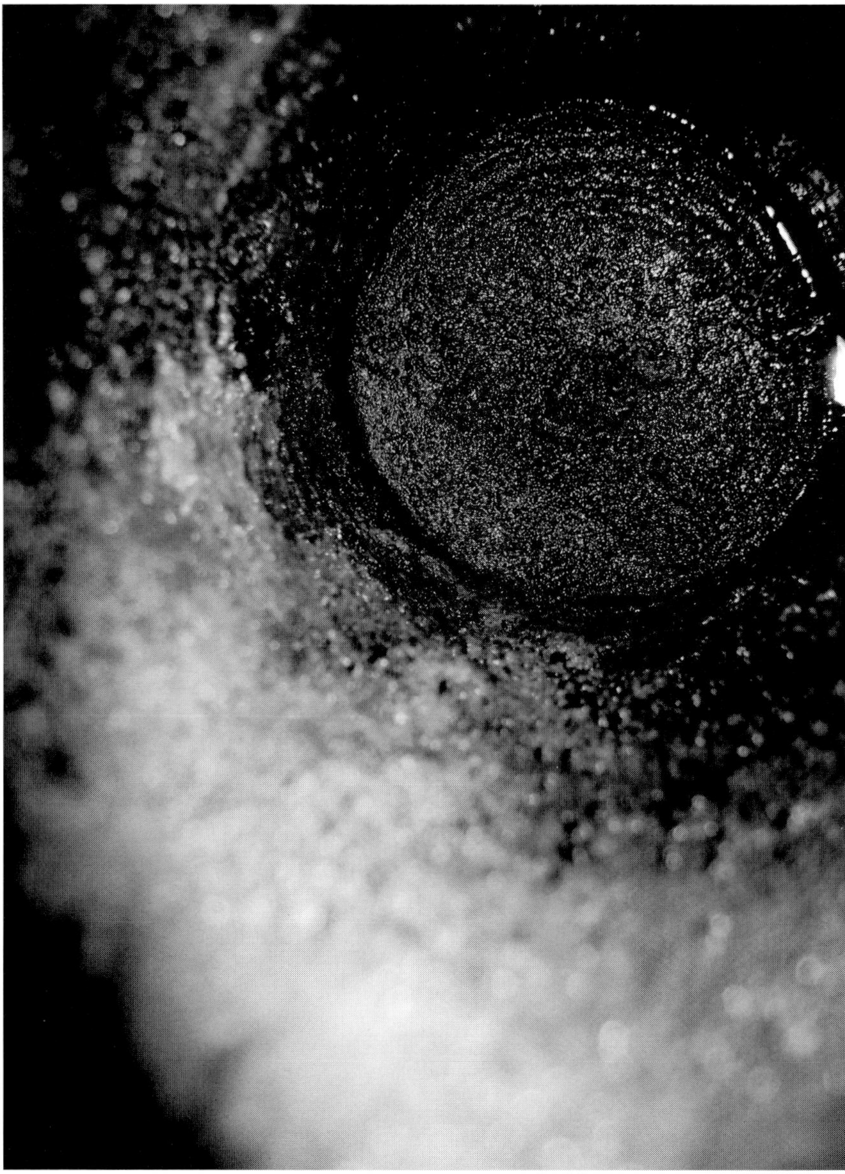

Yep and they are going to look inside the cannon by inserting a osteogram inside the small break in the side of the cannon and see if they can see the cannon ball that way.

Well at least we tried, and it will still be good to see the x-rays.

Yeh and now at least we can start to clean the cannon, which hopefully will help us to start putting some measurements to it and maybe even some age on it.

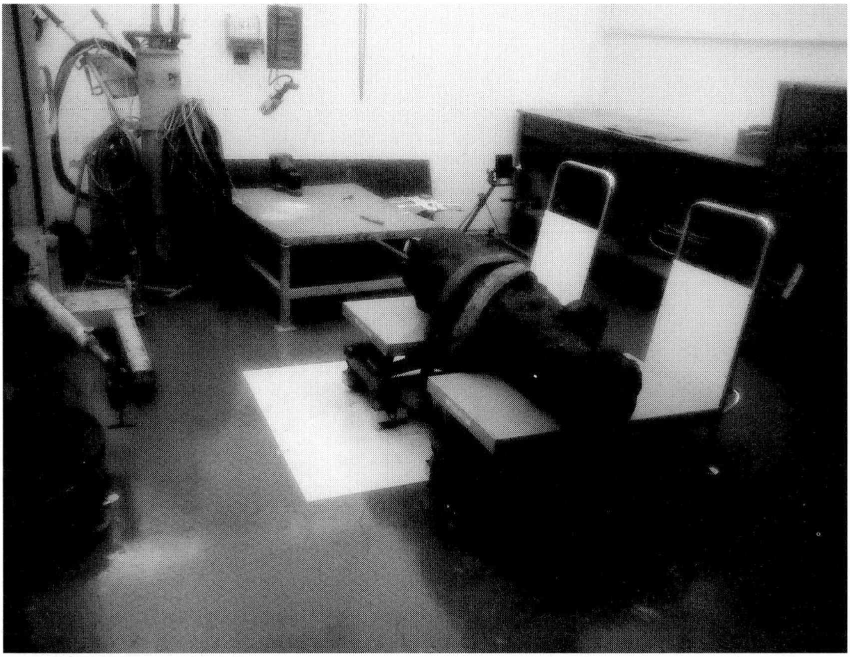

So what's the plan with our low tide beach search?

Let's see how the time goes, we might miss the tide or catch the end of it, but what we don't want to do is waste the whole day. If it looks we are going to miss the tide we need to scrub around it and put in a few hour grafts on the cannon.

I agree Captain Black let's see how it goes as we know time and tide wait for no man, not even us. And I quite fancy getting stuck in on the cannon.

We will both need to keep our eyes on Uncle Orange, you know what he's like with a hammer in his hands.

Yeh and he's half blind so he could end up twating your hand.

So what's the time now Mr Green?

12.40

And what time is low water?

13.40 So what are your thoughts?

I say we have missed the tide and if we try to get to the beach now, we are going to get stressed and get nothing done. Let's go home, have a cup of T and then slowly slowly start work on the cannon.

Sounds like a plan, are you OK to work on the cannon with us Uncle Orange?

Yes! Don't have to be home to about five o'clock.

That's a shame I was hoping to get rid of you, so we could do some real work.

Cheeky bastard, I'll can still show you a thing or two about how to use a hammer.

Yes that's what I'm afraid of, Mr Green you start on the back end and Uncle Orange you start on the big lumps of crud on the front and middle. We won't go any wear near the cannon metal until we get our hands in and get more skilled at what we are doing.

What about the tampion?

No Uncle Orange you stay way away from that, let's leave it in and untouched for another day.

What tools do we have at your house Captain Black?

Not much a couple of hammers and a mallet.

Don't worry guys I have got loads of tools in my van, chisels and hammers.

Have you got that tarps with you Mr Green, because if we get all that crud and stuff all over my drive my significant other is going go mad? Let's leave our selves enough time to clean up at the end before you guys do a runner on me. Also we need to put it back in the water, which reminds me I bought some Sodium Bicarbonate to put in the water. I had an email from someone at Plymouth Uni advising us on what solution to keep the cannon in.

What percentage of Sodium Bicarbonate do we need?

Only 1% to start with and change the water every three weeks. Right here we are then guys, you get the cannon out and start work and I will make us a nice cup of T.

There we are! Mrs Black is going to be well happy with that, all nice and tidy. All we have to do now is return the engine lift and where done. Tonight I might phone Evil Dr pork chop and see if he wants to come and see the cannon.

Is that a good Idea Captain Black, you don't think he might be able to identify it or know which country it came from as we know he is a clever guy with lots of knowledge. And the last thing we want him to say is its Dutch.

I think it will fine, it's still got lots of crud on it and there are no markings yet so any positive ID would be impossible.

The most he is going to able to tell us is its size, bore and the poundage.

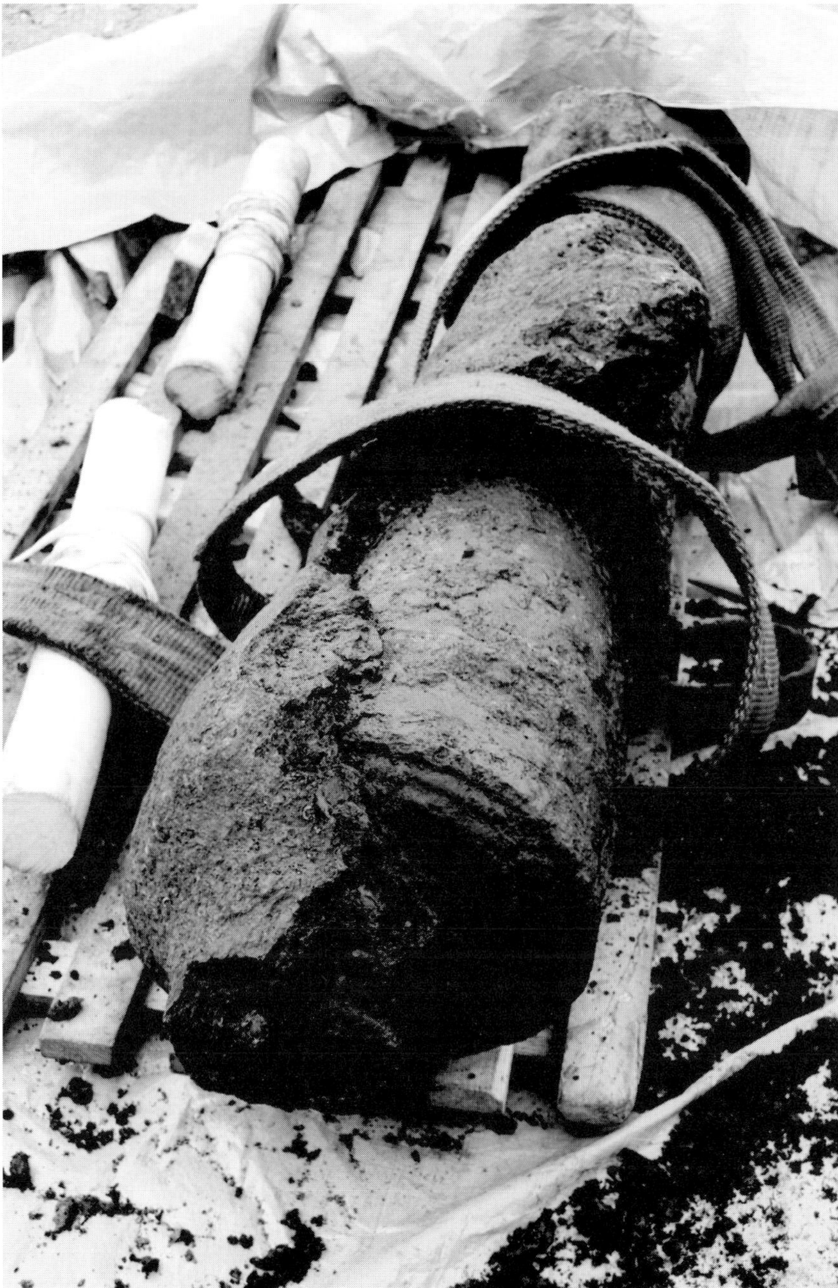

Ok but give me a call after he has been, and let me know what he says.

Yep will do talk to you later.

Oh just remembered Captain; I have finished the water dredge so we need to go to Bovisands Harbour and test it. It will need some adjustments and small changes but we first need to see how it runs.

Sounds good.

Also I saw an old VOC silver coin on ebay last night, it was in very poor condition and the date was not visible. It was silver, but covered in a hard crud. I wondered if I should buy it as it was only about £60 and it might come in useful.

Good idea, buy it if you want, but I thought you had one similar from the wreck in Scotland.

No not I.

Then it's up to you, see you later, bye.

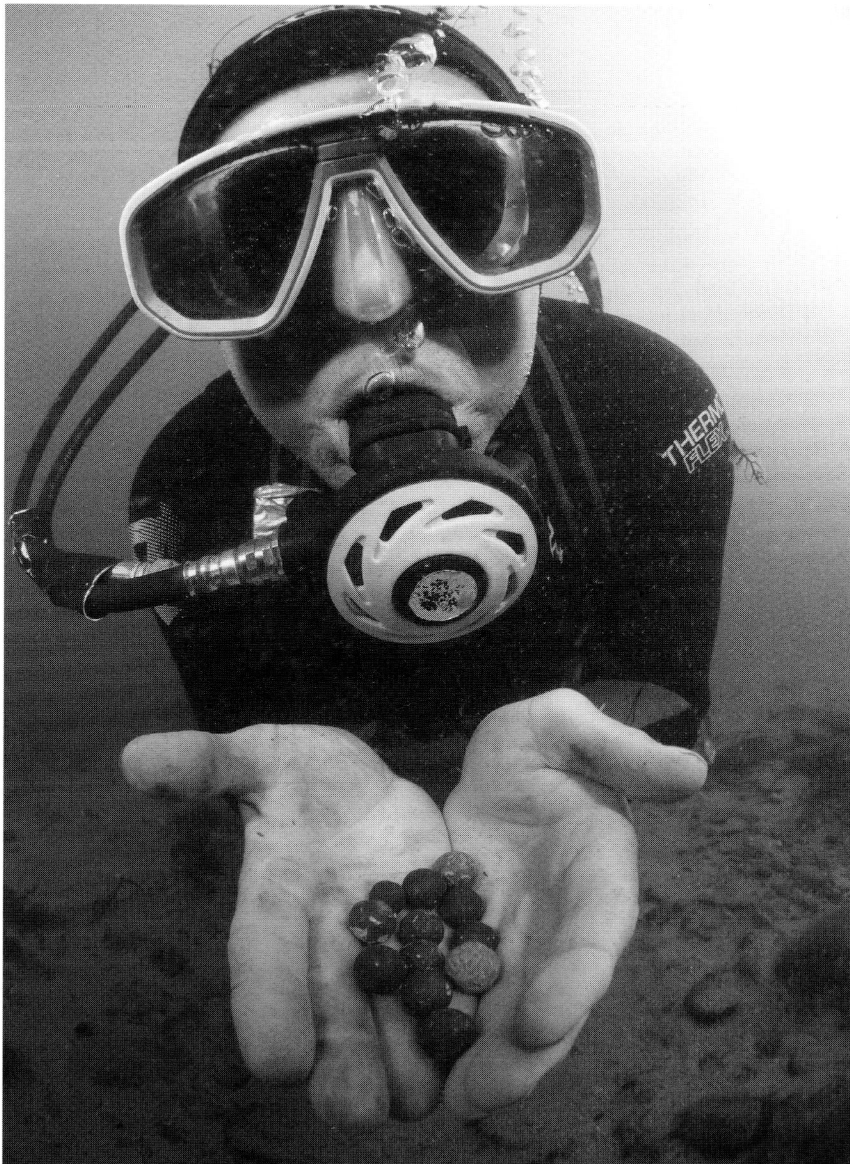

Photo: Dan Bolt

CHAPTER ELEVEN

TRUSTED FRIENDS INVITED FOR TWO DAY SEARCH

Dive Team

Captain Black, Mr Green, Uncle Orange, Chisseler, Marie, Kieth, Marion, Laura, Richard, Stevey, Dan.

The Objective

To survey the area, set ground lines for reference and to record position of any finds. To reach the area with metal detectors and mark any finds. To try and find the extent of the site piece together where the ship came to grief on the cliff and if we can figure out which part of the ship contacted the cliff and if she did as previously stated hit starboard side too.

To find and debris trail and locate an off shore site, if there is one. Through the recovered finds try to date and identify the shipwreck site. And through research on each and every find try and identify what the object is, what it was used for and which part of the ship it would of come from.

Only small objects are to be recovered and only objects that we knew we can preserve. Where ever possible we will take photos of the objects before their recovery. All finds where to stay the property of Captain Black and Mr Green and would join the other finds to make a shipwreck collection.

Time scale

Four days diving have been planned, some of the team can only do the first two days, so we would use these days for the wider area search.

Equipment

Two 6m ribs, individual scuba kit, two Aqua Pulse metal detectors, one Aqautech hand held magnetometer, 50m tape measures, weighted ground lines, hammers chisels, goodies bags, underwater camera, ropes and buoys.

Safety

No boat movement while any diver is in the water, no decompression dives, O2 kits and first aid kit on board as well as the VHF radio and the flag Alpha.

Depth max -12m
Vis 3m
Water Temp 16c
Air Temp 18c
Sea state Calm
Wind 4 knots, forecast good

The dive team was a very mixed bag, which kind of made it more fun and with very few egos on board the boats. There wasn't the completion to get in the water first, to dive the longest, or who came up with the best find, and as the people with the metal detectors where the searchers and not the diggers, they of course where going to come up with very little finds in there goodie bags. Some of the dive team where like me, used to following their noses and scrannying in a hole under some rocks like a dog digging for a bone. And some were new to this game and I am sure they won't mind me saying, to start with found it all a bit odd. Having been trained by BSAC and then over many years become BSAC instructors and taught hundreds of students the safe way to dive, how we did it was not in there manual. From dressing yourself, to not having a BCD but a back pack, to diving alone and no spare second stage regulator, things where not how their lifetime of diver training taught them they should be. But to their great credit, the rest of the dive team warmed to them and help them where ever possible. Plus they did come up with some nice finds all by themselves.

"I would of like to have seen their eyes as they swam passed the chisseler hand fanning in a glory hole, they told the story of while fining along the visibility slowly got worse and worse. And then they almost swam into a pair of fins sticking straight up in the air. They tried to see what was happening and looked down a huge hole to see what was being dug out and in the near darkness they could make out the chiselers eyes as wide as table plates and with a big grin on his face. He was in heaven, up to his neck in it, he had found what everyone was looking for a glory hole. And he was not going to move and come up until his cylinder was ringing. Never mind the contents gauge you can tell how empty the cylinder is, the tone of the ringing. But that's what it's all about, that's what I love the most there is nothing quite like it, you find a love trench or a glory hole and you start hand fanning or digging. You know when you're getting to the good stuff when the sand turns black and starts to smell like old oil. You have to dig down through the "layers of time" to get to where the bottom was hundreds of years ago."

"I remember once a long time ago when I was very new to diving and wrecking. The Dog took me up on a wreck site to have a good dig around and see what we could find. Usual routine for us one diver up one diver down. So the Dog who had been diving for many many years and had nose for it, just like the chiseler does. There are no courses for it, or things you can buy it's just a gift from the gods. Just like a gift for a sport or art they have a nose for the goodies."

"Any way after a hour I can hear the Dogs cylinder echoing from the bottom, and as the echoing went on and on it got louder and louder until it went on longer than I would expected, I was just about to put on my dive kit to go and check him out, when he pops up to the surface. Bloody hell Dog I scream at him, you had me worried then, you must be breathing water, you can't have any air left. So he looks at his gauge and says stop worrying will you I've still got a drop left in there. There lack of any figure tells me it's lower than low."

"So the Dog tells me he is in a glory hole and shows me some musket shot, and brass pin and a small knob off a draw. He tells me to keep digging in his hole and that he knows there will be something good in it soon."

"Off I go straight in his hole, its only 5m deep and fab vis, so I could see the crater he has been digging from the surface. I start hand fanning in the bottom of the hole, and within no more than three minuets I see the unmistakable glint of gold, and it's a beautiful 1759 half guinny that had been in the water for nearly two hundred and fifty years. It was it such good condition it could of been made yesterday. I put it inside my glove and go straight up to the boat. The Dog looks in my eyes and knows he is looking into the eyes of a man who has found his first gold coin."

After four days diving on the Ramscliff area, and having lots of fun with no accidents, we had amassed some great finds and had got to know are site a whole lot better. We now had a much better picture of where the ship was smashed against the cliff. We are even pretty certain we know which rocks the crew of the Aaketekeke climbed on to reach what they thought was the safety of land. And we can also see the path the rampaging mob hell bent on robbery and murder who climbed down to reach the cliff edge over looking this huge ship as it was getting smashed on the rocks while firing its cannons as a means of calling for help. Scared, starving Dutch sailors who were far from home. They must of been so happy to get on dry land, especially after watching some of the crew try to swim ashore only too drown and get smashed on the rocks. How desperate and hungry do you have to be to kill and rob another man after having just survived a great tragedy and who can barely walk. Pretty desperate maybe verging on starving I would think.

As the picture starts to unfold and the finds bring things to live it starts to get a whole lot more emotional and the reality of what we might have found starts to dawn on us. But for now it's time to take a step back from our thoughs, let the dust settle and then another exciting part. Trying to find out what the finds are, what they were used for and to see if there is any way they can positively identify the ship as the Aaketerkeke, which must keep reminding our selves we have not accomplished yet. Not beyond any reasonable doubt that's for sure! It could still all be in our heads.

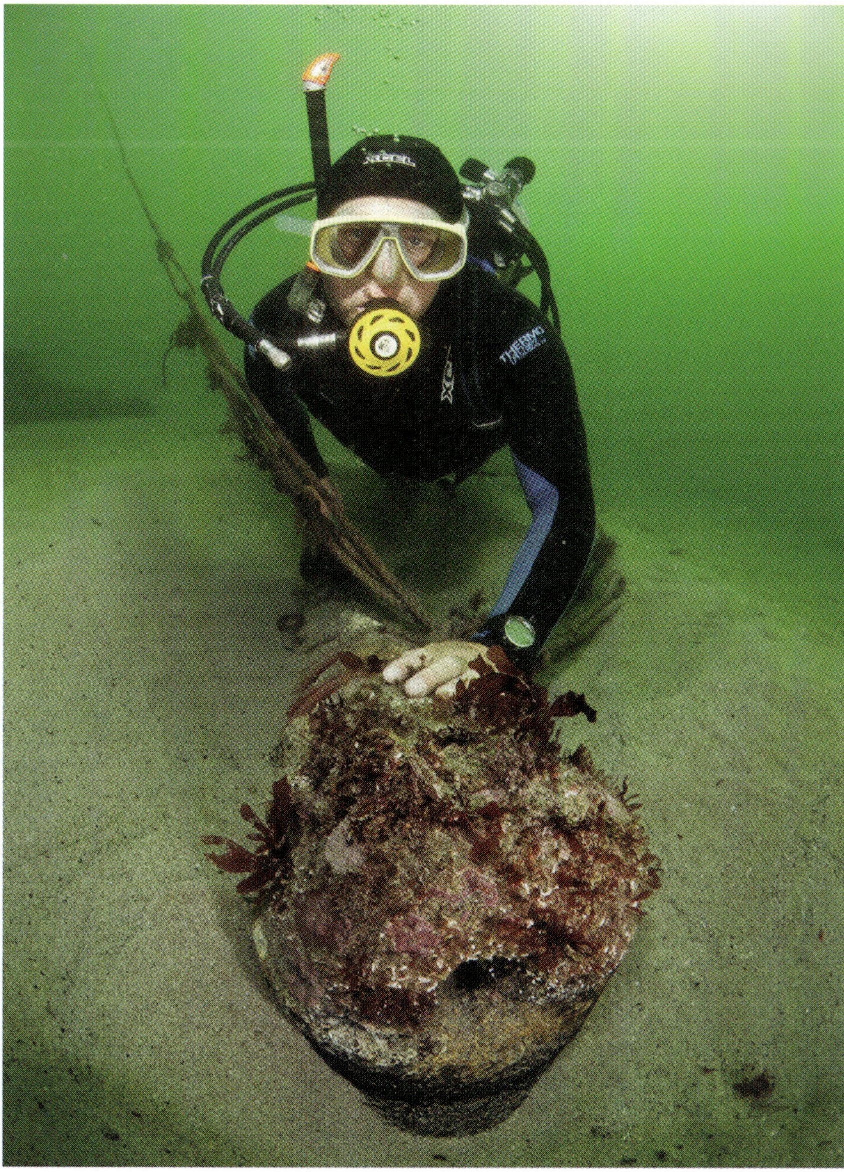

Cannon No.3. Photo: Dan Bolt

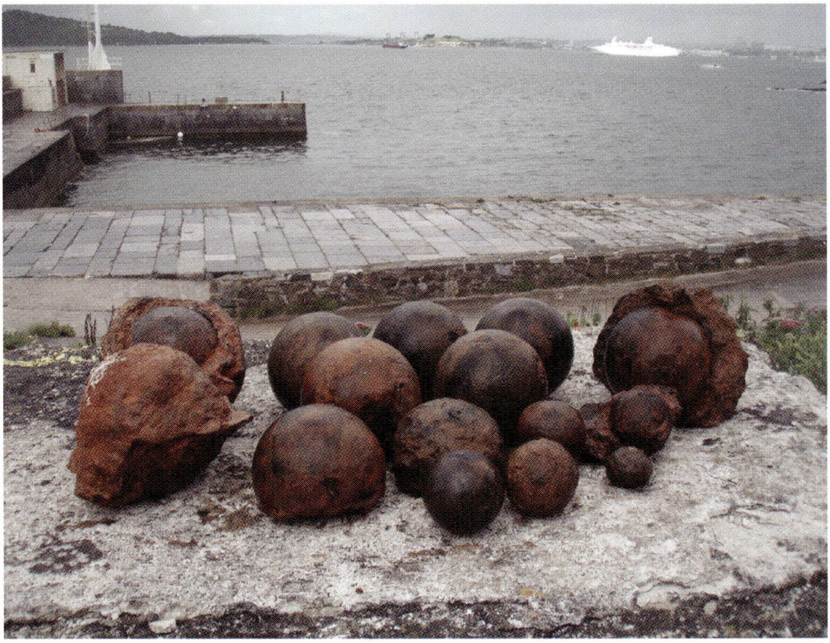

Various size sannon balls, some where found clean some in crud

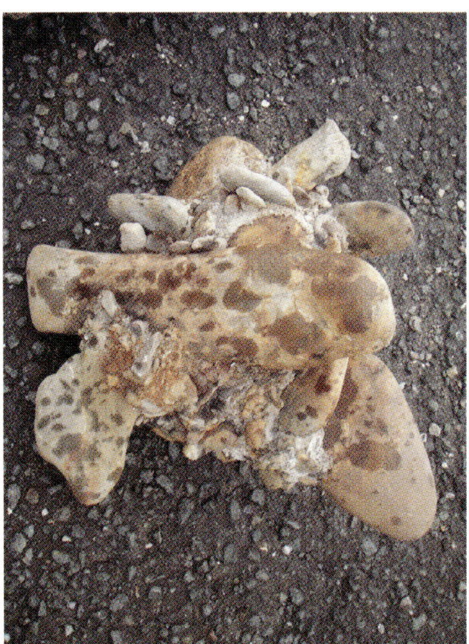

Lump of crud

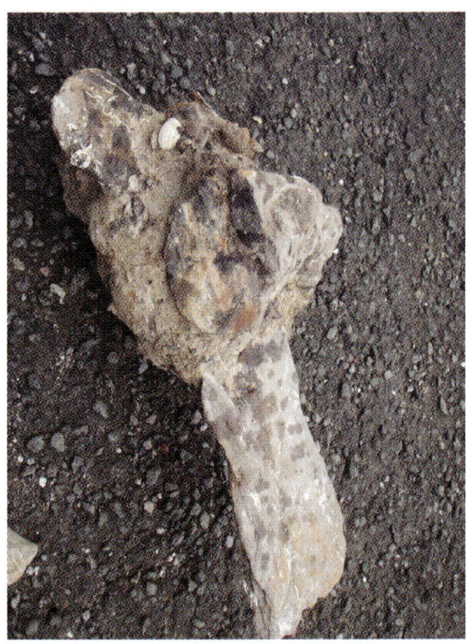

Lump of crud

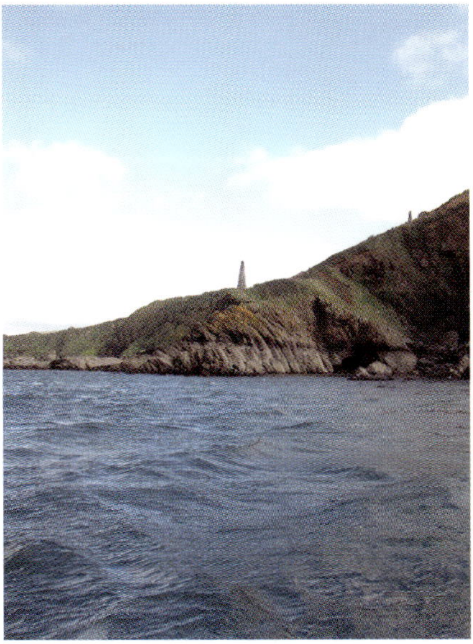

Ramsccliff Point: possible wreck site

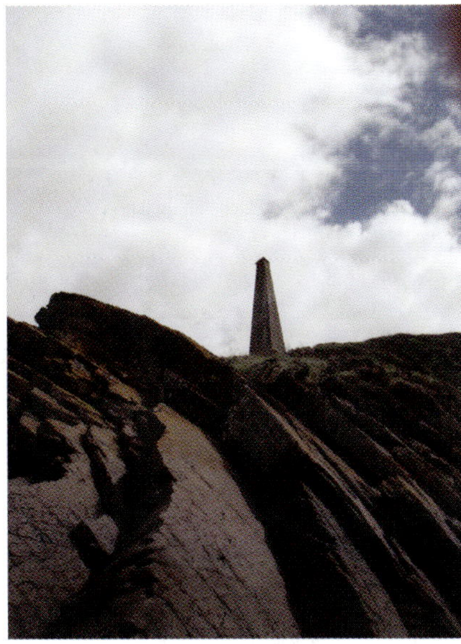

Tombstone? or witches work

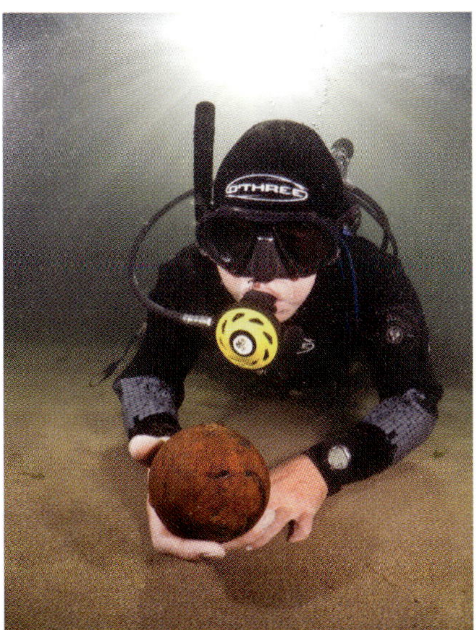

Another nice cannon ball. Photo: Dan Bolt

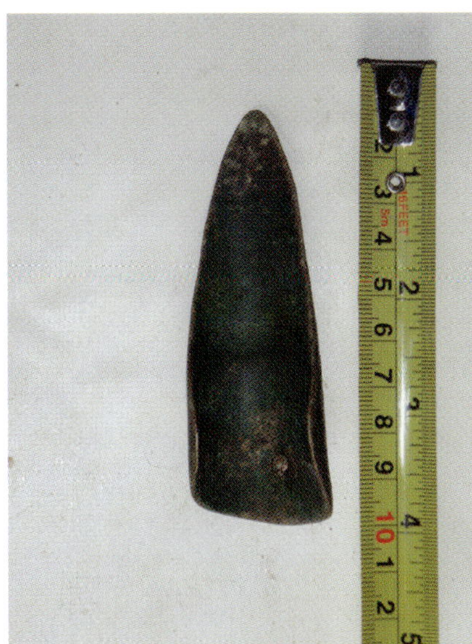

18th Century 'Swedish Fid' use to Splice Rope

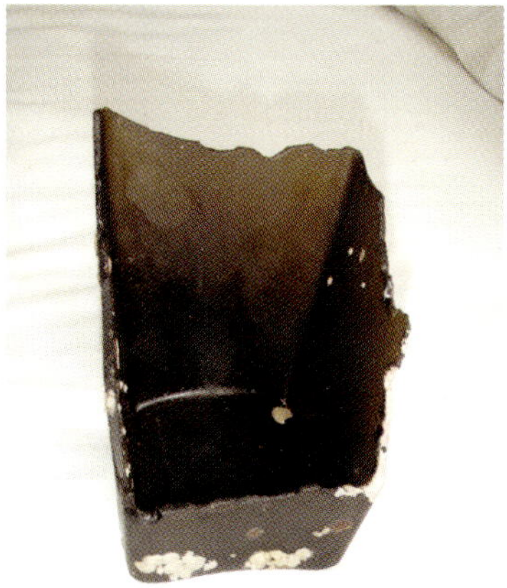

'18th Century Dutch Gin Bottle

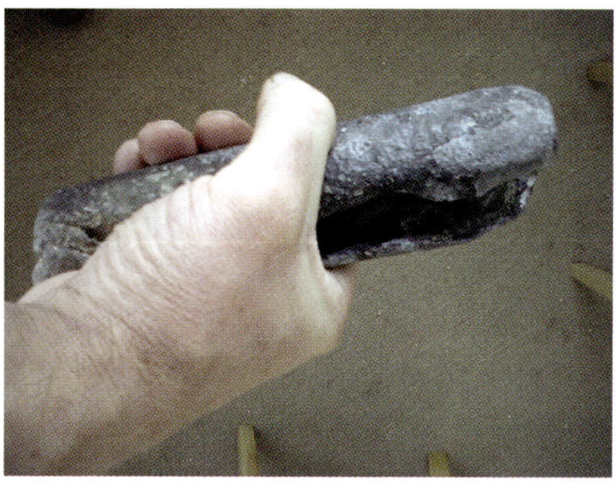

Ramming hammer

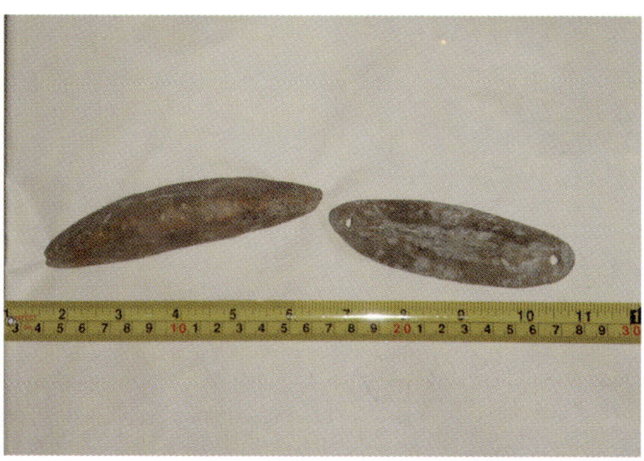

18th Century Dredgin net wieghts

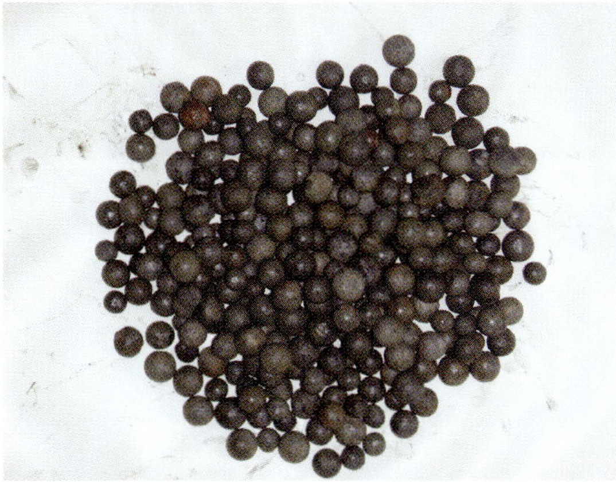

Hundreds of musket shots

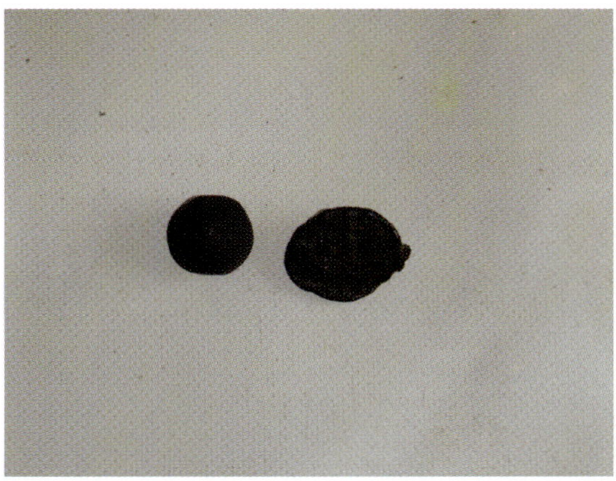

Fired musket shot

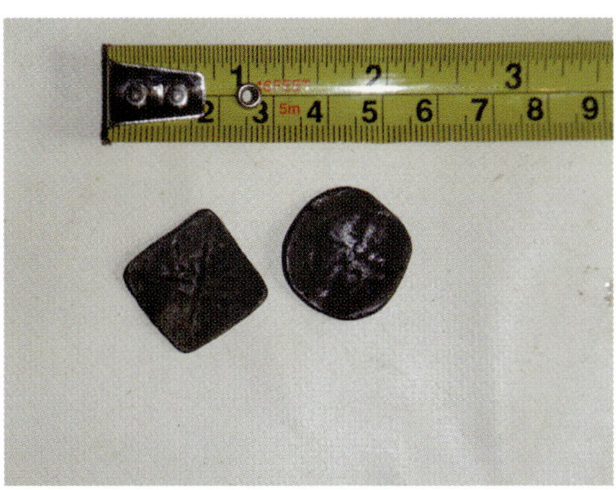

Lead Gold Coin Wieghts

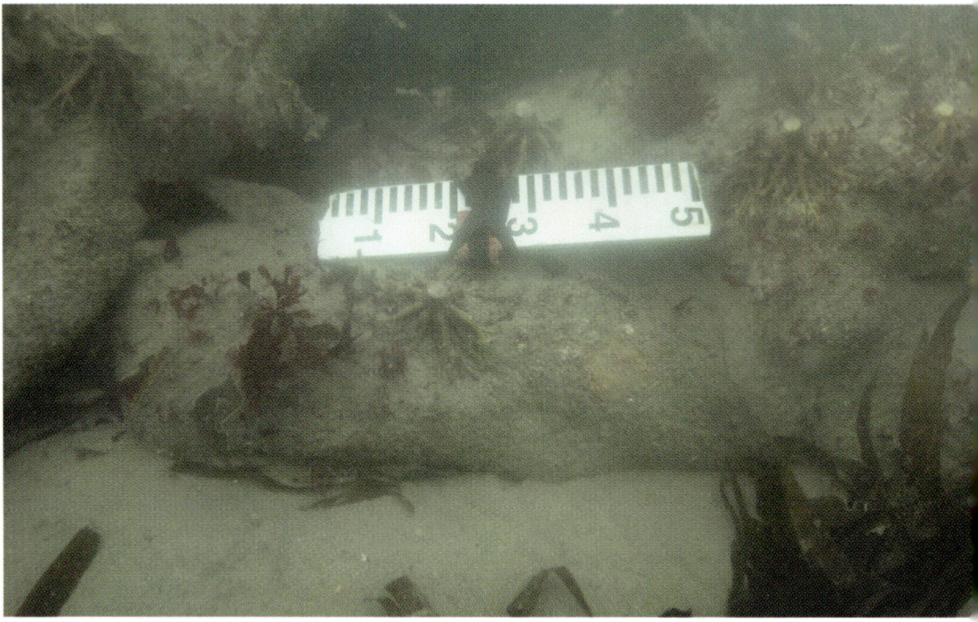

Cannon number 2: Photo Dan Bolt

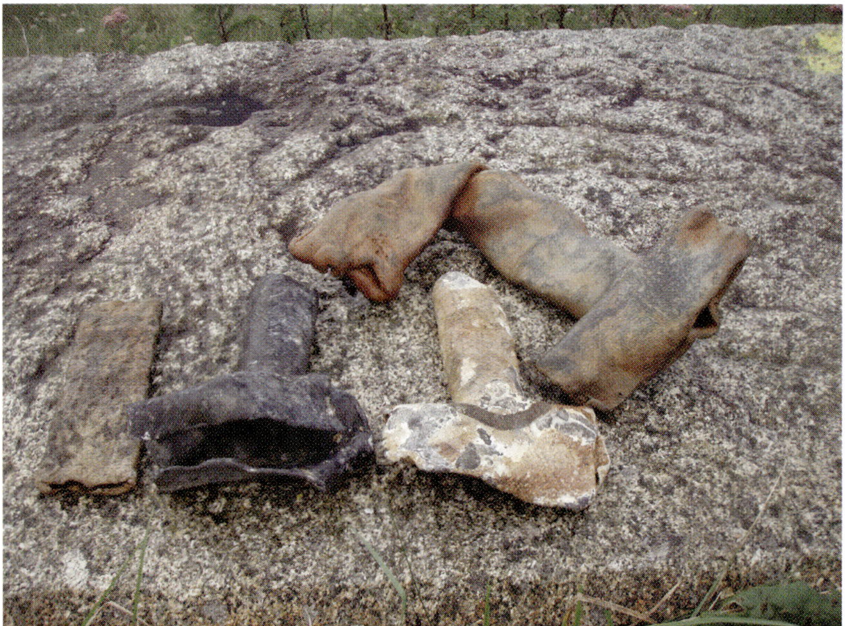

Lead pipes and scupers

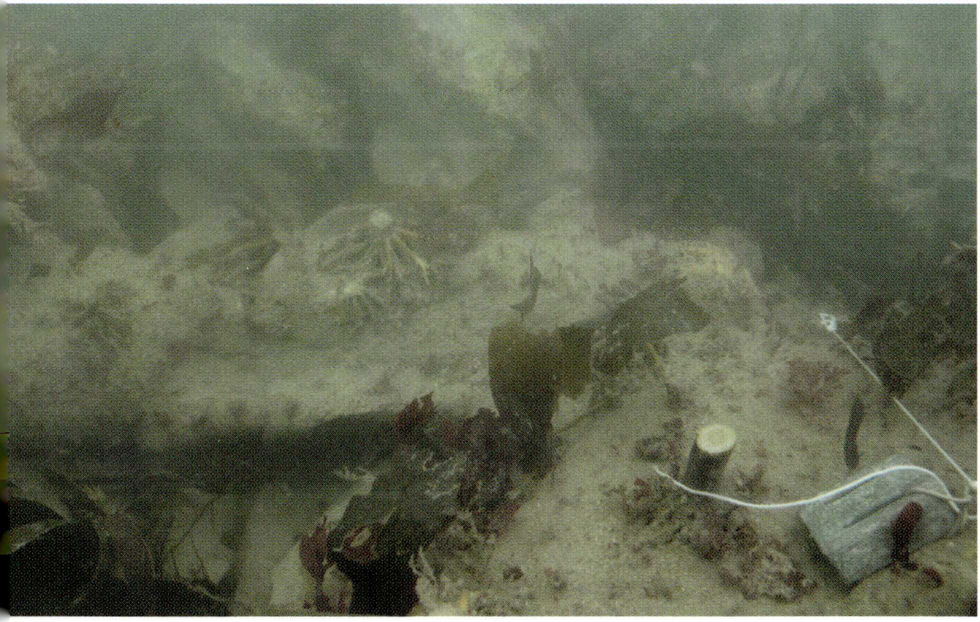

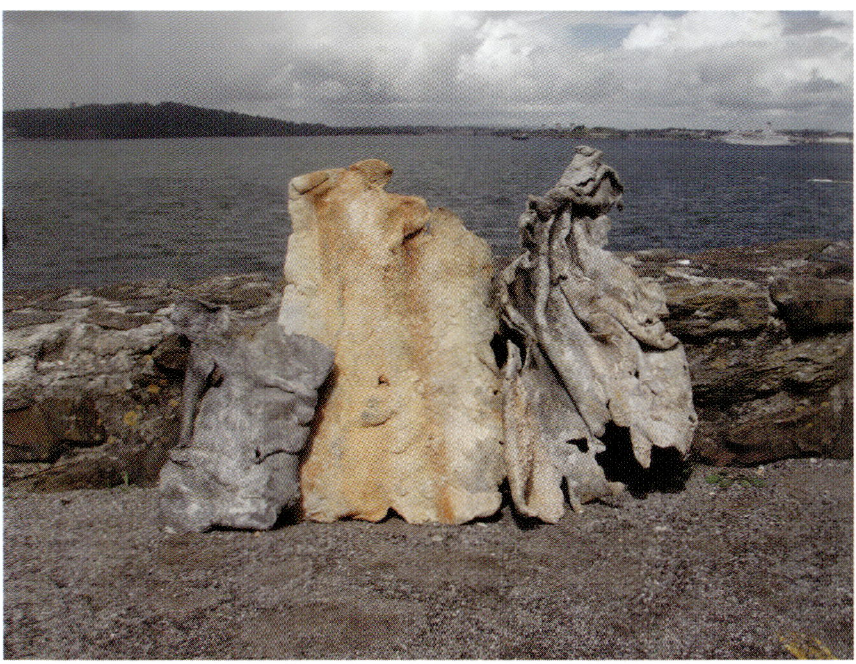

Lead Aprons from cannon 1,2 and one found in sand

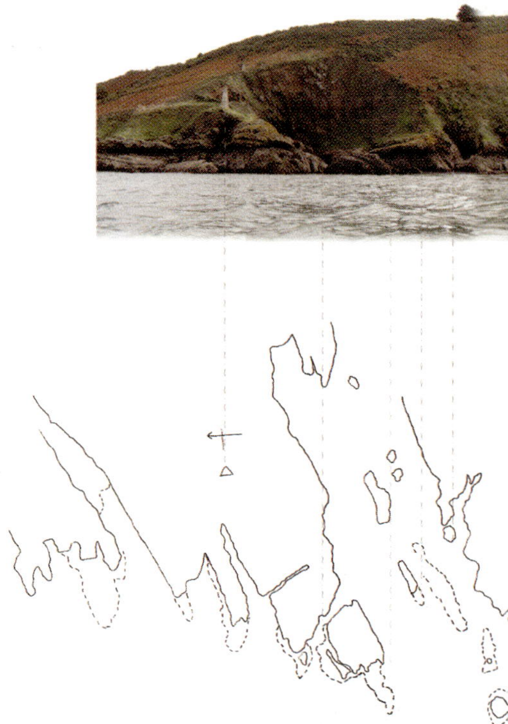

Photo and map: Dan Bolt

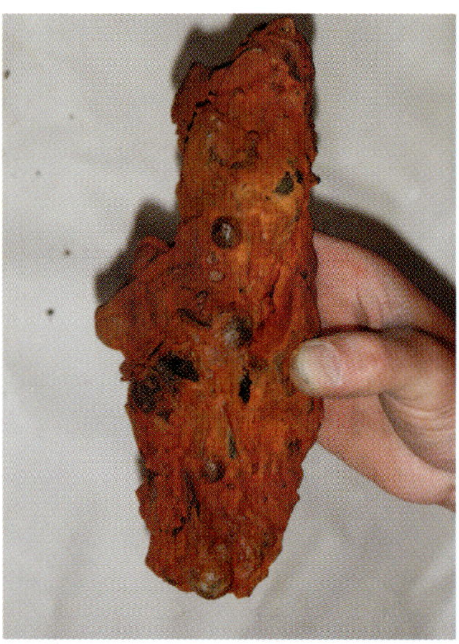

Musket shot in crud

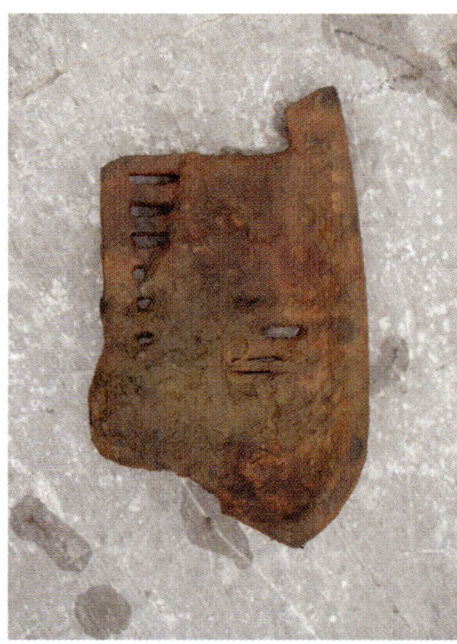

Fire Grate

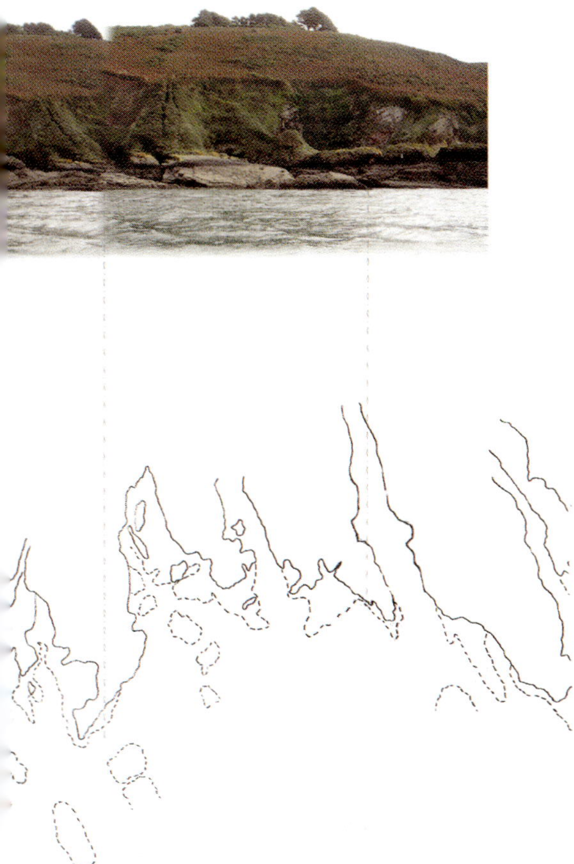

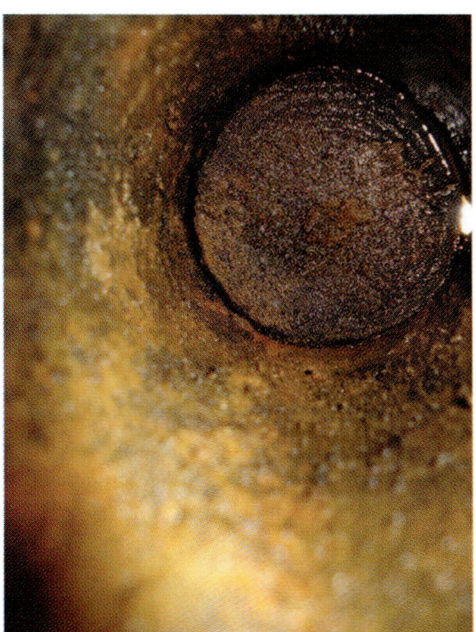

Inside cannon number 1

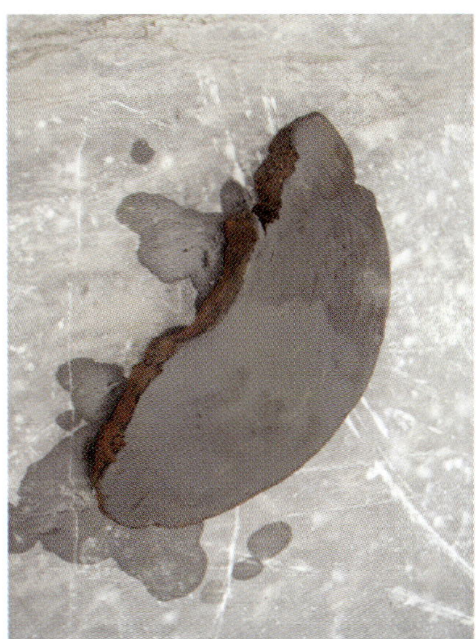

Part of a wooden block

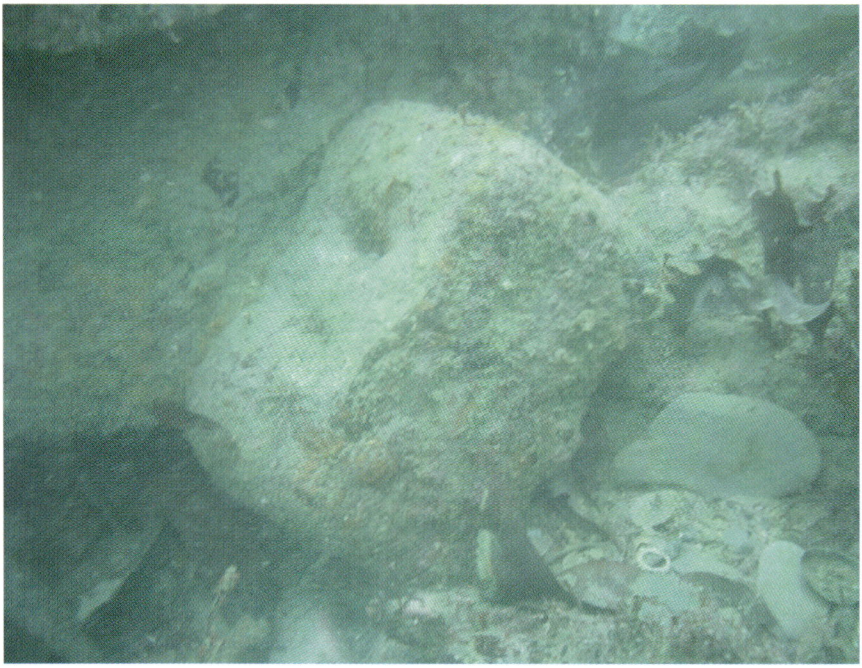

Ballast block in location: Namban Tetsu?

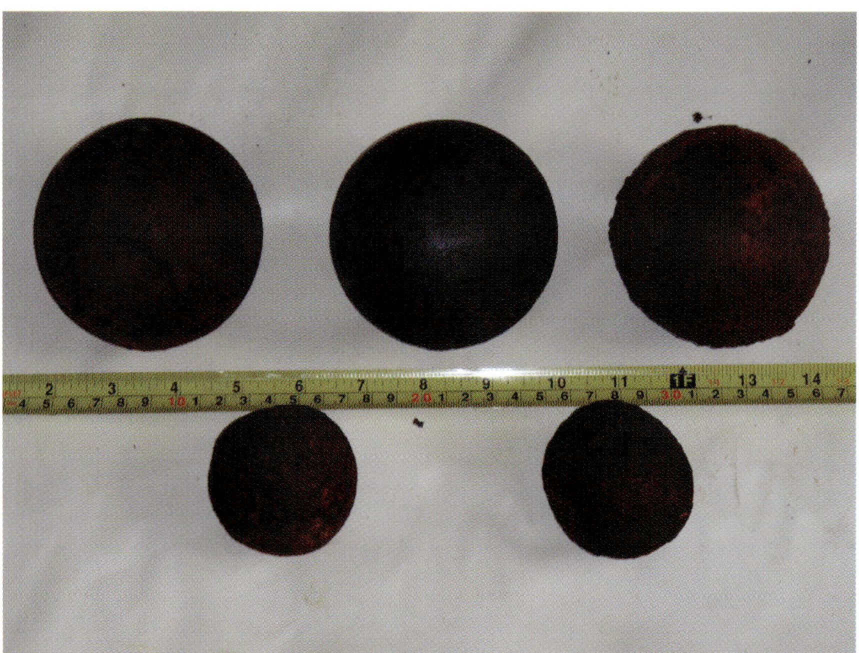

Small cannon balls

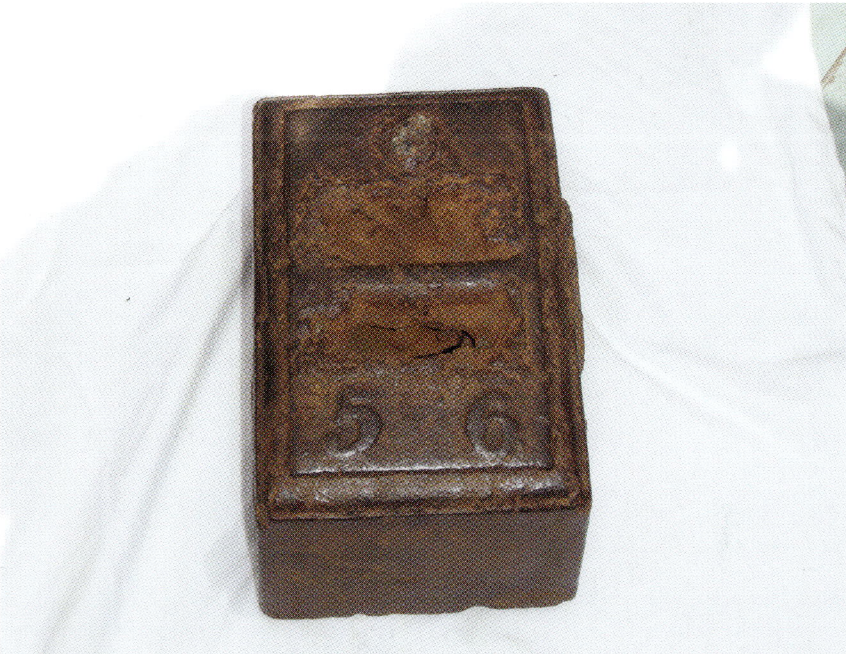

Worlds only VOC iron ballast block

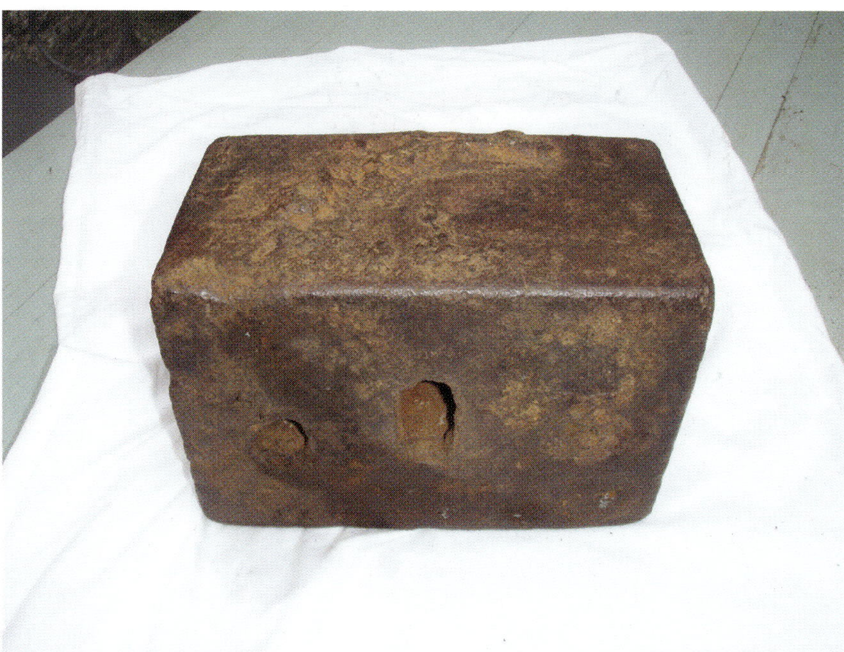

Keel locking pin holes in a 300 year old Swedish Iron Block

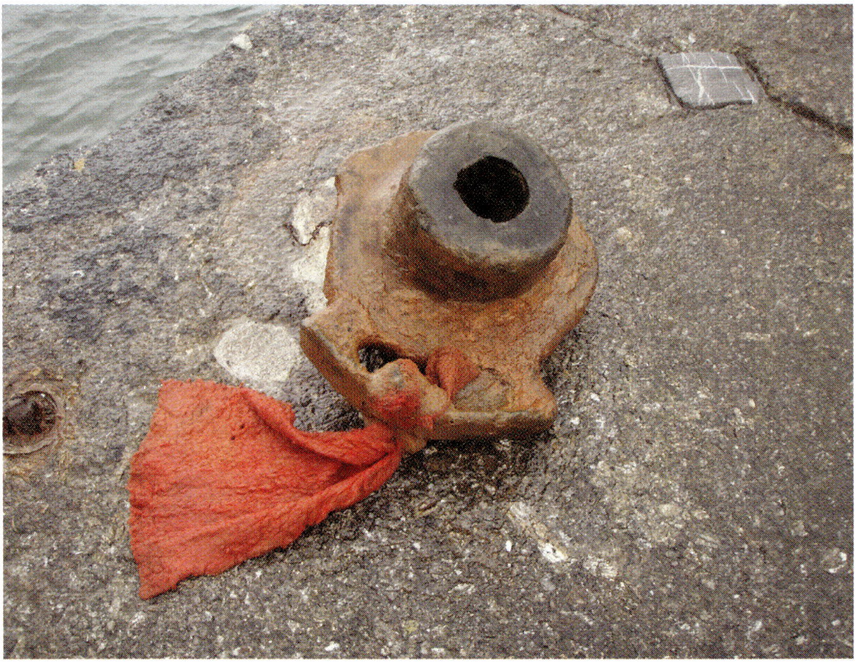

Possible gun carriage wheel

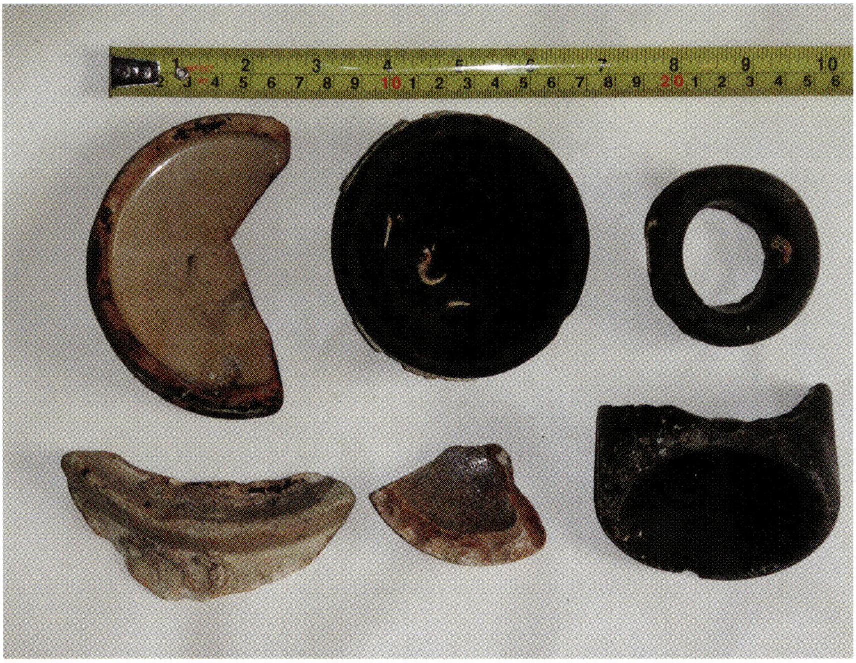

Crockery and Glass

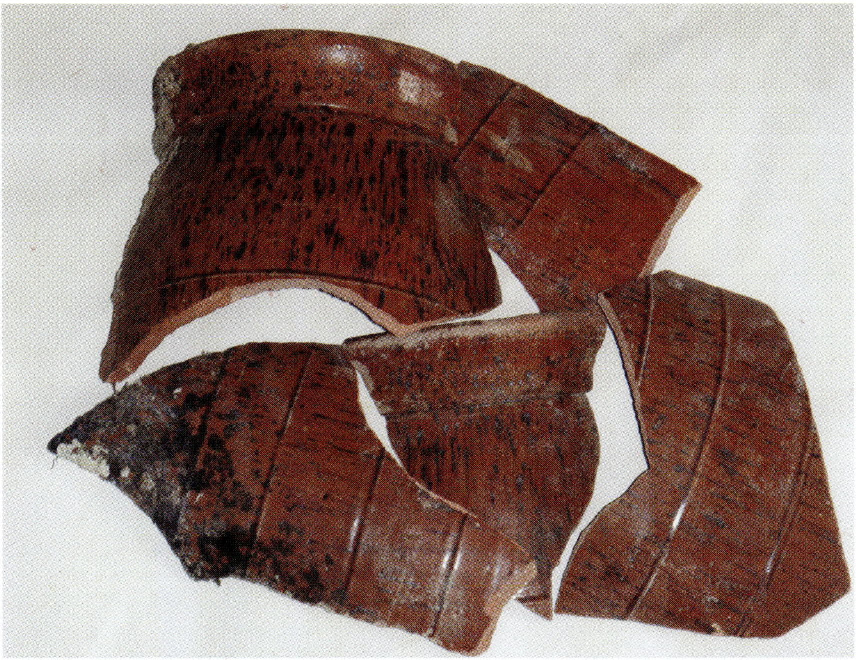

After 300 years of storms we find many parts of the same jar

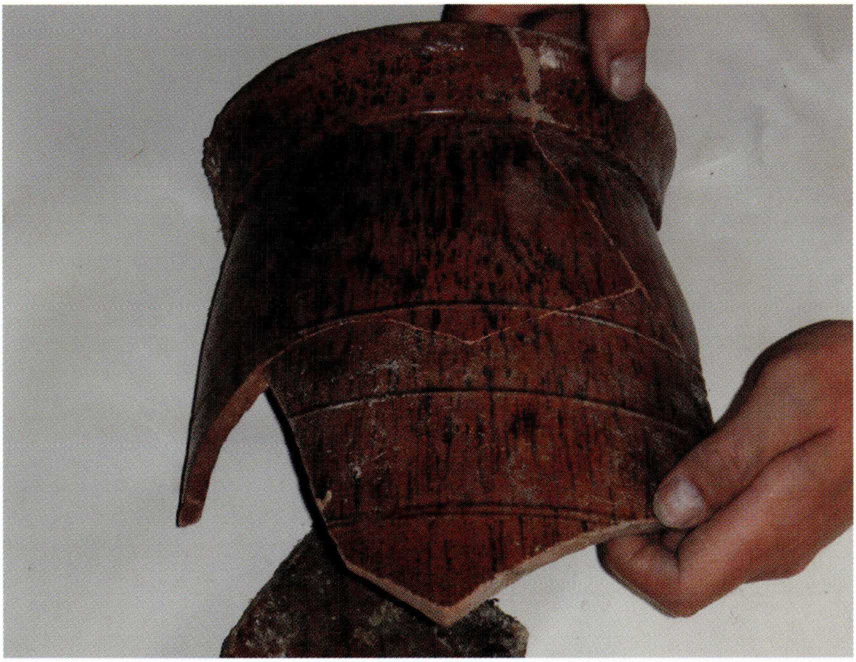

Now we have our own Ramscliff jar

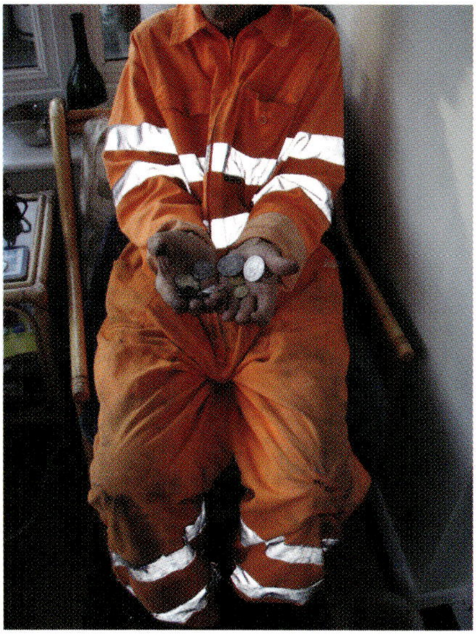

Uncle Orange

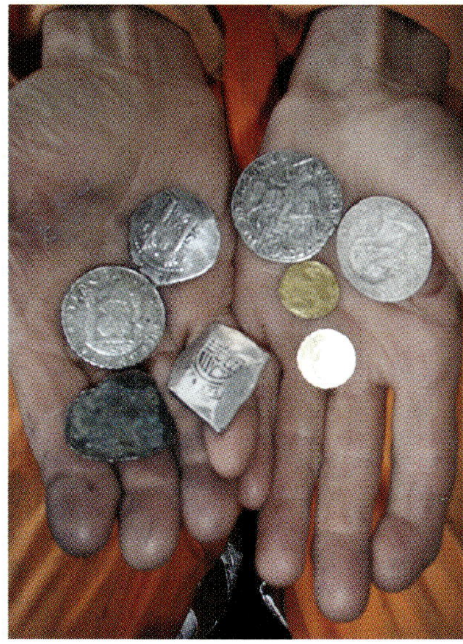

Uncle Orange's previous booty

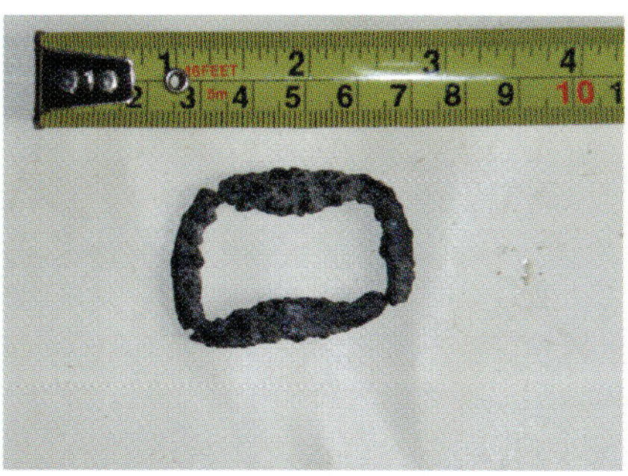

Shoe Buckel

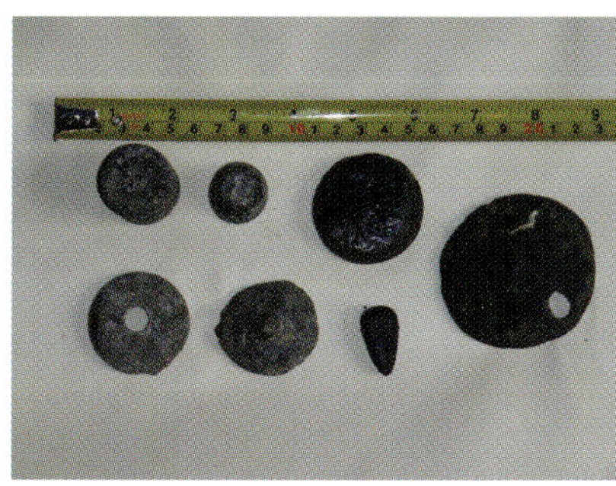

Load Wieghts

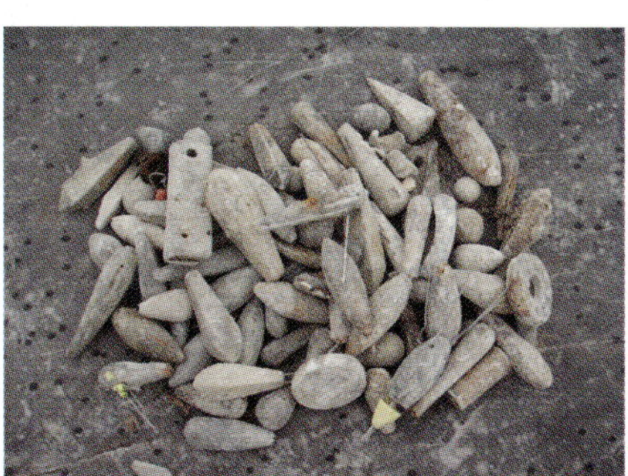

Hundreds of modern fishing weights

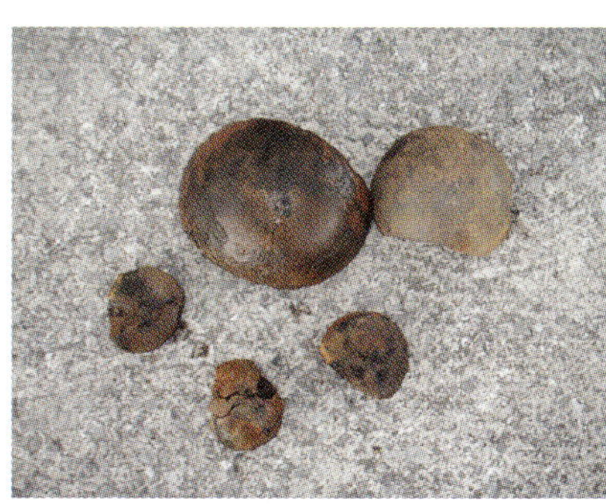

Broken cannon balls

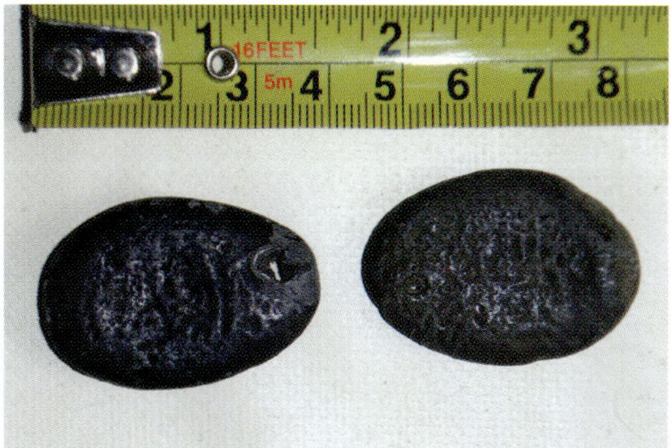

Tear drop powder weights

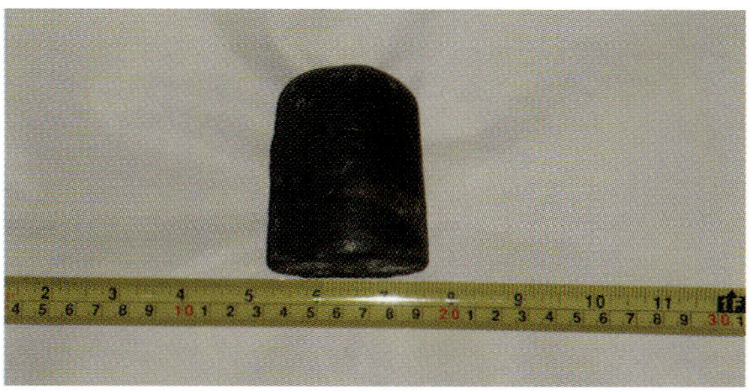

4 pound powder weight

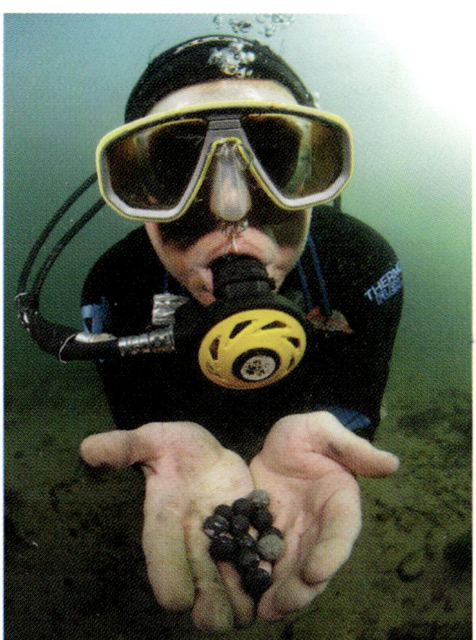

Musket slot a plenty. Photo: Dan Bolt

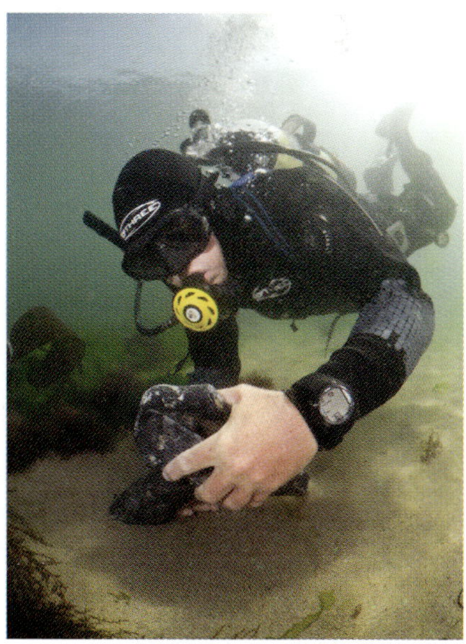

Diving recovering lead pipe.
Photo: Dan Bolt

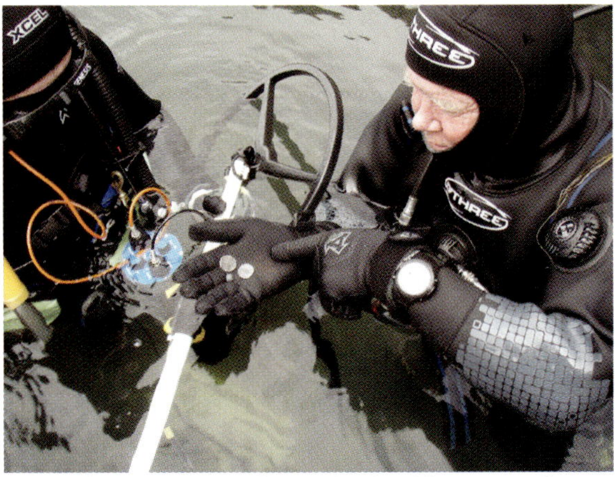

Shallow water finds two lead gold coin weights

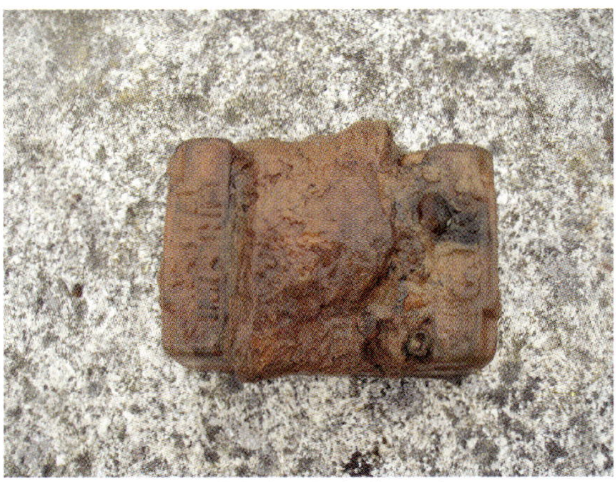

Small half cleaned weight

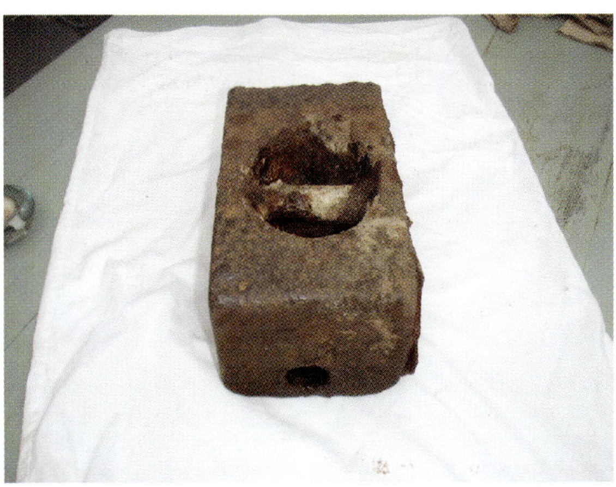

Half of a 112 pound ballasat block

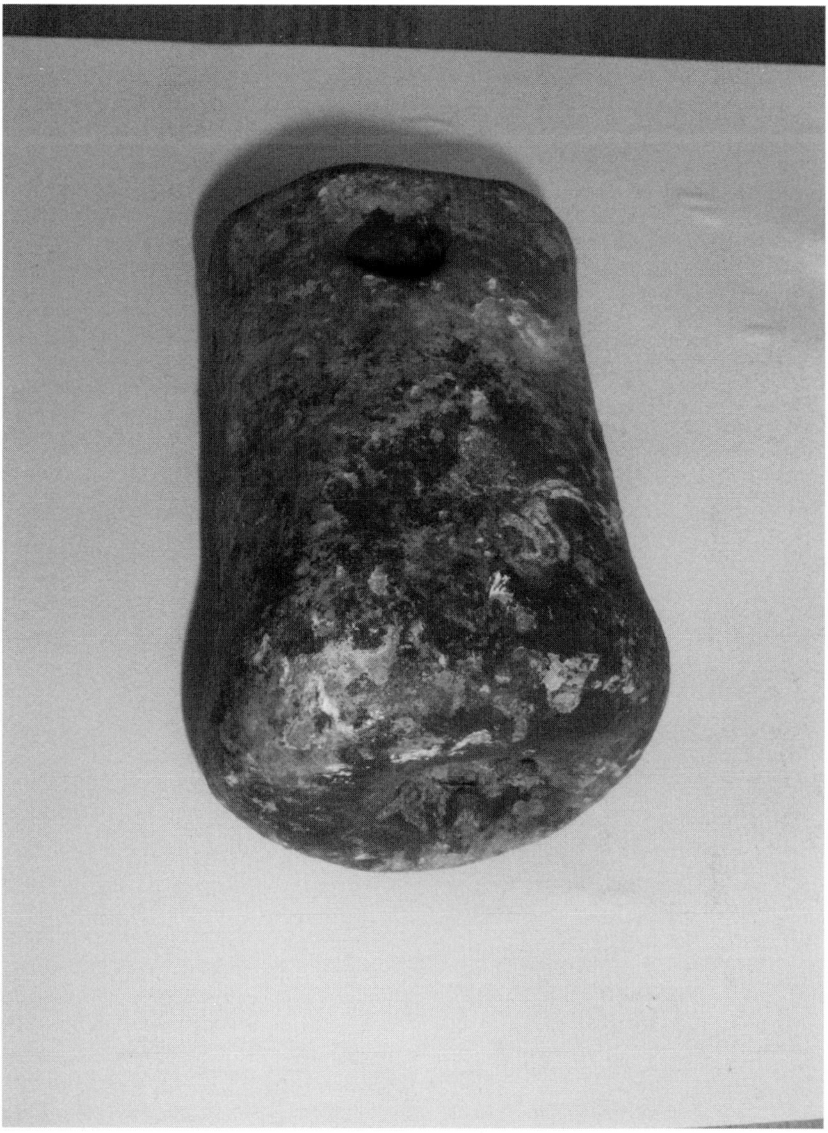

Ships sounding lead

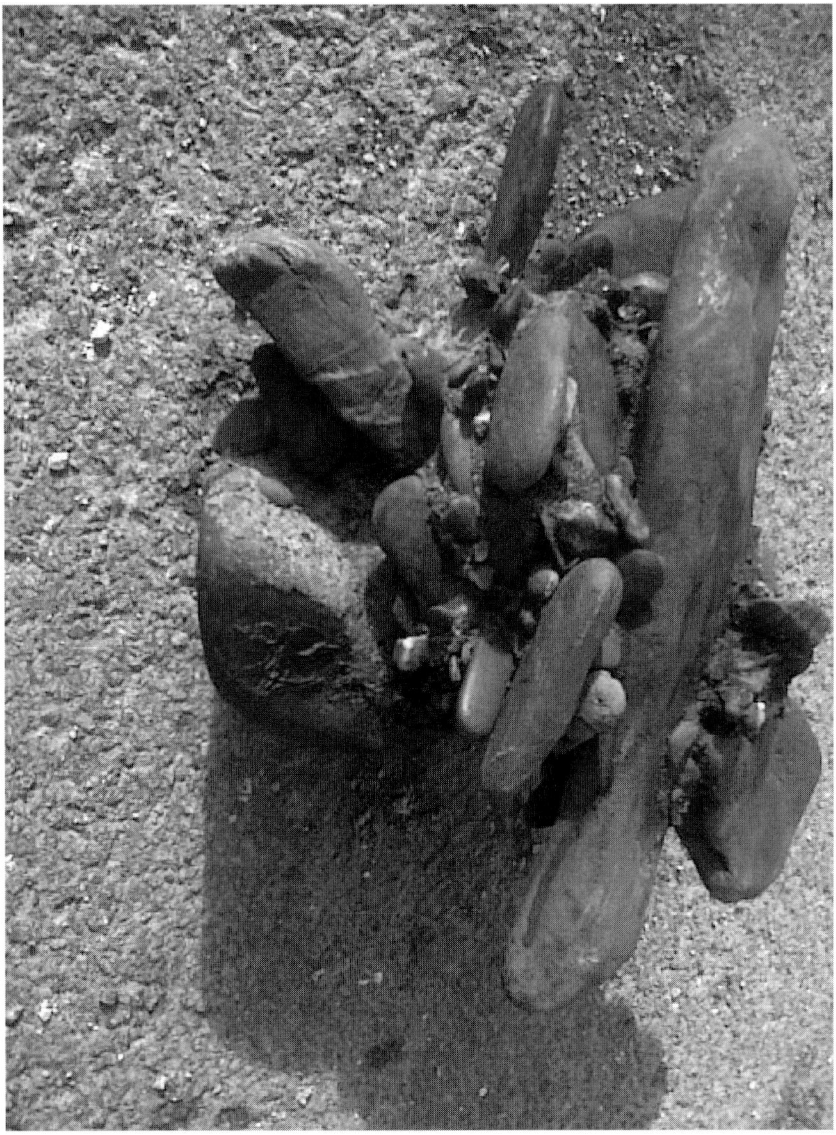

Lump of crustation

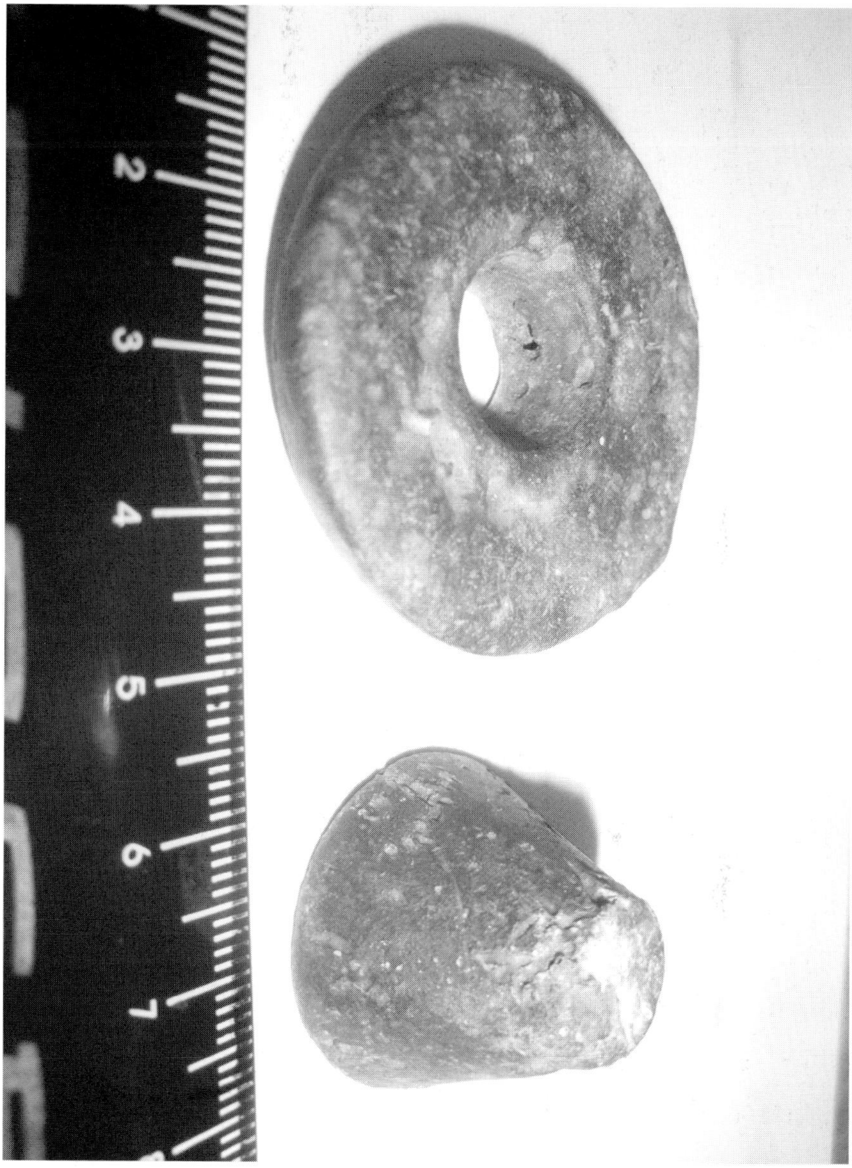

Lead weights, used to measure powder

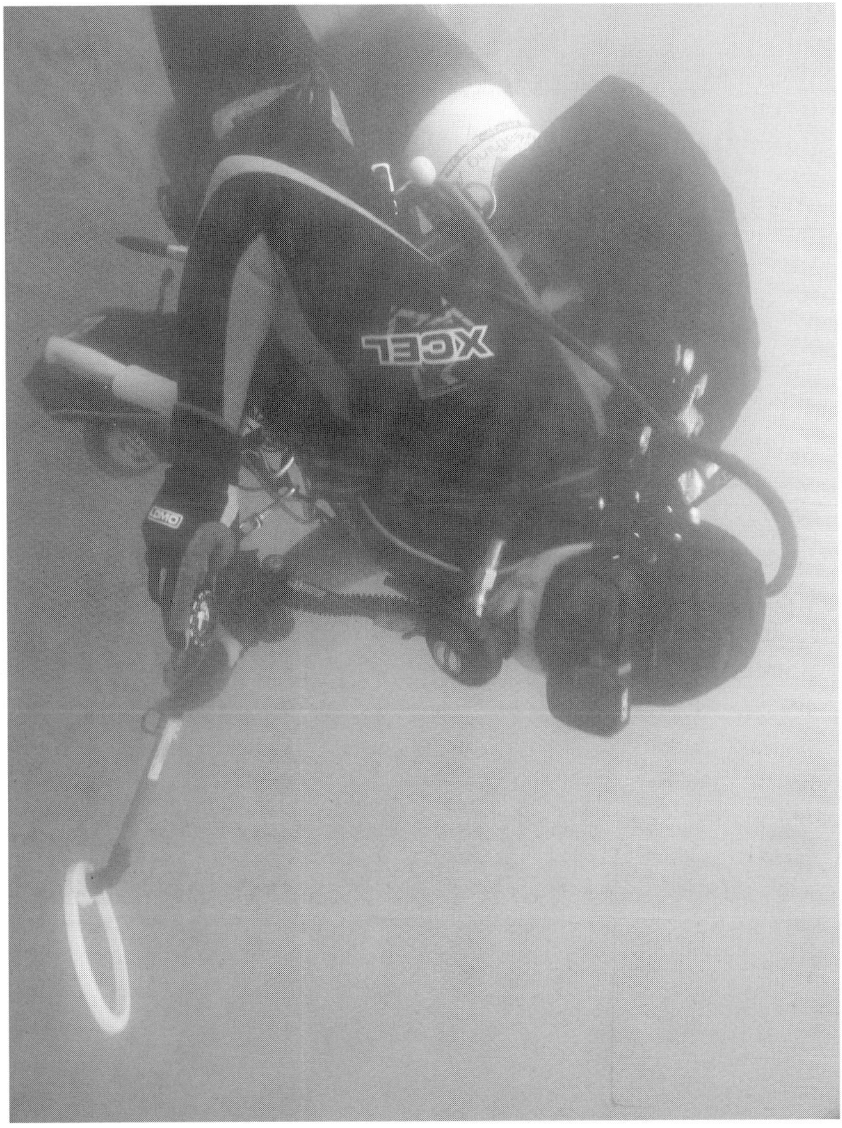

Mr. Green with his trusted Aquapulse

Chapter Tweleve

Research Back From Holland

Dear Captain Black,

Like you asked, I've carried out the research about the VOC-ship 'Aagtekerke', it's wreckage near Plymouth in 1721 and her cargo. Unfortunately, this ship belonged to the chamber Zeeland. From this chamber, a lot of archive material does not exist anymore. However, I've found some information about her cargo and the first moments after the ship wrecked.

The Aagtekerke was built in 1720 in Middelburg. It weighed 800 tons and its length was 145 feet. The Aagtekerke wrecked near Plymouth during it's first journey in December 1721. The captain's name was Nicolaas Rabodus.

In the resolutions of the chamber Zeeland (finding aid number 1.04.02, inventory number 7257), I've found the following information.

On January 8 1722 the chamber Zeeland received the news that the 'Aagtekerke' was wrecked near Plymouth. The captain Rabodus wrote this to the chamber. On the same day, the 'directors' of the chamber Zeeland decided that a plan must be made how to save the cargo. During the meeting of January 19 1722, one decided that some directors of the chamber Zeeland would have to advice their colleagues about this subject. A couple of days later, on January 22 1722, the chamber Zeeland discussed the advice some of its directors had come up with, and they decided to follow this advice. Meanwhile, on January 19 1722 and on February 2 1722, the chamber Zeeland received and read more letters, sent from England by Rabodus and some others, about the wreckage of the Aagtekerke. About the contents of this letters, almost nothing is said in the resolutions of the chamber Zeeland. On February 16 of 1722, the chamber Zeeland received lists, in which is summed up which cargo and how much money had been saved. The chamber decided that this cargo and money has to come back to the Dutch Republic. Unfortunately, the resolution does not mention what cargo and how much money has been saved. However, I've found some information about the cargo in other documents.

Most of the actual letters which do occur in the resolutions are either lost or hidden in the archives of the VOC. I've searched for them, but I did not find them on 'logical spots', like the series of letters, sent to the chamber Zeeland in the archives of the VOC. However, in the archive of the 'family Radermacher' (finding aid 1.10.69, inventorynumber 247), I've found the advice of some of the members of the chamber Zeeland about how to save the cargo of the Aagtekerke. The advice was to send a shipper from the Dutch Republic to London, where he had to find the shipper of the Aagtekerke, Rabodus. Thereafter, the undamaged, salvaged goods of the Aagtekerke had to be transferred to another ship of the VOC, the 'Samaritaan'. For the cargo that had become wet or damaged, one had to hire another ship, big enough to carry all these damaged cargo, and Rabodus had to take this ship back to the Dutch Republic.

Furthermore, in the same inventory number, I've found a list of some saved cargo and the value of this cargo of 1722. If this is the list, which is mentioned in the resolutions of February 16 1722, I can't say. In any case, according to this list, the ship contained in any case 13 boxes with, among other things, silver bars. The contents of these 13 boxes alone represented a value of. 197.736:5..

Furthermore, I've searched the series of incoming documents, concerning the 'VOC' and 'English affairs 'in the archives of the States General. This college was responsible for the policy concerning the VOC, so the chambers of the VOC corresponded with the States General. The incoming documents about the VOC (called liassen VOC, finding aid 1.01.02, inventory number 5743) did not contain documents about the wreckage of the Aagtekercke, but the serie incoming documents about England (called liassen England, finding aid 1.01.02, inventory number 5946) did. Luckily, two of them are in English, and the other's are in Dutch and one in French. The first Dutch letter contains, like the English ones, information about how the Aagtekercke was wrecked, (in a heavy storm, the ship was driven on shore not far from Plymouth), about the robbery of some cargo ('a large quantity of wine, brandy and some bale goods 'to be exact) and about the failed attempts to prevent this. Thirteen boxes with silver were saved. (It seems likely that these are the same boxes which I mentioned before, but I cannot be sure.) The second and third Dutch letter are copies of both English letters. The fourth Dutch letter does mention the intention to punish the people who stole some parts of the cargo of the Aagtekerke, and to prevent robberies from wrecked ships in the future.

Because in the last Dutch letter, two resolutions, of January 7 1722 and January 9 1722 are mentioned, I've searched for these resolutions. I have not yet found the second one, but the first one mentioned again that one must take care for the saved cargo, and that robbery of wrecked ships must be prevented in the future. So neither in the letter, nor in the resolution, concrete preventive measures are discussed; one only spoke out the intention that measurements had to be taken.

I did not found any information about the weapons on board of the Aagtekercke, and it is hard to say in what kind of documents information about this subject could be found. It's possible that documents which mentioned weapons of the Aagtekercke do not exist anymore.

I could search for further information about the wreckage of the Aagtekercke and the salvation of the cargo in the resolutions of the Chamber Zeeland and of the States General. However, because I don't know if these subjects came up in meetings later in 1722 or 1723, and if they did, on which date, this will probably become a very time consuming research, with a very insecure outcome.

The research, mentioned above, took 5 hours. The total costs for this research are 10 x 24,50 euro, plus administration costs (six Euros). You will receive an invoice with instructions on how to pay.

Kind regards,
Marjolein Jorna
National Archives of the Netherlands

What do you make of that Mr Green?

I need to read it through a few more times before I fully understand it, and to look for any clues. But the thing the jumps out at me, which I am sure is the same for you. Is that he states there were only 13 chest of silver on board, and that 13 chest of silver were salvaged.

I know that made my hart sink a little, not that all the artefacts and history isn't interesting but it's the treasure that's going to pay bills. I was hoping they would be able to find a complete infantry of what she was sailing with.

Ye so was I

When we have read about outbound VOC ships and there cargos, I have never heard of a ship of that size just carrying 13 chest of silver bars, have you?

No! I read about a VOC ship of a similar size and at a similar time sailing to the same place and that had 32 chests of gold coins and over 5000 silver bars.

In Patricks article he prints what he says is an insurance claim for the lost cargo, but I can seem to make head or tale of it, can you? Your eyes are much better than mine Mr Green have a read of it again.

To be honest Captain I can't make out anything for certain. At a best guess I would say there is 189720 Guilders still outstanding and being claimed for. But I think if you asked ten different people to read that document and give you there answer you would have ten different answers. If we based any of our searches or plans on that document that could easily be a forgery we are pissing in the wind.

I hear what you're saying Mr Green, but surely we have to believe something, some books some documents. I mean that's what keeps me going, that's what keeps my faith.

I know it does Captain, but sometimes someone can want something so bad they are willing to believe anything. If you watch every programme of the hustle on TV they always pick a mark, a person who is greedy or desperate.

So now you're saying I am mark.

That's not what I am saying; forget it I'm just meant it's very difficult to say with any certainty what the document actually says.

Hello Mr Green it's me you're talking to not some lawyer or what's his face from spooks

Harry Pierce?

Yeh that's his name, just tell me what you think it says.

I think the top half is goods recover 147, 736 and the bottom figure goods lost 153,720.

So that would mean that they sailed with more than just 13 chest of treasure on board.

Correct, and why would they sail to Batavia which took over ten months, on a ship that weighed 800 tonnes and was 145 feet long with

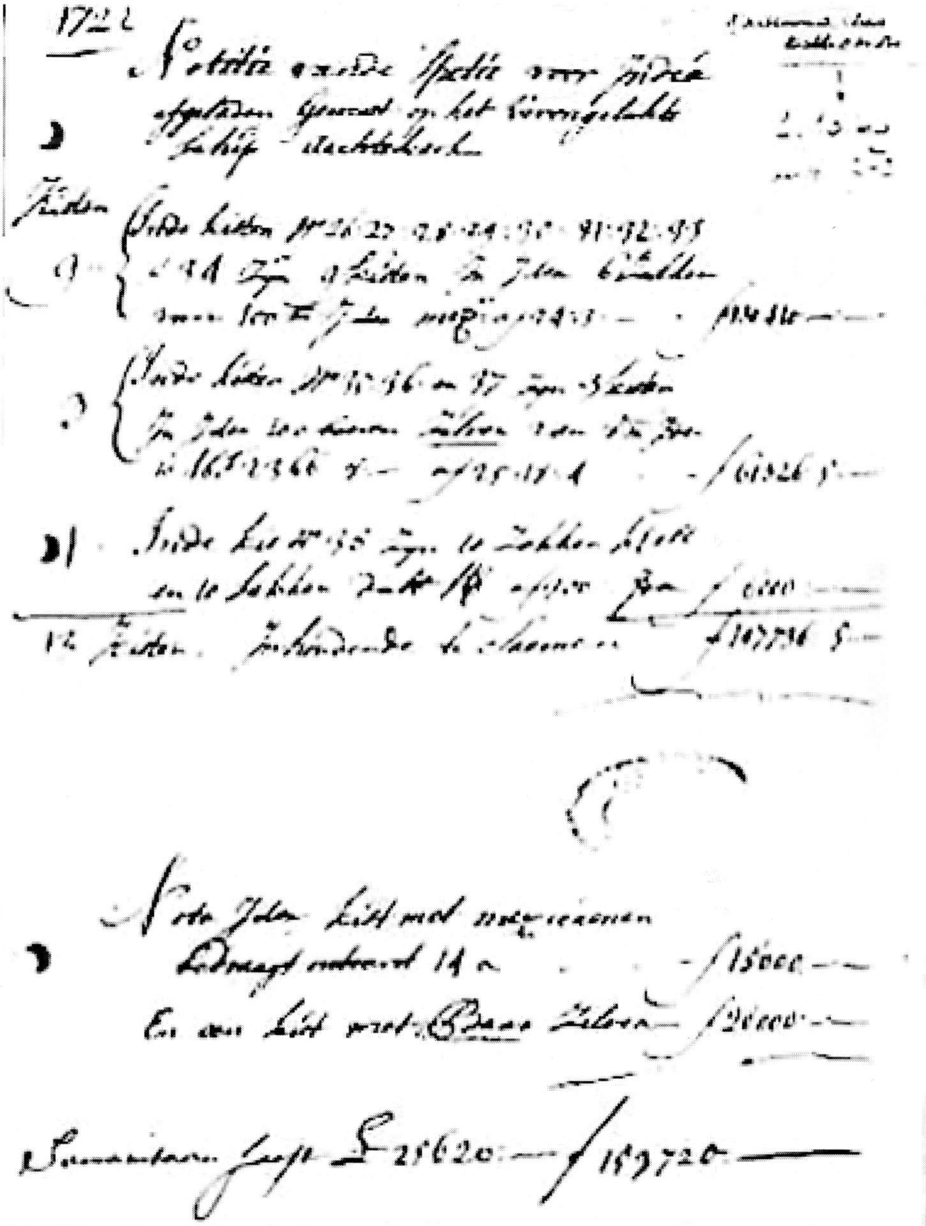

Document listing Aegtekerken's lost cargo
Source: Rademacher Collection, Algemeen Rijksarchief Den Haag.
Ref: 1.10.69 inventory no. 247

only 13 chest on board. We know they where creatures of habit and had very successful routines. Each ship of that size had the same number of crew, the same size and number of cannons, the same amount of swivel guns and two bronze cannons each. Also we know that VOC ships of that size and at the time making the same voyage carried way more than 13 chests. So I am putting a line in the sand and saying there is lots more treasure down there and probly silver bars. And I am sure that Richard Larns and his posy have got lots more information than us on what the Aaktekerke was carrying and what they managed to salvage.

Well I have got some new information on how the locals at the time might have tried to salvage some of that lost cargo mentioned in the above letter. Last might I was reading the book "Port Royal" By Robert Marx and he was discussing the methods use by contempory salvers back in the early eighteenth century. As it turns out one of the methods was to dredge the area with heavily weighted fishing nets and drag them along the bottom to dredge up any loose items.

That seems logical Captain, and if you remember that gully we dived in the Shetland Is was called "dredging gecko" which meant dredged gully. The same thing happened there in about 1712.

I wonder how successful they where?

Well as we know from our research in the Shetlands, divers where still recovering artefacts, silver and gold coins in the same gully they dredged hundreds of years later. And we have been recovering artefacts from the Ramscliff gully every time we go out there. Plus the fact we have now recovered lots of the weights they used on their nets, indicates that it was not so successful. I mean, having dived in that gully and seen all the sharp rocks sticking up, would you go anywhere near it with a bottom dredging net?

No! not a chance. You know that sand eel net I have, well that works very a similar way as their dredging net would of work. On the bottom there are small but heavy weights and on the top of the net are small floats. On each end of the net there is about 10 meters of rope from the top and the bottom. I choose a beach or river mouth where there is absolutely no rocks sticking up, and then one guy holds one end of the ropes and stays on the sand in the dry, and then I swim out and around in a circle with the other end of the ropes. I swim back to the sand about 20m away from where the other guy is. We then walk closer together and start taking in on the net. As we pull in the net the weighted bottom of the net dredges the sand to a depth of about 10cm. All the sand eels live in the sand and they get caught in the net along with the top layer of sand. And the point I am trying to explain

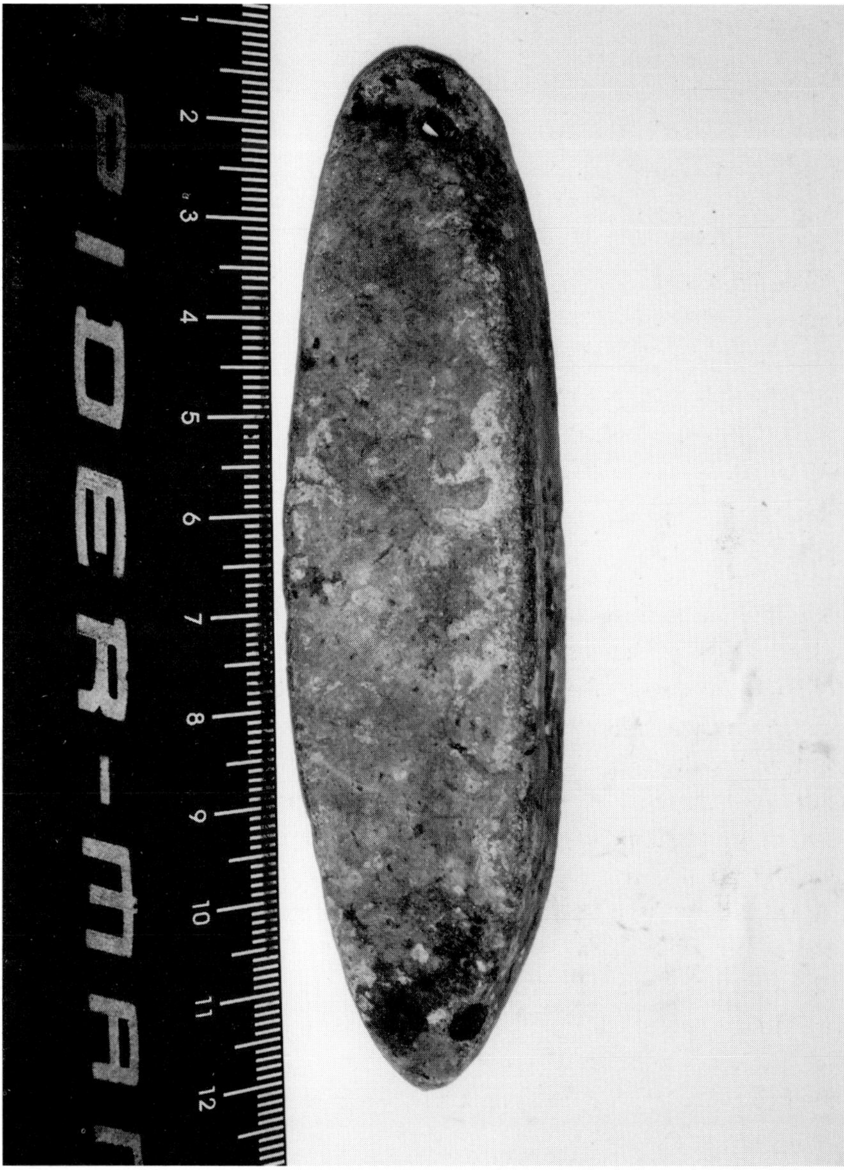

Contemparary dredging net weight

is that if there was one single rock sticking up above the sand I would never be able to pull the net in, and it would get ruined on its first dredge. So it's no wonder we are finding so many weights and all the things we have found.

Chapter Thirteen

A Visit From A Past Master

Hey Mr Green it is I, captain Black

Hi Mate how's it going?

Yeh all good.

Any news, anything happening?

Yeh a little something happened; you will never guess who turned up on my door step about 5pm last night?

I'm guessing its someone to do with the cannon, but no your right I can't guess.

None other than Peter McBride,

Cool that must have been a bit of a shock.

Yeh kind of, but I know he visits a friend of his who lives about 3 doors down, and I guess he has read about the cannon so not so surprising really. And as we know that once a great treasure hunter always a great treasure hunter, those old boys can sniff out a good lead anywhere.

How was he?

Yeh, he was very well and in good spirits

How old is he now?

Hmm I would say about late seventies early eighties.

What did he have to say?

Well he said he had read about the cannon in the paper and could he have a look at it, which I of course said that would be fine and started bailing out the water from the tank. And as I was doing this I handed him that broken cannon ball that we found, well his eyes grew wide open and asked if we had found it at the same place as the cannon. I could tell by his surprise at that find that when I started to show him the other finds, the large cannon balls and musket shots thought we would he be very very impressed.

And was he?

Totally, he was blown away and he was almost lost for words, almost. He said the cannon were pre 1730 and not British. He thought the large cannon balls were also not British and would come big calibre cannon.

He was desperate to measure the circumference of the large cannon balls but we could not find a tape measure. Did that stop a wisely old bird like him, not at all. We cut some string and put in around the cannon ball and then we cut it exactly to size.

He talked about ship wrecks near Plymouth and the size of ships that would have gun decks capable of caring cannons of the size that could fire the large cannon balls.

Did he say the words Aagtekerka ?

No he didn't, it was like he wanted too but could not bring himself to say it, but the worlds Dutch ship came out of his mouth a lot.

Did he ask where the site was?

Yeh of course he did he couldn't help himself, you know how it goes. Im a old man, I don't dive any more, I wouldn't tell anyone, you wouldn't mind telling me where the site is would you ? I looked him in the eye and said Peter you know I can't tell you it's just out there somewhere. I showed him all the finds so far and he said he thought we had a very significant wreck on our hands. We chatted for a while and then he left; he said he would call me when he had some information on the size of the cannon balls.

What size does he think they are?

He wasn't sure and nor am I either

Yeh nor me, let's see what he comes back with.

Ok see you next Monday for a day on the cannon. Let's try and get the tampion out if possible.

Good idea sees you then.

Oh just one thing, talked to the Ginger Witch last night and she said, we will find the answer to our cannon but not where we think, and something to do with the military.

Hope this doesn't mean British military or all our Dutch ship theories and hopes go down the swanny.

Well you know shes always right, but sometimes what she says is a riddle, so we will just have to see where things lead us, see you tomorrow.

Do you want to start emptying the tank and I will get the engine lift ready and we can get the cannon out and onto the pallet.

Sure thing Captain, where is the bucket?

Should be over there in the corner. I will get the kettle on and join you soon; by the way The Chiseller is coming to help us today.

That's good, because you always seem to slide off somewhere when there's hard graft to do, and don't come back at me with that usual line that you are the "thinker" the "marketer" the "Hype man" or whatever it is you call yourself.

Just get working Mr Green all I want to hear is tap, tap tap, you leave everything else to me. Im going to have a little lie down on my thinking couch.

Does the chiseller know what you're like, full of shit and making it all up as you go along.

No of course not, he is buying into the sizzle the same as everyone else, caught up in the dream dude, he see the dream and he wants in on it. You know what I always say "sell the sizzle not the sausage!"

Bugger off and lie down on that stupid couch, you're doing my head it, I can't believe I'm so stupid to listen to you, I'm going to meet the Chiseller and help him with the cannon

Give me 20mins to do some thinking and then I will come outside to see how you are getting on.

Hi Chiseller nice of you to join us it was great to talk to you on the phone and you are very welcome to join the "world's worst treasure hunters", you will be a very invaluable member of the team. Welcome on board, we will fill you in on all the details as we work, well as you two work.

I doubt he will tell you all the details Chiseller, I don't even think he tells me all the details, and I'm his bloody partner in crime.

Now now Mr Green, I was just coming to lend a hand, as all that noise was spoiling my thought process. Now you have got a better man than me with a hammer and chisel, I might as well make myself useful and make the tea?

Yes please that would be nice.

How about a cheese and ham toasty done on my George Foreman grill?

That does sound nice?

Sounds great we will both have one thanks.

How do you like the cannon chiseller?

Fantastic much smaller than I thought but very nice.

Do you think your get the tampion out today guys?

Yeh should do just going to finish off the cascable and the trunions first.

Cool be back with that sandwich in a minute.

"We call him the Chiseller because he does rock sculptures and arty stuff like that out of rocks. He is quite good at it and sells a few pieces now and then, many to people down from London. You know people with more money than sense. I mean he gets some old lump of rock, knocks it about a bit with a chisel, and then tells you some bullshit about it being a bird, or figure head or something"

"He stands about five feet seven, large build and a bit over weight, with kind of gingery hair, very little hair in fact. He has a completion of someone who would never be allowed in the sun without a wide brimmed hat. I think he would get sun burnt at a fire work display. After getting caught up in the race of running his own business, which has recently sold, he hasn't dived or had much fun in the last ten years. So he is very much up for it, mad for it. I remember diving with him about 12 years ago and he really had a nose for it. You don't come across people very often who just are blessed by the "Find Gods" but the Chiseller is one of those people for sure. I have met a few people blessed by the rugby gods" the "high board diving gods" Terry Marsh was a mate of mine and his was blessed by the "Boxing Gods" my youngest son is blessed by two gods "Gymnastic Gods and Football gods" "

"But it is rare to find someone the "Finds Gods" have blessed. The Chiseller has just got a nose for where to look. On land or under water he is the one that always finds the good stuff. I am really pleased he has joined the team. He is kind of the half way house between myself and Mr Green."

"Me being the forever optimist, and never let the rules or the truth spoil a good day out, and Mr Green keeping it real and keeping it (just) safe. Chiseller likes to dream a little, and knows he own limitations when it comes to dive time and depths. He knows he needs to shed a few pounds, and diving the way we dive, out of tiny rubber boats with lots of humping and carrying he is surely in for the fat boy sweats. But a better nose and persistence you will never find, reminds me a bit of a fatter, younger Uncle Orange. A big, kind hearted, teddy bear with two mad daughters, and a very welcome member of the treasure hunting brethren."

Here you go nice just a promised and big cheese toasty and a hot cup of tea.

Where the hell have you been? You said five minutes and been a chuffing hour.

Oh well I'm here now and that's what counts. Wow! You done a great job on the cannon you can really see the detail in the shape now.

Hey Mr Green haven't we seen that type of cannon somewhere before? You're not going to believe it, but I have seen the exact same cannon only in a larger scale somewhere before. Now you have clean the cascable I know I have seen the exact same shape somewhere before, I can see it in my mind now, they where huge compared to this one but exactly the same none the less. God I can't remember where I have seen them. I think it was in an old photograph or in a book. I'll go inside and see what I can find, back soon.

Is he serious Mr Green or is he just making it up to get out of doing some work and getting his hands dirty?

Well Chiseller, I wish I could stand here, look you in the eye and say, yes he is a lying son of a bitch. And that he is just full of shit and makes it all up on the hoof. And he is just trying to get out of some real work.

But you're not going to are you.

No! and it is bloody annoying and drives me bloody nuts, but having been his buddy, his work mate, his companion for many years now. The one thing that I have learned is never to take him for a fool, or underestimate him. When he says things like that, like he just said. And then he goes off to do something, god know what. I find myself hoping he is full of shit and he is just plain mad and lazy.

Umm I can feel a big BUT! Comming next Mr Green.

BUT! Chiseller he is maverick, and it might take ten minutes, or it might take a hours. BUT! He will come back out and blow us away with some news, or a clue or a book. He does it all the time, I'm telling you its stranger the fiction, you couldn't make the bloody stuff.

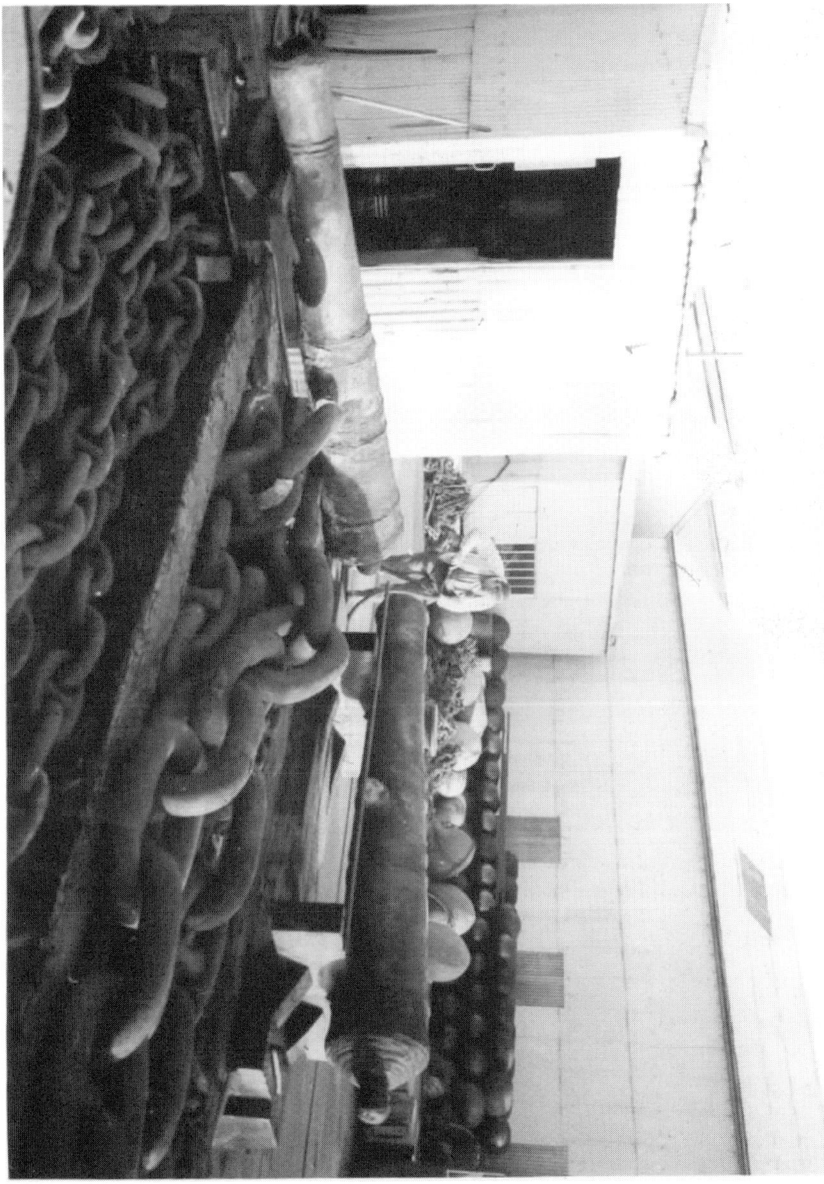

Are you trying to say he's got a gift from the gods, or maybe he's bewitched. What? What did I say, your face went a strange kind of blue like you had seen a ghost.

Nothing let's just get back to work.

Guess, who's the Daddy then guys, put down your hammers and lend me your pirate ears. Dunnarrrr here we go! What do you make of them bad boys?

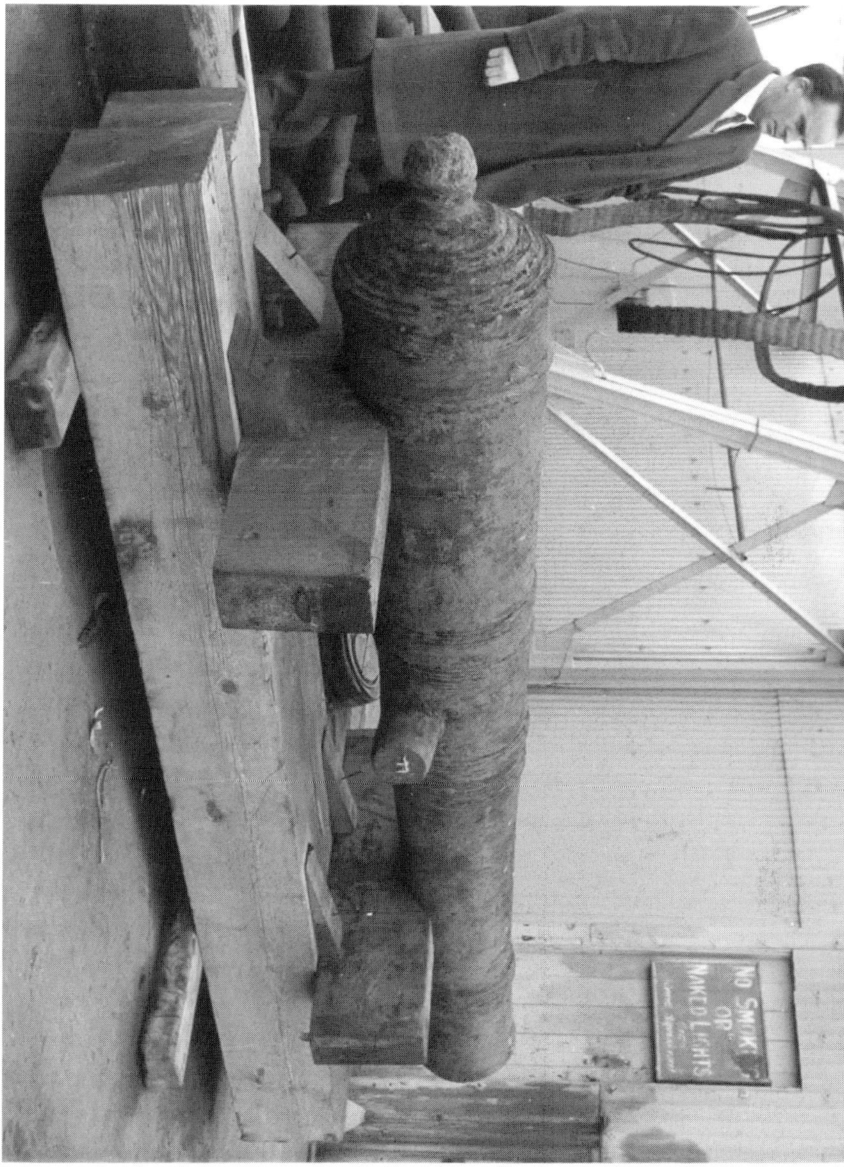

Well I take I would take my hat off to you if I had one Captain Black.

Thank you young Chiseller.

I have to admit I thought you were telling porkies and you where just making it up. But now I take that all back, they are definitely the same make of cannons, just huge mothers.

You agree Mr Green? Same cannons? You've spent many hours working on our cannon and know it best of all. Is it the same cannon?

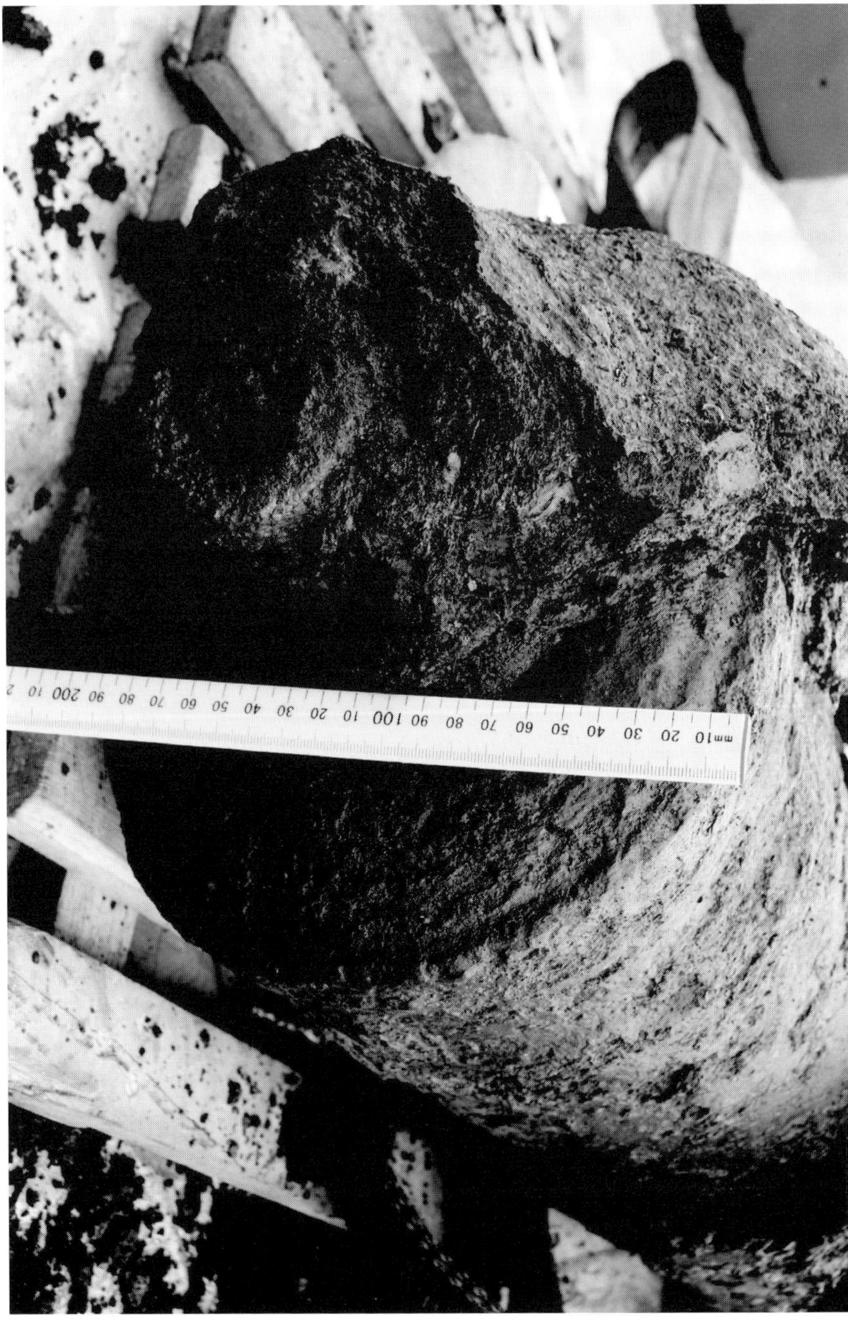

It defiantly 100% is, but the reason I am so quiet and the Chiseller is so excited is because he doesn't know you very well. I know, that like always your now going to tell us some crazy story about the cannons, aren't you?

Yes indeedey I am

See Chiseller, your learn that if you stay around him long enough, that he always bloody does this, and prepare yourself for "how the hell did he find that out mind fuck"

Listen in workers, I said workers not wankers. The photo was taken in Devon Port Dockyard in 1968, by the MOD photographer. The cannons came from a wreck site just off Milbay docks, between the pier and Drakes Island. There was about eight cannons there all about the same size, and in 1968 a well know salvager caked Silus Oats came along with his big steel boat and Crain and lifted those three cannons out of the water to weigh them in for scrap or sell them.

Only it turns out that someone already had dibs on them and was using them as a area to run underwater survey courses on, plus investigating the wreck site.

So when this person found out what Silus had done they went mad. Contacted the MOD and they were then kept away from Silus in the Dockyard. I believe that the guy who had dibs on them was so mad he made Silus put one cannon back.

What happed to the other two cannons?

The Dockyard didn't have the means or finance to conserve them, so they dumped them into the foundation of a new building that was going up.

You've got to be kidding!!

No that's the gods honest.

So do you know who this guy was who had dibs on the site?.

Don't give Chiseller that look Mr Green, he's new to this.

Of course he knows Chiseller, he always bloody knows, and I think you could be closer to the truth than you think, when you said he could be be-witched.

Mr Green knows what I'm going to say he just doesn't what to accept it. It was Commander Silver. And guess who did all the diving and survey work for him on this site?

Go on

His trusted companion, Peter McBride.

No shit, wow that is mad.

I will tell you something that is madder, I just came off the phone to him, thought I would ask if had any news for us on our cannon balls, and at the same time throw him a curve ball about the Milbay cannons.

What did he say?

He said they were made in Sweden but probably came from a Dutch ship, and he even said without prompting, the cannons were the size of cannons that would have fired the large cannon balls we have found.. And I am saying to you that they came off the same shipwreck that our cannon did.

That's a bit of a wild statement Captain; I can't see how you can say that. And how did he get from "cannons made in Sweden to a Dutch ship"

Right now you can give him that look Mr Green. Because I have the results of the surveys carried out by Mr Mc Bride and there's no wreck site. Nothing else down there just cannons

So what is it a dumping ground or something?

Enlighten him Mr Green.

What the Captain is saying or rather not saying, because you keep interrupting is that they where salvaged off our wreck by contemporary salvagers, which they where more than capable of doing. Loaded them onto a barge to take up to the Dockyard to unload and in the process the barge over turned or the cannons where lost over board.

So why wouldn't they salvage them again?

Because where they lay at the moment is deep, dark and very tidal, It's one thing salvaging them from our wreck site is, but not so easy from where they lost them.

Mr Green is right, where they are now is where wind meets tide and it's nasty and horrible.

Also when they grappled for the cannons they could only get the ones where the grapple or ropes would go underneath. And where they are now they would of had no chance it's a muddy shitty bottom.

And you're saying that Commander Silver had worked all this out?

No I'm not sure about that, because he never found our wreck site, the one he was looking for. He might have concluded that the Milbay site was the ships resting place. After all Peter Mc Bride just uttered the mortal words "Dutch ship"

How do you think he got from cannons made in Sweden to Dutch ship?

No idea on that I'm afraid Chiseller.

Thank god for that, for one moment there I thought you new everything.

No not I, only the Ginger witch knew everything, and that reminds me she did say that we would find the answer to our cannon mystery with the military. Ah but I can see by your face Mr Green, that you had remembered that already, and you didn't what to say it.

Chapter Fourteen

Lead Apron

Hello whos calling the mad house?

It's me the Chisseler, how's everything going Captain Black

Good thanks did you get my text?

Yes sure did and I will meet you at Morrisons at 11am, is Mr Green coming? Yep he will be there and he said to tell you it's your round for the cappuccinos.

I should have seen that coming a mile off, see you there.

Hey where's my chocolate sprinkles? You should know I like lots of chocolate sprinkles! Never mind sit down and I will give you the news on my latest dive into the murky world of unrecognisable bent up, rotten old iron that somehow, because its hundreds of years old becomes really exciting.

So in short you found some more info on our cannon?

Sure did, but that's not the best part, I also found something that in the article about that square piece of lead we found. But first the cannon. I was searching the net for hours on end and finally I came across this article on the salvage of "The Queen Anns Revenge" which was wrecked in 1718 off the coast of North Carolina USA. Which is only two years before the Aaktekerke was wrecked near Plymouth. So as I was scrolling down the article and looking at the photos, there it was our cannon, which they have called cannon number three. There cannon is seven feet long and a six pounder while we know ours is only

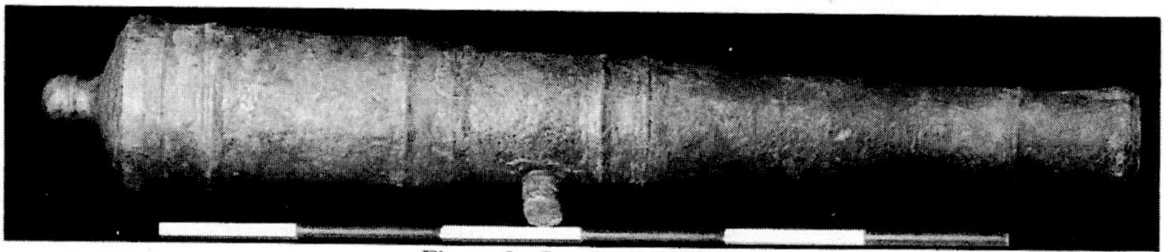

Figure 3: Cannon 3 233.001

QAR website

a two pounder. But when I show you the photo of their cannon you will definitely agree that is the same as our cannon. Here have a look.

Well Mr Green what say you?

You're right definitely the same cannon as ours.

Chiseller what say you young my young Padawan?

I agree, no mistake it's the same cannon. What do they say about it in the article?

They say

> "These guns are commonly called the Danish Descriptor "Finbankers" a general term that described a variety of Swedish guns associated with De Geers foundery at Finspound where they were produced. Quantities where exported to the Netherlands, ostensibly to arm VOC ships. But were also traded throughout Western Europe. It went on to say that." Ruth Brown forely of the Royal Armouries has noted a characteristic of the gun dating from 1660's to 1719. She stated that the gun was probably cast in Sweden most likely from 1660 to 1700".

Also it states in the article that eleven three pound "finbankers" where found on the Danish Frigate Myden (1718) with shape and mouldings identical to their cannon number three.

That's incredible Captain, a ship that was wrecked in 1718 has the exact same cannon as the ship we are looking for and the Aaktekerke wrecked in 1721. Also the cannons were no longer produced from 1717 onwards. Given that the Aktekerke would have taken many years to build, let's say they started her in around 1718 she could definitely have had brand new "Finbankers" on board.

What do you think of that Chiseller?

I don't think there can be any doubt that our cannon came off a Dutch ship that was built and sank between 17...and let's say 1730's. I mean the cannon three articles even said the letters VOC, so to me it's almost a cert that what we are diving on is the wreck of the VOC ship Aaketekerke.

I have some more info to tell you guys, but I will take a leak and one of you can get me a fresh cappuccino...and don't forget lots of chocolate sprinkles!

Cheers Mr Green and nice job with the sprinkles, in fact you've done such a good job I'm going to let you buy me one again some time.

Yeah Yeah get on with it, tell us what else you have found.

As I was scrolling down the same article and looking at all the photos I came across a photo of a square sheet of lead, and I couldn't believe it and just stood up and shouted out loud "hey I've got one of them"

You mean a photo of the old piece of lead we dug up from under the cannon after we lifted It.?

Yes the very same.

But I thought we agreed it was most likely just lead cargo?

We did and guess what, we were 100% wrong. It's in fact a "lead apron" ever heard of one of them guys?

No.

Me neither.

They were placed on top of cannons once the cannon was loaded and primed to keep any water from going down the touch on top of the cannon and getting the powder wet. They were square sheets of lead, heavy enough to stay on the cannon with the ship moving but not too heavy to man handle. They were tied down with rope through small holes and fansend to the gun carriage.

They were flat pieces of lead so they were easy to stow on the decks, somewhere more refined than others, and they had a raised mound somewhere near the middle which sat over the fuse.

Never heard of a "lead Apron" before and I have read so many books on ships and there fastenings etc. How do you know it's a "Lead Apron" and not a just a lead sheet.

Here you are guys, what is that a photo of?

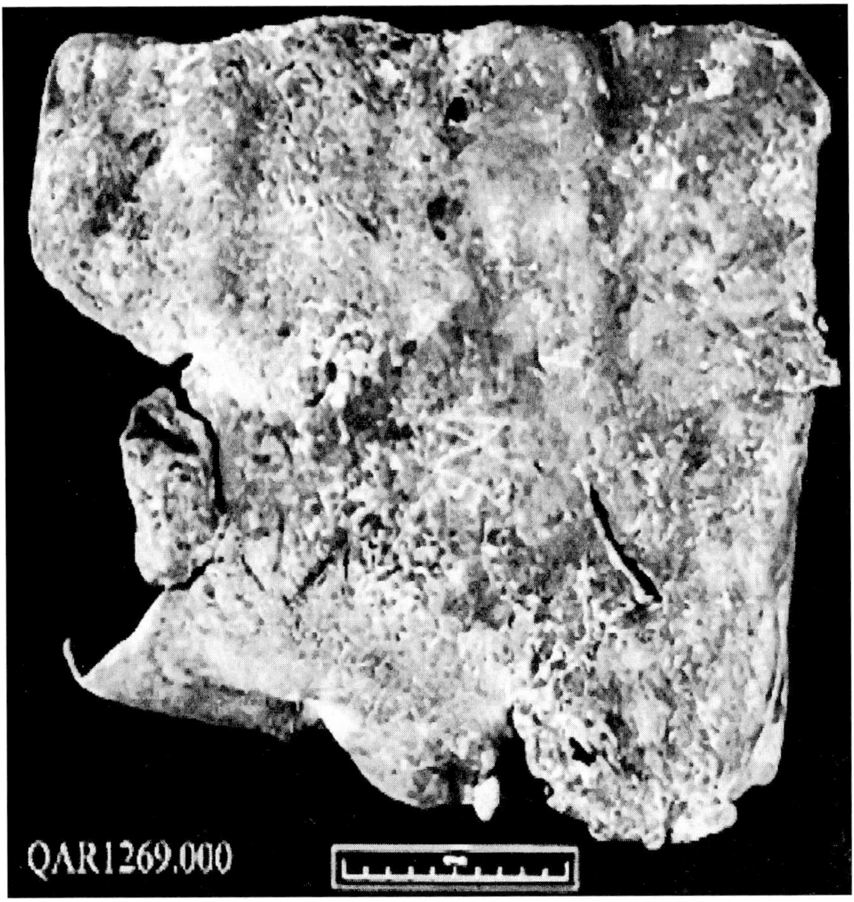

The piece of lead we recovered, the one we have just been talking about.

Yeh I agree with Mr Green, our piece of lead.

Both wrong, that my learned friends is the "lead Apron" recovered from the "Queen Ann's' revenge" 1997.

Here is the piece of lead we recovered from under our cannon.

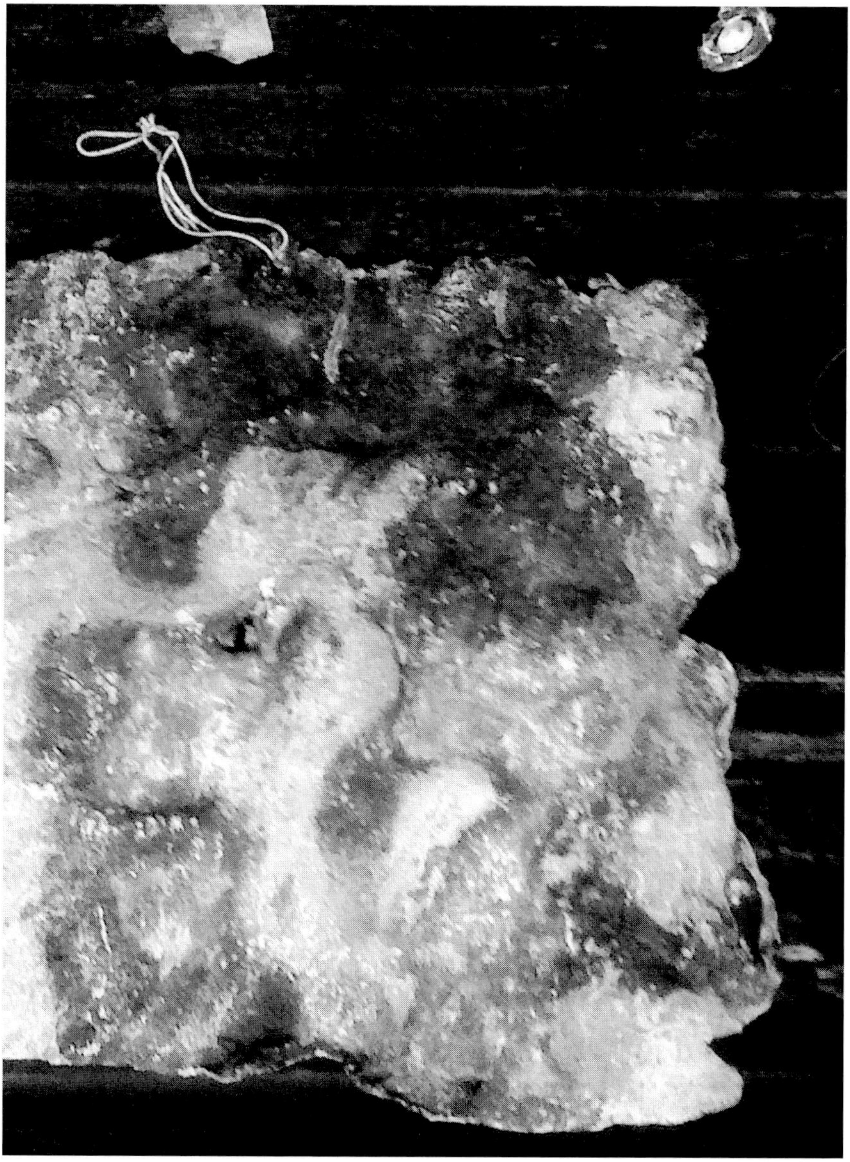

Again all I can say at the risk of repeating myself is that's incredible, if there's a "Lead Apron" than so is ours for sure, I can't believe I have never heard of them before.

I must say I agree with Mr Green, our piece of lead is the same as theirs, of that there can be no doubt.

Thank you both very much, and from now on you can't call it a piece of lead you have to refer to it as the "Lead Apron". And don't beat your selves up to much about never even heard of lead aprons, because Peter Mc Bride saw it when he came around and made nothing of it. Also I have phoned a few old divers, people you would have thought know everything and they had never heard of lead aprons either. And Uncle Orange who is like the oracle on stuff like that, had never heard of them either, and you would of had to bet money he would have one in his museum.

You didn't tell them all we had one did you?

No Just Uncle Orange, after all he is part of the team, and he knows how important it is to keep everything a secret.

Of course not, and on the "DROIT" form to the Receiver of Wrecks I just put down and sheet of lead as at the time that's all I thought it was. And if we informed her now that it was a lead apron she would probably inform "English Heritage" and then the pirates in suits would be all over us. I've spent hours on the net and believe me "Lead Aprons" are a very rare find, and if we can ever prove that our is a VOC lead apron than man alive it's a good find.

Plus the fact we have got the actual cannon that the apron came off, loaded, and primed with its Tampion in and its lead apron fastened on top. When you think about it the cannon was as ready as any cannon could be to fire. Which fits in with the story of its fate, if you have got local people from Plymouth killing and robbing on the cliff. Sure as hell you would want to keep your powder dry. There sure wasn't any Christmas spirit or good well to all men on the Cliffs of Plymouth on that Christmas day. I wonder if there even was such a things as Christmas day in 1721 and if they celebrated it?

Not sure would be nice to find out. Did you send the Receiver of wrecks a photo of the lead sheet?

No not yet but I might do in the future I'm not but what harm can it do, I mean after all to her it's just a sheet of lead. And when you look at it lead apron or lead sheet what's the difference, you could make one form any old lead exactly same in a couple of hours.

But why would anyone what to do that?

Good question Chiseller, why would anybody want to forge something like that, I'm just saying it could be done that's all, and if Uncle Orange wanted one he could make one. Also while where talking about lead, you know that lead tube like thing you found?

That thing that looked like a homemade sounding lead.

Yes, and here you are take another looks at it, right I have a little experiment I want you to try. Right hold this broom handle at its end and at ends length. Now try and get some weight behind it as if you where ramming the charge down a cannon at arm's length. How is it?

Not good, I can't get any weight or power behind it.

Ok now put said lead object over the end of the broom stick and try it again. How was that?

Incredible, a world of difference absolutely perfect for the job, and no chance of slipping or getting splinters.

What do you think Mr Green?

Made for the job I would say, just like the tool farmers use for banging in fence post, you can't hammer them in because there to high and you would not be able to get any drive with a hammer so you slide a post ramming tube over the top, then slide it up and down to drive it in.

As usual I showed it to Uncle Orange and told him what we thought it was, and he took it in his hand, did the ramming action and said, it was bloody amazing and reminded him when use to have to ram the charges down a six inch gun when he was serving on battleship many years ago.

He also said that he found it astonishing that we were finding stuff like the lead apron and now the ramming hammer and it was like writing new bits of history.

Re-writing history is a bit strong, but I do have to pinch myself some times as its along a bit surreal.

I am the same Mr Green and if I lay in bed thinking of the things we might find when we start dredging with that water dredge you are designing, there is no way I can get to sleep. How is the dredge coming on?

All done, and ready to test.

Good, then that is the next job. Test it and when it works well go out and dredge the wreck site.

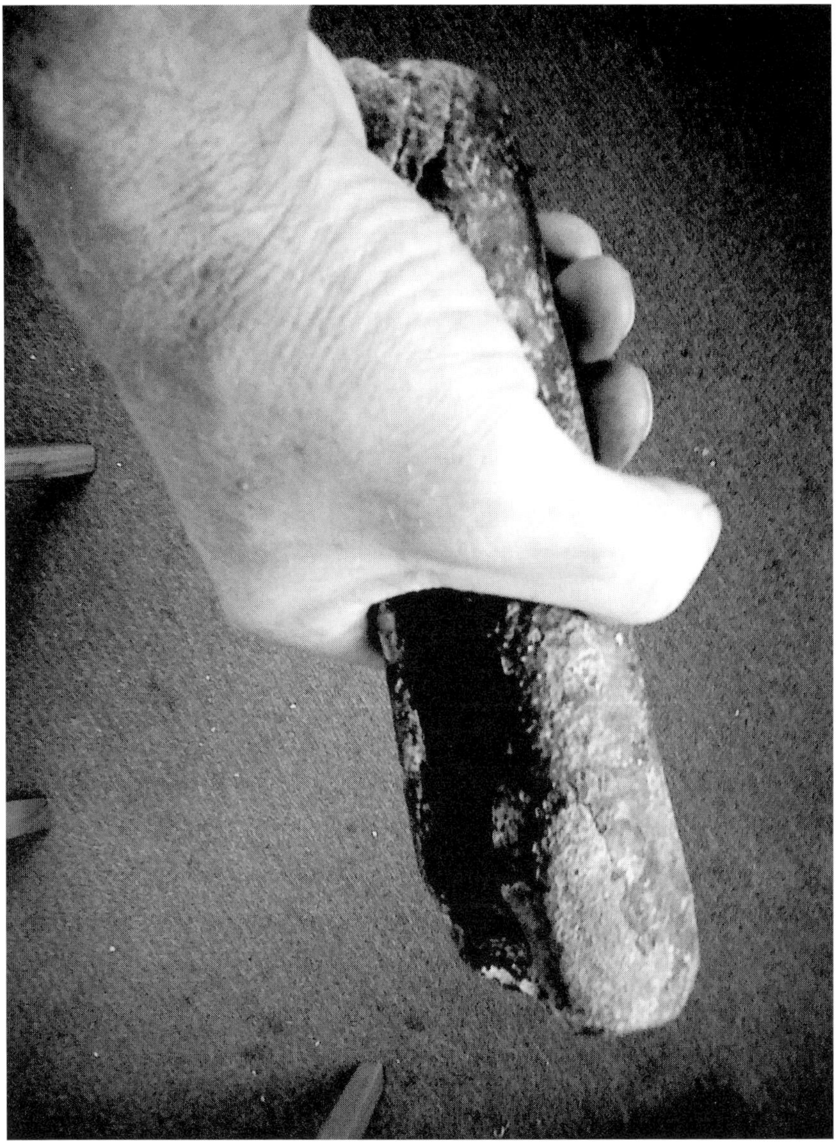

Possibly the only ramming hammer ever found

CHAPTER FIFTEEN

DIVING AFTER THE WINTER STORMS

Whose bright idea was it to go and dive today, we must be mad I spent thirty minutes de-icing my van this morning we must be mad.

I know Chiseller, I was thinking the same thing, I was watching the breakfast news and most of the country has ground to a halt with freezing ice and ten centimetres of snow. I have just had a text of Mr Green saying he is running late because of the ice. But on the up side, the sea is flat as you like and the visibility is going to be off the clock so perfect time for a good look around.

Yeh I know your right, but its just bloody freezing, no hold on my car display is telling me it's worse than that its actually -2oc.

Oh well let's get the boat loaded and make sure we have got everything ready for a quick dip and try and get back here before lunch.

As I desended down the anchor line the shock of the icy cold water hit my face and I had to swallow hard, I knew the pain would not last long and soon my exposed check bones would start to numb off.

"The water was so clear it was like looking trough vodka, no particles in the water whatsoever, no plankton and no sand particles. We had not had any rain for over five days and very little swell all week. The big question was, did the storms two weeks ago move any of the huge amounts of sand from the seabed and leave all sorts of goodies uncovered.

On the bottom now, just need to sort out my weights and take out my trusty green river knife, have a quick wee to warm up my brilliant XCEL two piece wet suit and I'm nice and comfortable and ready to search. I always like to dive alone and with my sharp knife in my hand gives me a sense of power and control over circumstances. The first thing I notice is that a huge amount of kelp has gone, ripped off the rocks and taken away by the storms. There is still some kelp storks left but they look like they are dying off. This is much better than in the summer when the kelp was out of control, and on every kelp leave was a fine covering of sand or dust. Which meant every time you brushed against some kelp you lost your visibility for a couple of minutes. This is much better and I can actually see the topography of the area we have been searching.

Now over to the sandy gully let's hope some of that sand has shifted. As I approach the gully I can see the bottom of the ocean getting lighter and lighter as well as getting flatter with every fin kick. And my hand and my knife sink into it, rich, golden, deep sand as deep as my arm will penetrate.

None of the sand had been removed it was just as deep as the summer, maybe more if that was possible, all of a sudden I don't feel so warm and cosy, maybe it was a bad idea to dive in this extreme weather. After ten minutes swimming over the sand with the occasional dig I decided to have a swim up the gully as far as I can, until my head hits the surface. To my surprise it looks like the storms might have moved some of the small rock and shingle further up the gully, and maybe there is something to find up here.

I can spot something that looks out of place in the distance at the bottom of a small pit, what is it it looks very black and like a tinny top hat. Wow that's neat, it's a pewter bottle top of some description maybe off a jar or a ink well, it must of been uncovered or moved last week, in the goodies bag it goes.

A few more minutes looking around and then that's me I'm cooked, 60 bar left and time to go up, think I will just stop finning for a second and have another quick piss to warm me up, ahhh that is so nice. Hey, what's that over there, I can see something that doesn't look natural, I mean it looks like a stone or piece of slate, buts its sides are to square and mad made. There we go, blimy that's heavy for a small object let's have a scrape with my knife, yep just as I thought a old piece of lead plate, bollocks never mind time to go, hope that coffee in my flask is still hot and Mr Green and the Chiseler haven't eaten all the biscuits.

My head breaks the surface and I can see the boat, only a ten metre swim, I'm sure I can manage it even with this heavy piece of lead in my hands.

Here guys take my goodies bag off me.

Anything Captain?

One nice pewter bottle top and a small piece of lead. Not much sorry guys.

That's OK get yourself in here and gets warmed up, and then the pros will show you how it's done.

Here you go Captain get some of that hot coffee down the hatch. Right let's have a look at what rubbish you've been picking up, open your bag. Nice, that is a nice pewter top, I would say off an ink well or something similar. And a small lead plate, not the best days diving ever but at least you didn't come up empty handed.

Hold on a minute, turn that piece of lead over a again, you see that raised area in the middle. Well I have seen a raised area with marks like that somewhere before; pass it to me a second. You're not going to believe this guys, but this is another "lead apron"

Are you sure Captain? Isn't it too small?

The lead apron at home has exactly the same size raised area for going over the touch hole. And look it's exactly the same just in miniature.

Bloody hell he's right you know, wow!! This must have been the lead apron for a swivel guns as it's so small. That's incredible I wonder if any swivel gun lead aprons have ever been found before.

I doubt it, I am certain they didn't find one on the Queen Ann's Revenge I know that for sure, and I have never seen any mentioned anywhere on the net.

Nice Find Captain

Thank you Mr Green, now you two get your lazy buts in there, and try and beat that if you can.

OK come up on the rope Captain nice and easy, it's going to be bloody heavy so take your time. And also you need to take this heavy goodies bag off me.

Christ that is heavy what the hell you got in there Chisselers?

Three nice cannon balls of different sizes.

Nice one and what's on the end of the rope?

A lead pipe from pump and another big bit of mangled lead.

How's Mr Green getting on?

He has found a lump of cast Iron, not sure what it is but it's been down there an awful long time.

Coooool very cooool

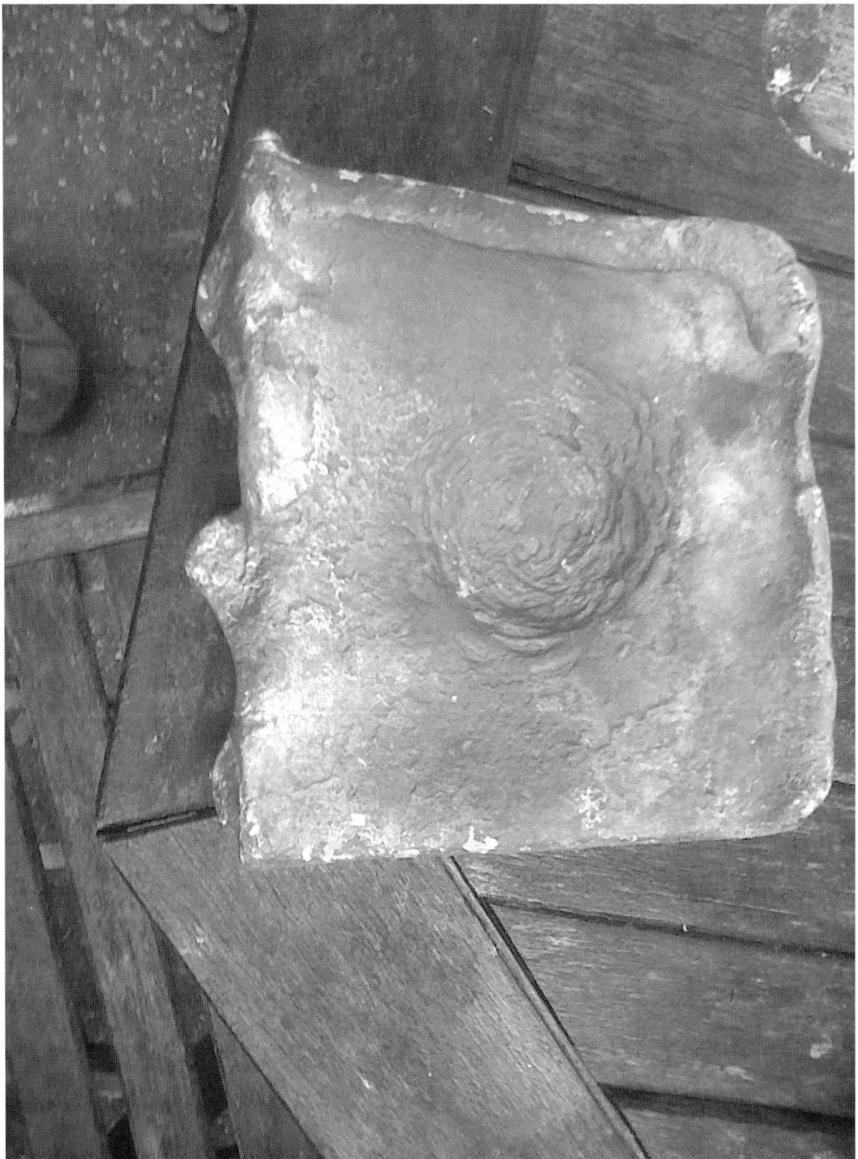

Very rare swivel gun lead apron

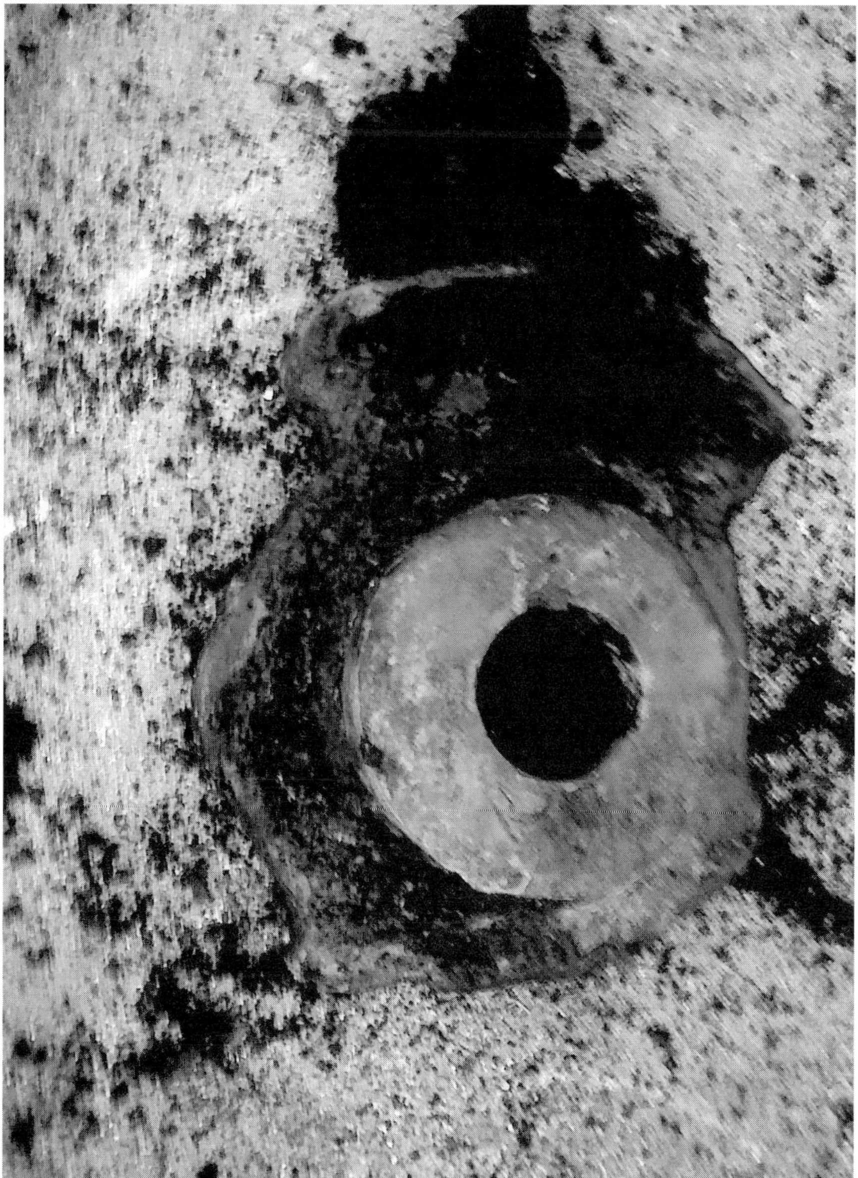

Gun cannage wheele and 300 year old cloth

Chapter Sixteen

Namban Tetsu

You know on the last dive yesterday, the one when we were digging out all those musket shots from under that big rock?

Yeh, the rock with the potato weight stuck to it.

Well you know that we have seen quite a few of those potato weights around the site, and we have always assumed they were the clump weights that would have been the previous divers who have surveyed the site all those years ago. As I have told you before, when I worked at Fort Bovisand teaching commercial diving there was lots of spud weights around and we used them all the time.

So it makes good sense to assume they are old potato weights, I mean they look like potato weights, and they are about the same size as the large weights. But when I was sticking my hand under that rock and grabbing hand fulls of sand and musket shots, my other hand was holding on to the potato weight. As I was gripping the weight tighter and tighter, my fingers managed to find some holes in the top of the weight which were perfect to get a hold of. Just as I was out of air, I mean really out of air, like none on the gauge but still sucking the last few breaths.

As you do, and as I have told you not too.

Well I had a quick look before I ascended all of 2 meters to the surface, and I don't think this one is a potato weight because it has at least three holes in the top that I can feel, even through the crud.

Having seen and used many potato weights, I can tell you this is not one.

So what do you think it is then Captain Black?

Well Mr Green I have, as you would quiet rightly expect of me be doing some research. I spent a few hours on Google and came up with this image. Here take a look.

That's fantastic, not exactly the same but near enough, and its got the holes it the top, or bottom depending which way it sits. Is it a iron ballast block?

Correctomondo Mr Green.

But isn't that bad news for us, because I always thought iron ballast blocks came way later than 1720.

Yeah so did I and that photo is of a ballast block from a ship about 1790 so much later than when the Aakterkerka was built. So I continued my search and found a article that said in 1737 a French ship designer when on a secret spying mission to dockyards of England and Holland to try and find out why there ships sailed better and faster than the French ships did.

In his report he mentions seeing bars of iron being used as ballast, both in Holland and England. He goes on to say that the blocks referred to as "kentledge" held the ship sail stiffer than stone or sand ballast.

So with eye witness proof that the Dutch were using some form of iron ballast around 1737, which is not so far from 1720. Did the article mention what type of iron/metal they used?

No! But I have seen the word "pig iron "used in a few cases, which I guess is just heavy old scrap iron.

A couple of things concern me though Captain, firstly wouldn't there be more of those ballast blocks be on the site, because we already know that a 1000 tonne ship needed about 250 tonnes of ballast.

And secondly, would they not be much larger? I mean if you have to add 250 tonnes of ballast I would have thought you would have used bigger blocks. I think those blocks can only weigh about 20kg

I hear what you're saying Mr Green, but I think all those round pebbles in that cave on the shore line are also ballast stones from the wreck, and she would had both. Some stone and some iron ballast. Iron ballast would have of help her sail better and also have saved and lot of space. Plus she might have been able to trade some of the iron blocks at the other end.

How many blocks have you seen Mr Green

I reckon I have seen about 3 or 4, but don't forget all I ever get to do is look down at the end of my metal detector as I sweep it from left to right, a bloody great whale could swim passed me and I wouldn't see it. How about you, how many have you seen?

I think I can remember seeing about 4 or 5, and I think one was much larger than the one we are talking about, and it was also stuck to a rock with crud. Come to think of it now, we should have known they couldn't of been 30 year old spud weight simply by the amount of crud on them, hind sight what a wonderful thing. So do we both agree that they are or at least could be iron ballast weights, and that they could be from a ship built in about 1717-1721?

Yes I think we both agree on that.

Good! So you put the kettle on while I take a piss and then I will tell you something that will really blow your mind. Here is something to think about while you make the tea. Have you ever heard the world "NABUM TETSU"

No what does it mean, make the tea then I will tell you.........

NABUM TETSU is the treasure, you know how we always thought treasure comes in shiny colours like silver and gold, well we were wrong "Nabum Tetsu "is the treasure.

OK so here I am at my computer, searching and searching the net for iron ballast block, stones, weights every which way you can. Then I type in "VOC iron ballast blocks" and it comes up with "Namban Tetsu Project"

And the aim of this project is to find out where the "Namban Tetsu" which means "foreign steel "in Japanese, came from to make samurai swords.

Apparently some very sort after expensive samurai swords have the inscription "Namban Tetsu" on them. Did you know that samurai swords have inscribed on the part of the blade that goes under the handle?

No! No I have No idea, all I know about samurai swords is that they sharp.

Well the guys who's project it is live in Holland and collect samurai swords, and one of them had in his collection a sword that when polished had the words "Namban Tetsu" on it, along with the swords maker and history and stuff.

So they set out to find out where the foreign steel comes from. And how did foreign steel get into Japan.

Some samurai sword web site I looked at referred to Namban Tetsu as "Foreign steel" or southern barbarian steel.

Is that because the steel or iron found locally in Japan was far superior to the iron from other countries Holland etc?

I guess that's what its suppose to say as we know things, and translations get lost and changed in time. Any way let's move on.

Their project says the only ships allowed to enter Japan for three hundred years was VOC ships, who they had a trade agreement with Japan. So the guys running this project believe the foreign iron ie Namban Tetsu had to come from VOC ships. So they looked at the possibility of the iron coming from cast iron cannons, and also cannon balls. But after further investigation and talking to metalogist they ruled this out. They then turned their attention to ...

Don't tell me "iron ballast blocks"

Got it in one Mr Green "iron ballast blocks" The next thing they did was to contact the Dutch Museums and archives and ask them the question about iron ballast blocks being used on VOC ships.

And what did they say?

They said that they had no record of iron ballast blocks being used on VOC ships and they were not used because the rusted.

Well that doesn't sound good for us.

Wait a minute, before you pull that long sad face. Like good detectives they did not stop there. They search and search the net and archives and this is what they had to say:

http://www.tokensugita.com/NT.htm

This was the start of what can be called now the 'Namban Tetsu Project'.

Of course there are some interesting questions like:

Why the special attention for Namban Tetsu ?

How did Namban Tetsu get into Japan ?

In our search for Namban Tetsu we have to go back in history. To be precise to the year 1600.

On April 19, 1600 the Dutch ship "De Liefde" reached the island of Kyushu with only 24 or 25 survivors from a total of 110 people. They are in a terrible condition. Only 5 men were able to stand on their feet. From these survivors, 6 men died shortly after. An inventory was made the next day by the local authorities. Beside the normal trading goods 18 cannons were found and 500 guns, 5000 bullets of cast iron, gunpowder and so on.

This was the first contact between Japan and the Dutch. The remaining survivors were free to go where they wanted.

Their ship " De Liefde " was confiscated by the Japanese. However, at the first trip sailing under Japanese flag the ship was wrecked in a storm.

One of the survivors was the helmsman William Adams. An Englishman by birth, but sailing in Dutch service. He gained confidence from the Japanese and later in the year 1600 he and the survivors of " De Liefde " were of great help for the Shogun TOKUGAWA IEYASU during the battle of SEKIGAHARA.

Battle of SEKIGAHARA.

This decisive battle on September 15, 1600 (on the ancient Japanese calendar, October 21 on the Gregorian (solar) calendar) cleared the path to the Shogunate for TOKUGAWA IEYASU. Though it would take three more years for TOKUGAWA IEYASU to consolidate his position of power over the Toyotomi clan and the daimyo. (= Local Lords)

SEKIGAHARA is widely considered to be the unofficial beginning of the Tokugawa bakufu, the last shogunate to control Japan.

During this decisive battle several records mention the use of cannons by TOKUGAWA Ieyasu.

*One source indicates that the 18 cannons coming from " De Liefde " were used with the help of the Dutch gunmen. (*1)*

*A 2nd source indicates the usage of cannons coming from " De Liefde ". (*2)*

*A 3rd source mentions: "and one of his generals, Shima Katsutake, (Sakon) was wounded, but his unit was equipped with several cannons, and managed to repel this attack." (*3)*

*A 4th source suggests the usage of the cannons from "De Liefde "during this battle. (*4)*

For TOKUGAWA IEYASU, (家康) this might have been a reason to pay special attention to these cannons, made of 'foreign steel', or Namban Tetsu.

This all took place in Keicho 5, (1600).

In the same year YUKI HIDEYASU, TOKUGAWA IEYASU's second son and founder of the Echizen Matsudaira family went to Echizen to establish a clan in Kitanosho. He patronized a sword smith called SHIMOSAKA ICHISAEMON.

Later around the 11th or 12th year of Keicho (1606 of 1607) this smith was summoned by TOKUGAWA IEYASU and HIDETADA, the first two shoguns of the Tokugawa Regime, and lived in Edo to make swords for them.

Owing to his contribution, he was permitted by TOKUGAWA IEYASU to use YASU, 康 one of the two letters composing the founder shogun's name, and changed his name to YASUTSUGU. 康継 *He was also given then the privilege to include the three-leaf Aoi crest. (= Tokugawa family crest represented by the hollyhock plant)*

And maybe it was on his order that YASUTSUGU, the first generation, had to make swords from this Namban steel. Maybe steel from a one of the weapons coming from "De Liefde" ?

It is for sure however that TOKUGAWA IEYASU was in the possession of the cannons from " De Liefde ". Naval cannons were used during the siege from Shimabara in 1638.

We will never know for sure what steel was used by YASUTSUGU. But Namban Tetsu must have had a special meaning for all that fought at Sekigahara.

This could be one of the reasons for the availability of Namban Tetsu in Japan. Some other sources however indicate that:." Namban-tetsu was a very precious imported iron in ancient Japan".

Therefore we studied the records from the V.O.C. (= Vereenigde Oost-Indische Compagnie) to see if iron or steel was mentioned for trading. But we could not find a positive answer on our question.

When the ships were leaving Europe the cargo was mostly bars of silver, some gold and copper coins. Trading goods were textile like linen and wool to be sold in Japan, China, Persia and to rich traders in India.

So the ships left partly unloaded to Asia. No mentioning of steel and iron.

But when ships are leaving partly unloaded, what was used for Ballast? (Ballast: Nautical, any heavy material carried temporarily or permanently in a vessel to provide desired draft and stability.)

*We raised this question to the "Nederlands Scheepvaartmuseum" in Amsterdam. A negative answer was given. ' No iron was used by the V.O.C. for ballast because of the rust '. (*5)*

But this did not stop us from doing more investigation.

*So we started to look at the various websites about the V.O.C. and on one of them we found the information we were looking for about ballast: ' Ballast is used to put weight to a ship, like cannons and anchors. Furthermore gravel and sand was used'. (*6)*

From the "Batavia Werf" also a positive confirmation was received about the ballast on V.O.C. ships sailing to the East.

*The ballast used for V.O.C. ships sailing on the route from The Netherlands to Batavia consisted mainly of stones and other building materials. Also lead was used and certainly also (old) iron. (*7)*

We found our definite proof of iron used as ballast when we looked through the wreckage report from the 'Geldermalsen'. The description of the cargo reads: 'The

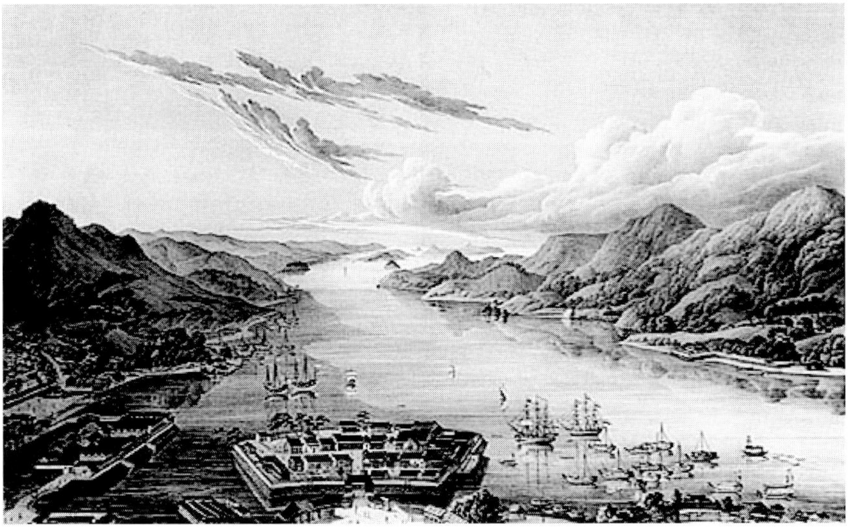

View on Dejima in Nagasaki Bay. Original published in 1832 in Leiden, the Netherlands

*boxes with chinaware came from the bottom of the ship, directly placed on the ballast of gravel, blocks of iron and tropical wood.'(*8).*

*Because the Dutch by means of the V.O.C. were the only foreigners allowed entering Japan, first through Hirado and later through Deshima (出島 literally 'protruding island') (*9) in the bay of Nagasaki the only possibility for steel entering Japan is by these ships.*

*Overall, 606 Dutch ships arrived at Deshima during two centuries of settlement, from 1641 to 1847. (*10)*

Source: www.tokensugita.com/nt.htm

Wow that is good news, those guys sure where determined to find out where "Namban Tetsu" came from.

Not just them but it seems all samurai sword collectors and samurai historians seek the answer to that question. When you have time you will have to read the whole Namban Tetsu project article on their web site its fascinating.

These blocks we have found might answer all their questions then?

It might indeed Mr Green, but I think they have been asking the wrong question, if you where a very skilled, very proud sword maker and you have just made a sword from inferior iron or as everyone seem to think "from southern barbarian steel.

Would you write on the sword "this is made from shit iron"

No of course I wouldn't

So why would you write on the sword something that is not usually found on samurai sword, I mean they wrote there name, there history and where they were taught. But what type of iron it was made from was never on the swords. So why would you put that extra information on it ?

Because it was made from superior iron and you wanted to shout about it and let people know this is a very fine sword.

A bit like a marketing tool?

Exactly like a marketing tool, and because you where very proud of it Captain.

And do you think a sword smith would know, when he was working with it that it was far superior iron?

Absolutely he would.

Yeah me to, but now comes the cherry on the cake, what to you think the quality of iron ore which is the basis of making iron is like in Holland ? To put it another way do you think the iron ore mined in Holland is very good quality ?

Don't know, tell me

Its low quality!

So what about the iron ore mined in Japan, is that any better ?

Yes it is. So there goes your superior iron theory straight out of that kitchen window, never mind Captain it all sounded good.

Before you scoff Mr Green, do you know where the world's best iron ore came from hundreds of years ago and still does today?

No But I have got a feeling you are going to tell me.

Sweden!!

Yes of course it does, I remember now. And that's why the armoured plating on the German tanks was better than our British armour because they used Swedish Iron.

And that's why the VOC got there cannons from Sweden, and that's why our cannon is a "finnbanker" made in Sweden for the VOC.

Yep and that's why the sword smith was so proud of his sword made from Swedish iron ore the best in the world that he wanted to shout about it "Namban Tetsu"

But the Japanese would not of known the iron ballast blocks where from Sweden they would of thought they were DUTCH the same as the ships.

That's why if you look at all the samurai sword web sites they also have a name for Dutch steel "Orlando Tetsu" but there is no world or mention of "Swedish steel" I mean why would there of been.

But how do we prove all this?

Well first we have to take photos of one of those iron block, bring one up and see how much crud is on it so we can confirm its been down there hundreds of years. Then clean it to see what we have got. Then I suggest we go back to the reference library in town and see if we can prove that the blocks are VOC and that they came from Sweden Sounds like a plan I will see you on Friday 9 o'clock ready to go.

My first thoughts are that I didn't expect it to so ornate, I thought, and I have read that iron ballast block where just old scrap iron, referred to as pig iron.

Yeah! me to Chiseller.

And I also thought that, its incredible how much work has gone into making that block just to be used as ballast. I never thought it would have a handle on it, plus to have the weight stamped on it is fantastic.

I hear what you are saying Mr Green, and I can also see your look, a look I have come to know as the doubting Thomas look. Tell us what you are thinking, what's wrong with it?

I just don't see how they would make ballast blocks only weighing 56 pounds, we know the Aaktekerka weighed 1000 tonnes and she would of needed about 200 tonnes of ballast, maybe more if she was sailing with a small cargo. So would they have made ballast blocks only 56 pounds? Could it not be a measuring weight for something else?

What about the holes in the bottom then Mr Green, they are exactly like the ones we have seen on the photos of other ballast blocks. The holes are there to pin the blocks in position.

Well said Chiseller.! I am certain it is a ballast block, and because of the thickness of crustation on it we all agree it's been down there a very very long time. Also we know that the measurement of weight in those days in Holland was hundred weights, 1 hundred weights is 112 pounds. So this is a half a hundred weight iron ballast block weighting, 56 pounds.

I agree with the captain, and you see that small lead plug on top. Well I think that was use to add lead after it was cast to make sure it weighed exactly 56 pounds. Whoever made that block took a lot of care and pride in their work. The handle is brilliant and would have been much appreciated by the dockyard workers or sailor who had carry them down steep ladders or to move them around in the hold with bent over backs. And as for only 56 pounds, well that would kill my back moving that around in a confined space.

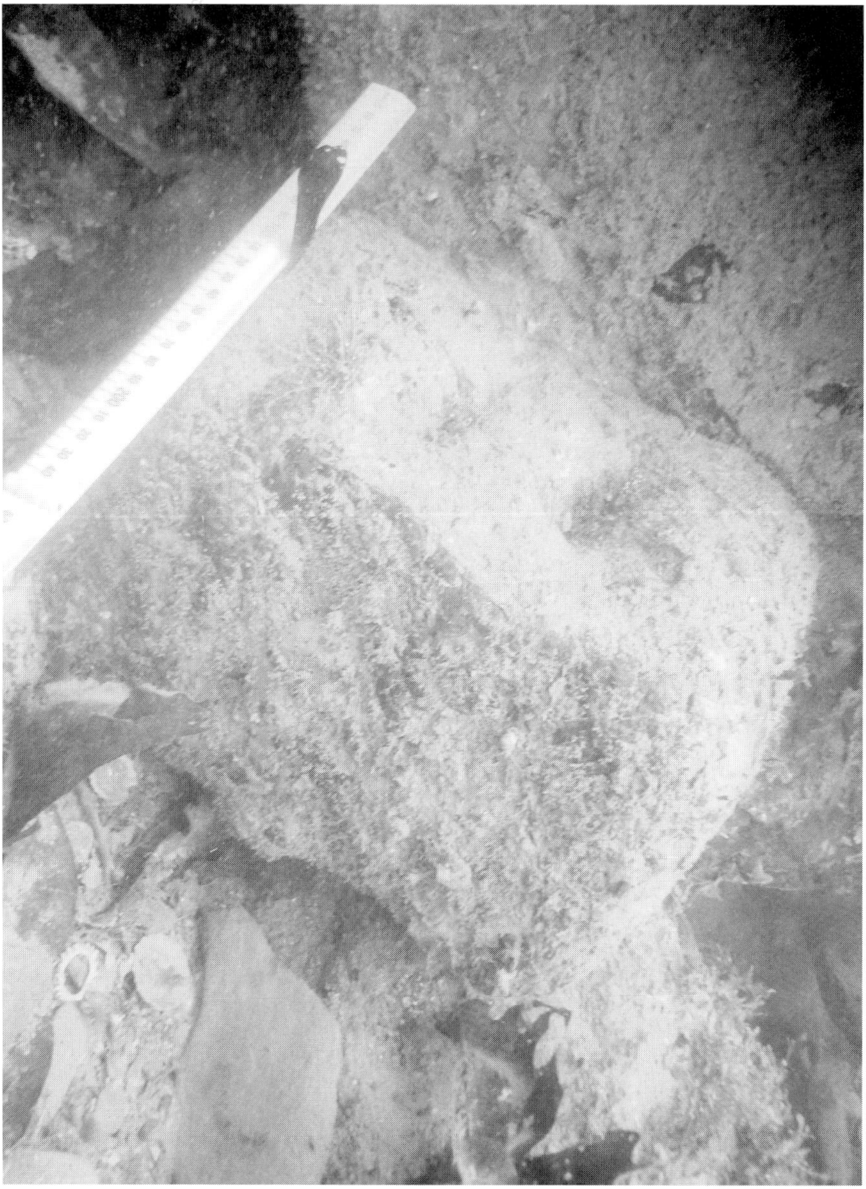

Worlds oldest iron ballast block in location

You have always shirked the heavy lifting Chiseller. Ha ha

I am surprised it does not have a foundry mark on it like cannons do, when its finished, weighed done and dusted. I would have thought it would of had a mark put on it to say "this one is complete"

Maybe it was on top of that lead plug?

Let's take a photo and see what shows up, sometimes you can see things on a photo that you can't see otherwise.

What does anyone make of that?

Could be an F, could be nothing.

And the foundry mark on the cannons?

We know Captain Black, a F

What we need to do if we find another one, is to take the crud off as carefully as possible.

Good point Mr Green, we will have to take off the crud very very carefully next time and see if we can keep and foundry markings intact.

Do you think we will ever be able to see a clear "F" on them like the Finbankers" cannons.

That would be very nice Chiseller, as that would be game, set and match. It would absolutely prove everything we have talked about. Let's get a tank to put it in and add the sodium Bicarbonate. Then we can get some lunch and head in to town to the library.

You don't want to carry on cleaning it Captain?

No I think we should leave it for a while we decided what to do with it, maybe we should hand it over to an expert to clean.

Not Uncle Orange with his big hammer hands I hope.

I was thinking more of someone who has done a degree in "conservation" but has never actually conserved anything.

Just go to McDonalds, your find loads working there along with all the marine biologist graduates.

Good idea McDonalds it is then, and it's your shout Mr Green seems how you had the smart alec remarks

Check this paragraph out guys, it absolutely nails it!

The Arming and Fittings of English Ships 1600-1815 By Brain Lavey

There is your 56 pounds Mr Green, black and white 340 to 56 pounds. 56 pounders being 10 x 4 x 4 inches.

And there is the evidence that they got the blocks from the same place as they made the cannons. The "tower" being the cannon foundry here in the UK"

It's exactly as I said, it was a brand new ship, ordering brand new cannons and at the same time placed a order for iron ballast blocks, from the same place the cannons where made.

Yep in the UK it was from the tower, and for the VOC would of also been there tower, and there tower, their gun makers where the Geers Foundery in Sweden.

PART IX

Internal Fittings

Chapter 34. Hold Stowage

Iron Ballast

One of the major considerations when stowing a ship's hold was to keep the weight, and therefore the centre of gravity, sufficiently low. Obviously the most efficient way of doing this was to place heavy weights as low as possible in the ship. Metal, in the form of lead and iron, provided the most obvious means of doing this. Lead, despite its cost, was the most efficient of these. Boteler and Mainwaring mention lead, but not iron, as a possible form of ballast.[1] In 1627 it was suggested that only ships with 'sharp and narrow floors, which carry much ordnance, and have three decks whereby the ordnance is carried high' needed iron ballast. Other ships could carry coal instead.[2] Iron ballast does not seem to have been used much for at least the next century, and there is little contemporary mention of it. The *Royal Katherine* of 1664, for example carried 145 tons of ballast, but this was evidently stone or shingle.[3] In 1676 the Admiralty decided that the new galley frigates should have 'iron ballast out of the Tower if it can be had'.[4] This seems to indicate the rarity of its use; it was discussed by the Admiralty itself rather than treated as a routine matter, and it had to be obtained from the Tower, rather than from stocks in the dockyards. The galley frigates were designed for fast sailing. As late as 1752, a list was produced showing ships with only one type of ballast, which it can be assumed was to be shingle. But by 1756 another list shows nearly all the ships mentioned carrying large quantities of iron as well as shingle.[5] Lead ballast was also in use at this time, but only for the royal yachts, which were regarded as very fast sailers.[6]

Iron ballast, sometimes known as 'kentledge', came in the form of strips known as pigs. These varied in size, from 3ft × 6in × 6in, to 1ft × 4in × 4in, and in weight, from 320 to 56lbs, but the largest of these sizes was by far the most common in the late eighteenth and early nineteenth centuries.[7] A pig had a hole at each end, to make it easier to lift. To be efficient, the iron had to be laid as low as possible in the ship, but it could not be put right in the centre of the hold, because the keelson and limber boards would lift it too high. Burney suggests that it should be at least 5in away from the limber boards, and kept from sliding inwards by strakes of fir nailed to the internal planking.[8] But some plans show it brought right up to the limber boards, stowed diagonally on top of them, and even on top of the keelson. Others show it outside the line of hatchways and the well of the pump, perhaps to allow room for the movement of stores. In general, frigates seem to have had it closer to the centre than ships of the line, probably because their floors were less flat.[9]

The bottom level of the hold was already divided into sections, known as 'rooms', by the athwartships riders which were part of the structure, and were known, for this purpose, as 'sleepers'. Within each room, several rows of pigs ran out from the centre of the hull. Close to the keelson, the pigs were piled two high; the top ones were known as 'riders'. Where they were three high, they were called 'double riders'. Most pigs ran fore and aft, but some ran athwartships where the shape of the ship dictated it. The greatest quantity was usually placed forward of midships, where the floor of the ship was widest, and the ballast could therefore be kept lower. The rows tended to reduce in length and depth towards the bow and the stern, and the ballast did not extend very far towards the extremities of the ship. On frigates and smaller vessels where the run aft was very fine, little ballast was placed aft of the pump well. A few tons were kept spare for shifting about, to alter the ship's trim.

The quantity of iron ballast was usually decided by the ship's designer. In the 1750s the amount seems to have varied considerably, even among ships of a similar type. For example, in 1756 four 90-gun ships, the *Prince*, *Ramillies*, *St George* and *Prince George*, carried 102, 50, 98 and 50 tons respectively, while the *Cambridge* and *Newark*, both 80s on the 1745 establishment, carried 71 and 150 tons respectively.[10] In the same year, Captain Rodney of the *Dublin* had a dispute with the Navy Board about the amount to be carried, and later removed some iron and shingle, against its instructions, but to the improvement, he claimed, of the sailing qualities of his ship.[11] By 1796, the amount of iron ballast was standardised for each type of ship.[12]

Shingle Ballast

Even when iron ballast was carried, a ship usually carried on average about four times as much shingle, though the proportions

Let me read you that article from the Queen Anns Revenge web site again...

"These guns are commonly called the Danish Descriptor "Finbankers" a general term that described a variety of Swedish guns associated with De Geers foundery at Finspound where they were produced. Quantities where exported to the Netherlands, ostensibly to arm VOC ships. But were also traded throughout Western Europe. It went on to say that." Ruth Brown forely of the Royal Armouries has noted a characteristic of the gun dating from 166o's to 1719. She stated that the gun was probably cast in Sweden most likely from 1660 to 1700".

That all make perfect sense to us three Captain, but there is nothing there to show that Dutch ship builders use Iron as ballast, maybe the English where years ahead of them. I am not trying to piss on your fireworks, and your research is first class and must have taken a long time. But some none believer from Holland might say where it shows Iron was used in Dutch Shipbuilding in the eightieth Century because as we have already read, the VOC say they have no records of their ships using Iron ballast.

That's why you are on the team Mr Green, to dot the I's and cross the T's. And I knew you were going to say that so I have saved the best for last.

Read this

18th Century Shipbuilding by Oliivier Blaise 1737 Translated by David Roberts Published 1992

"Navy warships. The exploitation of this medium during the Georgian era remains a matter of some confusion. T.R. Blanckley's A Naval Expositor of 1750 explained that "Ballast – is in great Ships generally Beach Stones, and in small Iron, laid in the Hold next the Keelson, in order to keep the Ship stiff, so that they may bear more Sail." This preference is similarly conveyed by the chronicles of Blaise Ollivier, Master Shipwright at France's foremost Royal Dockyard at Brest. Ollivier undertook a secret mission to all of England and Holland's major naval dockyards in 1737, when HMS Victory was just being completed in her dry-dock at Portsmouth, to report on methods of shipbuilding by France's maritime rivals. His five-month mission resulted in a

360-page manuscript accompanied by 13 sheets of diagrams and plans. The shipwright (Roberts, 1992: 167, 169) agreed that the English ballasted ships with what he termed 'earth':"

They stow it in a straight line and parallel to the keel from the main forward bulkhead to the main after bulkhead, and also in a straight line athwartships. They do not use iron kentledge to ballast their ships save for long commissions, and in those ships which have insufficient space in the hold to accommodate earth ballast. I confess that when I saw at Deptford Dockyard that great quantity of kentledge of which I spoke… I believed that the English knew how to make good use of it… I have asked the reason of several officers; they replied that iron ballast stiffens all the movements of the ship, especially the rolling. Upon receiving this reply I enquired as to how the ballast is stowed, and was shown it on either rise of the keelson to larboard and to starboard of this timber. We used to find the same inconvenience in our own ships when we stowed the ballast as the English do, but now that we lay it along the rungheads our ships have an easier motion. The English admit that if iron kentledge did not make the movement of their ships so harsh it would be more advantageous to ballast their ships with kentledge than with gravel or earth, since the weight of the iron is farther removed from the centre of motion, and because the weight of the stores stowed atop the ballast is carried lower down."

"Ollivier's argument is inconsistent, however, and contradictory to follow. By his own eye-witness admission (Roberts, 1992: 55), he also reported how he "found next to one of the docks at Deptford a very great quantity of kentledge which they [Royal Navy] use to ballast their ships. The iron pigs are about 36 inches long and 6 inches square, and with these dimensions they must weight 350 pounds. I will say nothing about this sort of ballast: its usefulness is sufficiently well-known; I wish that no other were employed in the King's ships. The pigs which I saw at Deptford are pierced diagonally by several holes along the edges"."

I'm sold Captain

Me to Captain that shows us that the French wanted to know why Dutch and English ships sailed stiffer and better than the French ships did, and he put it puts some of it down to their ships having Iron Ballast.

Cheers Guys that's just what I needed to here.

So what the hell do we do now, how we can answer so many people's questions about all sorts of shit?

No not people questions Chiseller, countries questions, countries history, countries heritage. You think about it, we have got Swedish history, Dutch history and Japanese history, awesome! Here is another little jem that helps us understand why they could re-forge a ballast block as appose to other iron items. I found this on a Samurai sword forum of which there are hundreds.

> "Nanban-tetsu is a steel which was imported into Japan by Portuguese or Spanish merchant ships in the end of Muromachi period(1392-1573). The steel was produced in India and called "Wootz steel". Nanban-tetsu steel was shaped in some forms of a gourd called "Hyotan", a oval called "Koban", a square timber called "Saijo", a semi-cylinder called "Tajo" and others. In 1613, one of the Japanese sword smith, Echizen Yasutsugu 1, first produced a sword using Nanban-tetsu steel. Since then, many sword smiths who lived in Echizen area (Fukui Prefecture) had used Nanban-tetsu steel as a material of Japanese swords. The steels produced using the "Nittoho-Tatara" furnace in Shimane prefecture has been examined by forge-welding as a function of phosphor content in the steels. It is concluded that "Hyotan" shaped Nanban-tetsu steel is not good for forging, "Saijo" shaped Nanban-tetsu steel is good for forging, "Koban"-shaped one is difficult to forgeweld and "Tajo"-shaped one is intermediate."

So I would definitely say out of all those shapes the ballast block is "a square timber shape called Saijo"and as it says "Saijo shaped Nanban Tetsu steel is good for forging"

Maybe we should go out and buy a samurai sword with "Namban Tetsu" on it, so when we tell them that Namban tetsu was the highest quality iron ore on the planet, the swords go up in price and we make a killing.

And have you got £50,000 kicking around to buy a sword Captain Black?

No! I would be lucky to put together 50 pence.

So bang goes your plan.

Bollocks!

So Mr Green, take your time and us some well thought out, unanswered questions please.

Ok I will.

If the ship needed 200 tonnes of ballast, where are all the other blocks?

Are we going to find blocks of different sizes?

Are we going to find a foundry mark on one of the blocks?

Do we clean all the blocks or do we leave some in crustation?

What do we tell the Receiver of wrecks and when?

Good questions, I will take number one. I think she would have had a mixture of stone ballast and iron ballast. I also think with the blocks having a handle on and holes in they would of been quite easy to salvage. Especially with a grapple or a pole with a hook on the end. So I would say most of them where salvaged by contemporary salvagers.

Over to you Chiseller for question two, you look like a kid in school who is going to piss his pants unless you speak up.

I am sure I have seen a larger block somewhere down there. Not sure if it was twice as big as the one we have, but pretty sure it was larger.

Next answer, I think we will be very lucky find one with a readable foundry mark on. And we leave some in crustation, maybe for an expert to clean we will have to wait and see.

The last question is the easiest one of all to answer; we do exactly as Professor Blue advices us to do. We do it by the book and 100% legal. That is the only way that some day we might get just rewards for all are effort and expenses. We fill in the Driot forms and put on them exactly what we know to be fact!! So far this is all ifs and maybe's. We have found nothing with VOC on it and nothing with a date on it so we just report what we have found.

Now it's time to move up a gear and get back in the water, it's the perfect time of year, the weather gods will shine on us I am sure.

Spring is here and we need to dive our asses off and get all those blocks videoed, photographed and in my back garden. Regulators move out!!

Just a quick one captain

Yes what is it?

Well me and Mr Green where wondering what the Ginger witch makes of all this, you know the Namban Tetsu and stuff?

She is dead!

Dead?

Dead!

Bloody hell what happened?

Well apparently along long time ago she did this mean old wizard in France a favour, and in return he gave her as a present the best set of boobs and women could wish for.

Yes sir they where fab I remember checking them out several times.

I don't blame you Chiseller, but I bet you didn't know they where fake and dangerous. Turns out that when this French guy gave made them, he hid inside a small explosive device that he could detonated whenever he choose too. Any way she went to some witches and wizard ball kind of gig thing, and after a few potions he tried to get in her pants. But good old Ginger, she was having none of it. And apparently he was so pissed at her that when she was on her flight back to blighty BANG!

OH my god that's terrible.

That is some way to go, talk about a blow job; I am never going to let my significant other have a boob job, especially if it comes from France.

Well it's done and it's over and I don't want to talk about it anymore, let's go diving the sea is as flat as a witches tit.

Chapter Seventeen

The Freediving Swimthrough

I bumped into one of our old freediving students in Morrison's the other day, remember Catweasel he used to work at the fort he also used to help me with the freedive courses and come spear fishing with us.

Yeh I remember Catweasel, quiet a short fat dumpy guy with a funny little goatee bearded. He always wore the blue two piece wet suit you sold him, the one you convinced him was a perfect fit, but in fact it was always to tight on that little pot belly of his.

Would I do that to Catweasel, never Mr Green not I? Any way me and Catweasel went for a coffee and had a good old chat. And one of things he brought up was a swim through that we found and we would take the students there to let them have a go at swimming through the cave. Catweasel must have a better memory than me because he could recall how beautiful it was, how long it was and more importantly where it was.

That sound good Captain wouldn't mind having a go at that myself when we get the chance.

Well you're going to get the chance sooner than you think, because Catweasel god bless him, and his memory also talked about a old broken ships wheel that we found half buried at the entrance to the swim through. He remembers we dug it out and it was about 5 feet across, a broken cast iron rim with a brass plate in the middle.

Where is this swim through?

It's along the same stretch of cliff we are diving

Can't you remember more exactly?

No I can't and I didn't want to press Steve too hard on the subject. I got his mobile number off him and we can always meet up in the future to pick his brains or even take him back out there. I would like to try and find it ourselves first if we can. But since our cup of coffee I have been doing some research on ships wheels. So when do you think ships wheels where invented?

Oh' I would say about a thousand years ago.

No! They are a relatively new invention, they where only invented about 1710. I read in this book that the first ever recording of a ship having a wheel was on a wreck of a ship that was build in 1710. They did not find the wheel but there was fixings on the wreck to suggest it had a wheel as well as a whip staff. And here it what it said in

If that is true than there is a good chance the Aagtekerka could of had a ships wheel. We know she was being built from about 1718 -1721 so there is a good chance she would have had the new invention.

That's right Mr Green and if we look closely at that photo we have of a VOC ship built in 1725 you can see a ships wheel. And hold on to your pants, if we find the wheel and it has VOC on it or the makers signature and date inscribed on it, that will prove it came off the Aaktekerka and drum roll druuuuum it will be the oldest ships wheel in the world!!

Holly maloney that would be off the clock!!

Yes it would be off big ben!! There are still a lot of ifs and buts, if I can find the swim through, if it's close to our wreck site. If no one else has found it and taken it, and if the storms haven't move it or smashed it to bits.

How long ago did you and Catweasel dive it?

About 11 years ago.

That's a lot of storms and stuff.

I know but I remember it was only by luck we found it, if weren't spear fishing really shallow, we would never have been there on scuba. And if some divers had found it before us I think they would have lifted it, if only to weigh it in as scrap. So we have to keep the faith and go look for it.

So that's today's dive plan?

Yep as soon as the chiseller gets here we will take the rubber boat out from Fort Bovisands and go up and down that area to see if anything comes back to me. Then if the vis is good I will snorkel that whole area while you two can continue work on the wreck site.

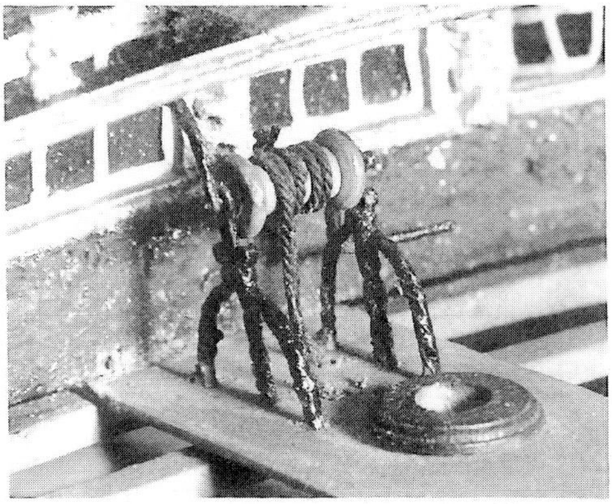

An early eighteenth century model showing the earliest known version of the steering wheel – a windlass set athwartships. NMM.

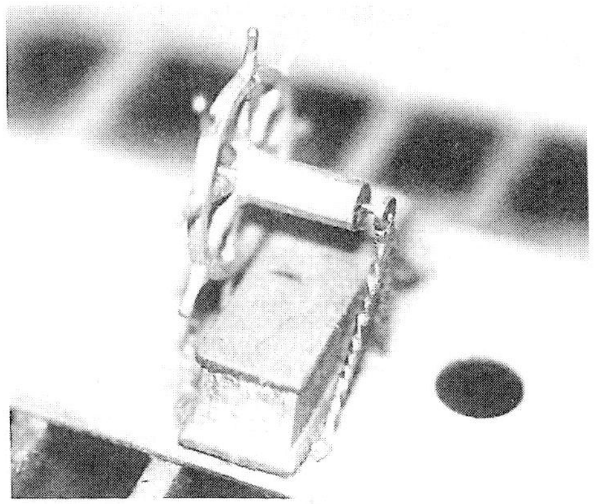

The oldest known model of a fully developed steering wheel, on another model at the National Maritime Museum. Author's photograph, courtesy of NMM.

The Date of the Wheel

It has often been remarked that the wheel came surprisingly late in the development of the ship, and that the inefficient whipstaff was retained for a long time. But, as we have seen, it had only just been discovered, or rediscovered, how to operate the tiller through a wide angle, and the wheel followed this development remarkably quickly. Though the invention of the wheel is rightly credited to the British Navy, no trace of any order to introduce it has ever been found, despite extensive searches in the archives. This suggests that it was developed by sea officers and the artisans in the dockyards, rather than by the central administration.

Much of our evidence about the early wheel comes from two models in the National Maritime Museum at Greenwich.[1] The earliest of these, already mentioned, shows a windlass with its barrel running athwartships. The other (above, right) shows a ship fitted with a fully developed steering wheel, but still with the rowle for the whipstaff fitted below. Both these models are considered to date from about 1703, though the evidence for this is based almost entirely on their decorations. It is conventionally believed that decoration was greatly restricted by an order of 1703, and that ships built after that year were much plainer. Both these models have dimensions which suggest a later date than 1703, but decorations which, according to this theory, can only have come from before that year. Therefore they are dated as 1702' and 'circa 1703'.

All these theories are based on rather flimsy premises. Many orders were issued to restrict carved works in the late years of the seventeenth century, and the early years of the eighteenth. Most were almost completely ignored by the master shipwrights, and there is no reason to believe that the orders of 1703 alone were effective. It is more likely that the orders had a cumulative effect over the years, and it is rather dangerous to single out 1703 for exclusive mention. Moreover, it is believed that the second of these models, the one with the fully developed wheel, was made for or by the Master Shipwright of Plymouth, and was not an official Navy Board model. To decorate his home, he might well have requested a model with carvings which were no longer fitted to real ships. The other model is also very unconventional in style, and does not have the look of a true Navy Board model. Nevertheless, both models do date from the early years of the eighteenth century, as one bears the cypher of Queen Anne, who reigned from 1702 to 1714, and the other has a partly obscured date which reads '170–'.

More precise dates can be found from other sources. It is clear from her contract that the *Russell*, an 80-gun ship begun in 1707, was intended to carry a whipstaff.[2] On the other hand a plan of the *Ossory*, a 90-gun ship launched in 1711 shows a 'steering rowle' in exactly the right position for a steering wheel. Another ship of the same date, the 50-gun *Gloucester*, had a companion for the whipstaff.[3] All this evidence tends to suggest that the wheel was invented a little later than usually believed, nearer to 1710 than to 1703, and that it was applied first to larger ships. This is no surprise, for larger ships suffered worst from the disadvantages of the whipstaff, its bad location and relative weakness. No First and Second Rates were used between 1697 and 1702 because they were rarely employed in peacetime. On the other hand, they saw heavy service in the early years of the War of Spanish Succession, which began in 1702. It was probably during these years that the wheel was developed, on active service. Its use spread fairly rapidly after 1711, and it seems to have been a standard fitting on warships by 1715.

Early Improvements

The early wheel was situated directly above the end of the tiller, and behind the mizzen mast. This of course was inclined to restrict the helmsman's view, and during the 1730s there was a tendency to move the wheel forward of the mast. This presumably involved a slightly more sophisticated system of rigging the tiller ropes.

We anchor the small grey boat right over the top of our work site, it's a stunning day. The sun is out and the sea is flat as it ever gets. Visibility is good and our peregrine falcons who keeps watch on us has two young off springs, today is a good day. The boys are kitting the selves up and I slip off the small grey boat and into the flat sea. It's about 1 hour off low water and its quite a big spring tide today the water is going to go a long way out. Which is good because I haven't been freediving for while and my breath hold is not what it used to be when me and Catweasel used to come out here.

Got my Xcel 7mm suit on, my rubber weight belt and my sharp knife in my hand. I have spat on my mask and adjust my snorkel; fins are on nice and tight and off spit into my mask I go. I was thinking of taking my spear gun but decided against it. When your spear fishing it really heightens all your senses and you are much more focused and aware off things around you and any movement, but I knew there is lots kelp around at the moment and if I am going in very close to the rocks to look for a small cave or swim through I didn't want the gun getting caught in the weed.

My ears are feeling good and I equalise with ease as I head for the bottom of the big green ocean, no big blue in Plymouth that's for sure.

I decided to make my way closer to Fort Bovi as I don't think I would have taken students much further the other way or much deeper.

I can remember the entrance to the cave was on the sea bed its self and not halve way up in the rocks so each dive I get to the bottom first then swim along where the sand or weed buts up against the rocks. There are places where the rocks go in, but they do not open out into a cave. I find some deep cracks in the rocks, but again they do not turn into a cave or swim through. The sea is a greeny colour and the weed is very brown, there is little or no plankton in the water so I am able to look in-between the large storks of kelp and can see for about 4meters which is very good for this time of year.

The good thing about doing this search snorkelling is every time I come up I can take a look around and check my bearings and see if anything comes back to me. Two hours pass and I have searched all the way back close to the harbour and all the way back again. Mr Green and Chisler are both sat in the boat with their kit off and enjoying what looks to be a nice cup of coffee out of my flask, bastards.

They show me their finds and are a little disappointed in my reaction to say the least. But half as disappointed as when I tell them I can't find the swim through. And no matter how many suggestions they have and ideas where it might be, and no matter how many times they say just think back to when you and Catweasel were out here, I can't bloody remember where it is.

Two weeks later there is an even bigger tide, a spring tide 5.8m H.W *and 0.43* L.W *the weather is shit, wet and miserable par for the course, a normal day in British summer time. Mr Green can't make it today so the Chiseller and I decide to paddle the grey dingy out to the wreck site. He is going to walk on the rocks at low water and I am going to paddle the boat close to the rocks and see if I can recognise any rock formations or any reference points to give us a clue to where the swim through might be.*

I get my snorkelling gear on just in case I see anything worth a dip to investigate. We get half way out and the Chiseller says he has forgot his glasses and we have to paddle all the way back because without them he is as blind as bat, not a good start to the day.

I drop him off on the rocks and we start our search, after an hour of going over the same ground I snorkel that time we stop for a short coffee break. Chiseller suggest that we search the other side of our wreck site even though I am pretty sure it's closer to Bovisands and not further away. But what the hell it's worth a look so I drop him off on the rocks and we start the search again. By now the tides is rock bottom and at its lowest point. I shout to the Chiseller that I reckon we have about half hour search time left and when the tide starts to come in on a spring tide its races in.

Some time passes and we have struck out again and by now the tides is starting to make, it's time to look for spot to collect him off the rocks safely. I paddle it to a suitable place and call Chiseller over. As he carefully makes his way over to me stumbling and slipping on the infamous green sea weed he freezes and puts his finger up to his lips to give me the sssssssh sign. All is quiet, we are both still and then I hear it, we stay quiet and then is comes again. It's the sound of air being compressed and then being blown out of an opening. Unmistakeable if you have heard it before, if you live near the coast and spend as many hours in the or near the ocean as we have.

In between myself and the Chiseller is a large rock pool about seven meters long and four metres wide, we can see how deep the rock pool is because the vis and light are not good. We watch the surface of water in the rock pool every carefully, we don't need to talk to each other and ask any questions we both know what we are looking for. We watch and listen, we watch the next wave make its way to the outer rock face and then as if my magic the surface of the water inside this rock pool which is cut off from the sea "rises".

We both know this can only mean one thing; somewhere below the rock face is an entrance to the open ocean, a tunnel a swim through.

Even though the visibility in the sea is very poor and the tide is moving quite fast I have to go in and have a look. Chiseller is trying to persuade me to leave it and come back another day but I am having none of it. The lost swim through has been driving me nuts even giving me sleepless nights, so I am going in shit vis or no shit vis.

First dive was crap; I come up after only about 20 seconds disorientated and confused and my mask full of green yucky snot. Down again and not much better, Christ its dark down there today, next dive was a bit better, and I start to get my lungs. I take my time; hang on to the boat and this time gets a real good lung full of air. Duck and dive and my ears clear like a well oiled machine. Once on bottom I can see what looks to be a lighter colour of something a metre or so in front of me. I swim towards is and there she blows, and entrance to a cave. Now do I risks swimming through it or do I go up? Have I got enough air in my lungs to make it all the way through? How far is all the way though? Bollocks go for it now I decide. I gently kick my fins and keep my arms in the close, my knife is out of its sheaf and in my hand, don't want to get caught on any fishing line while I am under six meters of rock.

The light is always a tiny bit bluer in front of me which helps me follow a line, then it's all dark and eerie I must be like the grand of Duke of York's men neither half way up or down, that sound starts playing in my mind"the grand of Duke of York he ten thousand men he marched to the top of the hill and marched them down gain.......... So dark now and that bloody song is getting louder and louder in my head. Don't say that of all the great songs in the world the last song I'm ever going to think of is the Grand old Duke of York, I try to get it out of my mind and try to hear a great song like "Bat out of hell" Bat, Cave, hell oh my God I'm going nuts.

My lungs start to tighten and I get the swallows which having taught hundreds of freedivers and see plenty of them suffer shallow water black out is not good, it's the time to come up. But which way is up and where is up. Turn back or keep going? Which is the shortest route, no idea bollocks just keep going how long can it be and is the tunnel wide enough for me to turn around in any way. One more verse of the Grand of Duck of York and I can see light coming out of the darkness, three more fin kicks and I am there. I get to the surface and my lungs are burning, I rip out my snorkel and gulp as much air as possible, cold sweet fresh air.

I can only see the top of the Chisellers head sticking up over the top of the rocks, he's still looking down into the dark green sea. Hey fat boy, over hear I shout at him, he looks around and can t see me. Oy fat boy over here, this time he sees my waving hand. What the bloody hell you doing over there you nutter he screams at me. Come and pick me up and I will tell you all about it I shout back.

So now we have finally found the swim through I have been looking for, I think! The visibility was so bad there is no way I could look for a ships wheel or anything, the next thing we do is plan for a scuba dip in the swim through and this time we will make sure we have some cleaner water and hopefully Mr Green and his metal detector. A week passes; the wind and rain have stopped and today is a good day to dive for treasure.

Its only two of us Mr Green and myself, we take the small grey boat out and throw the anchor right at the bigger of the two entrances' to the swim through. Mr Green hops over the side of the boat first and I follow short behind him the boat is left empty and is our giant marker buoy. Not quite want the PADI or BSAC training manuals say, but hey sometimes you have to live on the edge.

The water is nice and clear and we can see the entrance as a lighter shade of green in front of us. It's about one meter high and one metre wide plenty wide enough to get through. As we pass through the entrance it starts to get darker but we are still able to see all around us. The bottom of the cave and swim through is full of small hand size pebbles with no sea weed cover whatso-ever, everything is so still and calm it's like tunnel that time forgot and void of time. As we swim further into the semi darkness there is sign of light above our heads, but also a small circle of light ahead in the distance, I signal to Mr Green to surface where we are and we both fin up slowly. As we break surface we both look around to locate the boat so we can get are bearings, but there is no sign of the boat. We are surrounded three hundred and sixty degrees by rocks. Mr Green takes his mouth piece out as do I "Wow how cool is that we are in a rock pool. It was very cool, a rock pool cut off from the sea and accessible from a swim through tunnel.

We go back to the bottom and progress towards the other circle of light. As we get closer we can see that this entrance is much smaller than the one we swam through to get into the swim through, but it's still big enough for us to squeeze our selves through. As we are just about to fin through the entrance here aloud buzzing noise a noise I have heard many times before, it's the unmistakeable sound of Mr Greens metal detector going off. We swim throw the light and I signal to surface, Mr Green acknowledges and we both slowly head for the surface. We are both blown away at such a beautiful exciting cave and even though it's only about 10 meters deep it's a really good buzz going throw it. Mr Green asks me which entrance was the ships wheel located and

I can't remember is the honest answer. Well I only got a signal at this end he tells me and it was a big signal, big enough to be a ships wheel. So we make a plan to have a good look at where the signal is, king of get some rough marks and start digging.

What we did not account for was as soon as you broke the seal of the pebbles the hole area turned really dark with silt, and as there was absolutely no tide or current passing throw the tunnel the silt did not clear. We took turns digging and passing the pebbles through are legs to the other guy as there was not enough room for two to dig. We made some good progress but by the time are cylinders where empty, the end of our fingers where cut to ribbons, tinny little razor blade cuts. We both knew that as soon as I hands warmed up they were going to hurt like hell. We made plans to come back the next day but this time with work gloves and a plastic drum with holes cut out and a weight in it to make it sink, then we would put the pebbles in and drag them out of the tunnel.

The next day anchored we the small grey rubber boat right on top of the entrance where we had be digging the day before and both went in together. Everything was going well and we were getting quite deep now, the plastic bucket worked well, the visibility was not great but workable and the metal detector told us the target was still there, so we just kept digging. Then without any warning someone turned the lights out, I went black as the ace of spades, I mean black. One of us must have moved a pebble above an iron target that had been buried for ever, the seal must have been broken and the blackness had been released

I would have signalled to Mr Green to surface if I could have seen him, I couldn't even see the inside of my eye lids, I could even taste the oily stench of the darkness. It was impossible to tell which way I was facing and which way was in or out, up or down, it was less black with your eyes closed.

I scrambled around on the seabed feeling what I thought was the walls, I made a decision to make my way in one direction and kept going, after about 7 metre's I knew I must of gone the wrong way we were not digging the far in and it must be less than that to get out. I turned around and kept my hands on the side of the tunnel and felt my way alone the tunnel. Slowly the blackness turned darkness and then semi darkness and I knew I was out. Where was Mr Green? Absolutely no idea.

I headed for the surface and boy was I glad to see the big blue sky, "you took a while" said this smiley voice from over my shoulder. Mr Green was right it had taken me a while and he found that quite amusing. Bastard!

We have a bit of a chat and decided to carry on with the dig only this time one stay just outside and the other dig with their fins pointing towards the entrance. I dig at the coal face with my eyes closed and Mr Green stays out side, I start passing him what I believe to be stones, and then the next stone is far heavier than a stone.

I keep digging again and every 5 mins pop out side to sneak a look at my contents gauge just to check I have some air left in my tank.

Soon I dig out another really heavy lump of stuck together pebbles, I pass it to Mr Green and take another look at my gauge only 40 bar my work here is done, Mr Greene comes to the surface with me and has the big lump in his arms. Together we lift it in to the rubber boat being careful not to puncher the tubes on the boat. 70bar left in Mr Greens tank so he waits a while for the blackness and goes down to give the now big hole a once over with the metal detector and to check if there is any more targets left in the hole. There is still another target in the hole; I can't make up my mind if that is good news or bad news.

We get back to Fort Bovisand and unload the boat, and stow everything away. Then we help each other get off are Xcel wetsuits which are stinking and full of tiny bits of black grit that scrapes our cold soft skin off. Once everything is clean and we have had a cup of coffee we get out the big boys lump hammer.

No the secret here is to find the right pitch to hit the lumps of crud, not too hard not to soft, get it right and they open up like a chocolate orange.

Whack whack, touch harder, whack whack the crud spits open and inside is a medium size cannon ball about a twelve pounder I would guess and it's in tip top condition, so amazing it's like brand new. I know it's just another cannon ball, but it's our cannon ball of this size, we have twenty two pounders, six pounders, four pounders, two pounders but this is our first twelve ponder. And everything we find tell us a story and gives up another piece of the puzzle, we now know that arter facts from the Aaketerker washed up in this swim through, and help us keep the faith that we will find that ships wheel.

The next few days we go back to the same place and this time the Chiseller comes with us. After a short time digging in the big black hole he comes up and tells us it's like diving in ink and it's not for him. Which is perfectly understandable and he decides it's best for him to do a good search of the wider area. During the next few days we find another 3 cannon balls in the massive hole we have now dug, and one copper kind of nut thing with locating lugs which we talk ourselves into believing might of held the wheel in place. The

Chiseller find six bits of broken crockery, which in itself is not amazing. But at a much later date and when we had a wet and windy after noon we get the six pieces out of the booty box and hey presto they all fit together. 300 years getting smashed by storms and tides and we find six bits of broken crockery in different gullies and they all fit together.

And you've guessed it; we now have our own "Ramscliff Jar"

CHAPTER

ASK THE EXPERTS CHAPTER AFTER NAMBAN TETSU

It was driving me nuts, just sitting there in the back of my brain having a little scratch now and then. The little nagging thought of was the block of iron really "Namban Tetsu" and how much was it worth. Even when I was really busy doing stuff with the kids, football or netball it was always in my mind having a tiny scratch at my skull. Who would be interested in buying the block, and how much would they pay. Perhaps the VOC museum or the Swedish science museum. Maybe the Samurai museum in Tokyo or even the British maritime museum. Would a private collector be interested be they already had a Namban Tetsu sword worth thousands of pounds.

I needed to find out for my own sanity and shear curiosity I needed to get an idea of how much it was worth. Money was getting real tight and Unlike Mr Green and the Chiseller I needed to know there was going to be some reward, I was not just in it for the love. I know I promised them both that we would just sit on everything and stay under the radar, but I Couldn't.

Call it weakness call it greed; call it whatever you god damn want but I needed to know if I was sitting on some sleeping money pot. I thought if someone in authority, and expert or something to give it their seal of approval, there stamp on it as "Namab Tetsu" 18 century VOC ballast block. And then if they could value it and come back with a very nice valuation I would get my mojo back, my smile hell maybe even my swagger.

I know myself pretty well, and I knew that once the thought was in my head there was only one way to get it out. So why delay let's get it done.

About a year ago I was watching a programme on TV called "Dragons Den". A panel of five potential investors sat on their thrones while entrepreneurs pitched them with their business ideas. The dragons and some of them could not have been more accurately named questioned them. The dragons individually would decide either to invest or not. Great programme I love it. I'm a big fan.

In one episode I remembered a guy came on from a auction house and presented and idea about getting antiques valued on line. The customer sends them a brief description of their item and some photographs paid a tenner and hey presto, they got a valuation emailed back to them with 48 hours. Each item would be pasted to the relevant expert to comment on a value, and all in strict confidence. Perfect! Just the perfect web site for me to use. A quick search on the good old net and I found the name of the company the guy was pitching. Valuemystuff.

I went on their site and filled in all the forms, name address usual stuff, then it ask for a brief description and age of the item to be valued. This was the tricky bit, do I put down everything I think it is or just some of it. I went back to their page on confidentially and read it again. It all seems to check out and everything was above board, so I decided to write all the information I believed to be true.

18th Century iron ballast block.

Found on a shipwreck.

VOC

Namban Tetsu steel.(used to make Samurai swords)

Cast in Sweden.

6 Inches by 4 inches by 10 inches deep.

And I attached two photos of the block, one under water and one after cleaning.

I guess you pay's your money you takes your chances; I paid my money and hope I haven't done a deal with the devil. I hope it wasn't the devil in me that was giving me all that brain ache and sleepless nights.

Too late now I had hit the send button and it was off to be valued by an expert, and I was quiet excited to see what they came back with.

Now I had another dilemma sent from Satan to deal with, do I tell Mr Green and the Chiseller what I have done or not. One half of me says its only right that I tell them, after all we haven't had any secrets from each other so far, well maybe one big one. But I have already squared that away in my subconscious and it sat pretty well there, so I was happy with that choice.

If I tell them that I had sent the Namban Tetsu block off to be valued, and then the valuation comes back as only several hundred pounds, they will be gutted and probably a bit less motivated. And if they value it as many thousands of pounds or even more they will be very happy with what I have done. I hoped!

So by telling myself that for their own sake it's better to keep in a secret from them, then that will be right thing to do and in fact I am being a good friend. Yep that works

And when the valuation comes back with some really good news, I will tell them then and everything will be cool and we will all be even more motivated. And at least I will know that at some stage I will be able to put some money on the table and not be the total waste of space that I am sure some of my wife's friends must be thinking I am.

All I had to do now was wait a couple of days and I should have their valuation back, I think what happens is they have different experts in different fields.

An expert in let's say fine art, one in furniture another in crockery and I assume they have one in militarily or naval items. So I cross my fingers and my legs and look forward to a good night sleep.

Two days pass and my brain strain has been pretty good, a couple of lovely night's sleep. I am in a good mood with the kids, lots of laughter in the house, fun and games, even sat down and played a board game with the family, and It's been a long time since I did that.

I woke a bit early on the third day after I had submitted my valuation form, bit excited, and tiny bit cautions. Checked my email and nothing yet, checked it every ten minutes that day, all day but nothing. Then just as I was waiting to do his teeth before bed I thought I would have one last check. And by the love of god it had arrived 18.59pm. I'll have a quick squint before I carry him up I thought, then he will get an extra big cuddle.

Description:

A cast iron weight of rectangular section, cast with a hoist bar in the top and the numbers 56.

Measurements:

Height: 6 inches, Width: 5 inches, Depth: 10 inches

Date:

Mid 19th century.

Value:

£20 - £30

Additional Comments:

Your claim that this has connections with the Dutch East India Company but there are no photographs provided of the expected VOC symbol. You also claim it to be early 18th century but the type-face used for the numerals was not in common usage until the early 19th century. Steel was far too valuable an industrial commodity to be used for ballast until the Bessemer Process made it much cheaper to produce in the mid nineteenth century. Stones, earth, sand or gravel were the most usual materials used for ballast as they could be tipped out into the harbour when not needed.

Without details of where and when this weight was raised from a wreck and that it was legally obtained, its relationship with Japanese swords and the use of Namban Tetsu is tenuous to say the least.

Having discussed the matter with colleagues in the Token-kai it is safe to say that there is little or no commercial value from the collector point of view. It is possible that there might be academic interest, from a museum or other similar institute.

Thank you for your custom.

We look forward to valuing some more items for you soon!

Value My Stuff

Valuation Report

View your valuation's online certificate: www.valuemystuff.com/my-account

Description:

A cast iron weight of rectangular section, cast with a hoist bar in the top and the numbers 56.

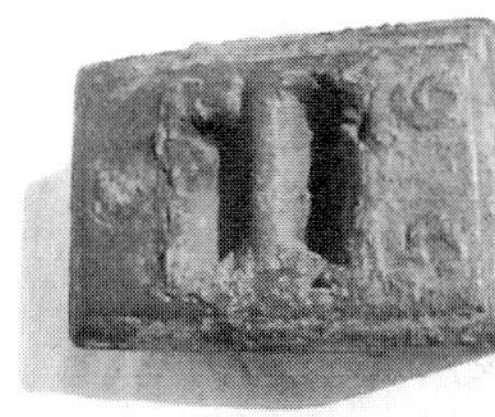

Measurements:

Height: 6 inches, Width: 5 inches, Depth: 10 inches

Date:

Mid 19th century.

Value:

£20 - £30

Additional Comments:

Your claim that this has connections with the Dutch East India Company but there are no photographs provided of the expected VOC symbol. You also claim it to be early 18th century but the type-face used for the numerals was not in common usage until the early 19th century. Steel was far too valuable an industrial commodity to be used for ballast until the Bessemer Process made it much cheaper to produce in the mid nineteenth century. Stones, earth, sand or gravel were the most usual materials used for ballast as they could be tipped out into the harbour when not needed.

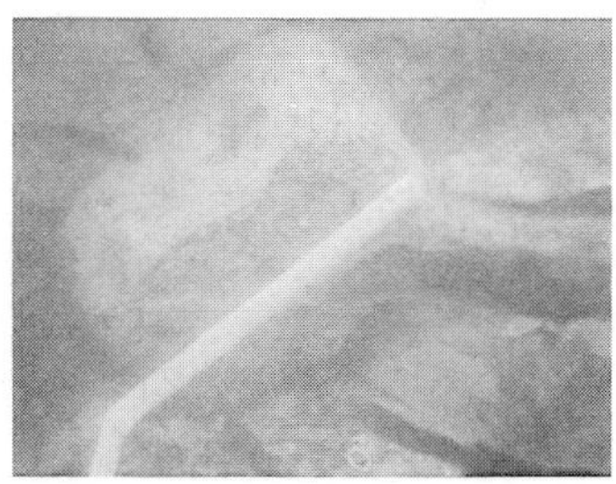

Without details of where and when this weight was raised from a wreck and that it was legally obtained, its relationship with Japanese swords and the use of Namban Tetsu is tenuous to say the least.

Having discussed the matter with colleagues in the Token-kai it is safe to say that there is little or no commercial value from the collector point of view. It is possible that there might be academic interest, from a museum or other similar institute.

Thank you for your custom.

We look forward to valuing some more items for you soon!

Value My Stuff

Notice:

This valuation is addressed solely to the person named above and no other person and consists of two pages of which this is the first page and the estimate of the value stated above is given on the basis of and subject to the Conditions of Business set out on the second page of this valuation.

View your valuation's online certificate: www.valuemystuff.com/my-account

Howard Jones : V34076-1 Page 2 of 3

Chapter Eighteen

The Search Widens

One day in mid winter I promised I would take oldest son surfing on the North coast of Cornwall. He went in and I had a few hours to spare, with three young children that does not happen very often.

After pondering what I going to with my valuable time, when I remembered there used to be a small dive set up nearby. Kind of a scuba school/ charter business. It didn't take me long to find and was easy to spot with all the junk outside, just like a good old fashioned dive shop used to be.

I knew straight away I was going to get on well with whoever was inside, and the proprietor of this outfit. As well as all the old scrap and dive cylinders scattered up against the porter cabin there was this nice 7m rib, on a far trailer attached to a four wheel drive vehicle.

Inside was a mirror of the outside, more scattered dive kit and stuff everywhere. The one thing that caught my eye was a very shiny yellow torpedo shaped object attached to an equally impressive coil of nice shiny wire. The code must of been at least 100m long, I could see it was rigged to go on the rib outside, easy to deploy and recover.

A well built big guy sat behind the desk, he had a well weathered face, with a deep permanent wind tan, with squint lines under his eyes which came from screwing up his eyes when driving the fast rib I had seen outside.

He introduced himself as the Hamster and we shook hands, man grip to man grip, though rugged hand to tough rugged had. The

Hamster kindly made me a cup of tea and we started to swing the lamp, telling stories and swapping ideas.

After several cups tea and several pisses behind the porter cabin we started talking about the elephant in the room. The beautiful bright yellow magnetometer which is used to tow behind a boat and located large iron objects such as cannons and anchors.

At the end of a lengthy discussion two things had happened, one was I now knew the Hamster new his onions when it came to doing mag surveys and all the electronics that involved. The second thing was we had agreed a price for him to bring his rib and mag set equipment up to Plymouth to do a mag survey on a certain area for me. All I had to do now was convince Mr Green and the Chiseller that it was a good idea and a very good price.

After months of waiting and keeping in contact with the Hamster we finally had a weather window and a date that suited all four of us.

The first area we wanted surveyed was about the size of six football pitches, the Hamster told us this would take about four hours. And second area myself, Mr Green and the Chiseller had agreed upon was a much smaller area but a much harder area to navigate as it was very shallow and there was lots of gullies and panicles.

The first area was several miles away from our wreck site and was a completely new target for us, a target we had carefully selected, and was going to be our next project after we had completed this site. The second smaller area was where we believed the Painted mans lost cave was lost.

The Painted man had told me that twenty years ago he had found a cut off cave with cannons and cannon balls in it. He told me it was very difficult to find as lots of kelp guarded the entrance. A rock had fallen down to almost cut the cave off at spring low water. He told me that it was very tight and only one diver at a time could fit in.

This had puzzled me and the three of us for ages and we had spent many long hours looking for it, we couldn't figure out how cannons and cannon balls could have got stuck in such a cave.

We did the full Monty search, spring low water dives and snorkels, high tide good vis dips, metal detecting you name it we searched for it. We hate being defeated and what made it worse, is that someone had found it in the past even if it was by luck, and we couldn't find it. We where pretty sure it was in an area about 150-300 meters from our wreck site. The Hamster was good to his word and turned up at Mount battern slipway with his nice big rib in tow, bang on 9am. The weather wasn't great a force 4 South Westerly, it was doable, just wasn't going to be a very comfortable day in a rubber boat.

All loaded up with ropes, buoys and one set of dive kit we head off out to sea, I watch the change in Mr Green and the Chisellers expression, and here it comes, at the same place every time. It is so reliable you could set your watch by it, two minutes in a boat, wind in the hair water underneath them, they are at sea! Peace and quiet, no mobile phones, no children, no wives no traffic no shopping world's best internet divers! They are at sea, and this is where these two men are very happy, very confident, and very knowledgeable.

We give the Hamster a general direction and he gently eases the throttle down, the engine starts to sound sweet and the boat is on the plane. Just as you would expect from a good Pirate the Hamster asks us for the lat and long of where we are going so he can put it into his chart plotter. Even though he knows he will be on site in less than ten minutes, he still has to try and get the marks from us. This does not annoy us, far from it, it shows us we have chosen a good man for the job we would'nt expect anything less from a fellow treasure hunter. As he would have no doubt expected he got the reply "it's a case of need to know Hamster, and at the moment you don't need to know, follow my arm and I will point you in the right direction, good try any way mate"

Imagine if the boat had broken down, or we hit a long, or had to go to some ones aid. And we had passed on the marks of our new site and which was now in the Hamsters' GPS and we never even got to do are survey. Of course he was going to know the area eventually and he would have all the results on his soft ware. But by the time that had happened we would of been with him all day, built up a Pirates rapour with him, and paid him good hard cash for the job. We would have had an accord, a contract.

The first area we surveyed took about 4 hours, up and down, back and forth towing the fish at about 2 knot, and the time looking closely at the screen to spot any spikes, any changes in the magnetic field of the sea bed below. Cold and wet, sandwiches and crisp gone, flask of coffee empty we decided to head home. The results were not as we were hoping for and we were a little disappointed to say the least. The Hamster tried to raise all spirits bless him, and told us that once he got home in a nice dry office he could analyse all the data we recorded and we would be surprised what showed up."Bloody surprised I replied!"

We stowed the equipment away and hit the throttle to get the hell out of Dodge, the weather was worsening and we were homeward bound. As we got close to our good old wreck site we found a bit of shelter from the wind, we had a lee from the cliffs. A quick decision was made and we were going to run a quick few survey lines with the magnetometer up and down our site. As we knew exactly where a cannon lay on the sea bed we used that as our first target to get a scale of what a single cannon would look like on the screen.

First run showed a small spike, not that impressive. The second run must have towed the fish straight over the top of the cannon and wow we had a fantastic spike like the Eiffel tower. Cool now we're good to go, this was exciting for us a good chance to widen our search just to see if there was anything we had missed after our years of swimming up and down the whole area.

Ten minutes into the search and about 250 meters from our known cannon the Hamster gives out a squeal, and says we have a target on our port side. All three of us stare at the screen to check it out. Yes it is a signal, but not as large as the previous cannon signal. We go ahead and then do a one eighty turn bringing us back to where we got the signal, this time is on the starboard side, same place as last time. Good news!

The Hamster tells us that he believes its a good target, possibly cannons and the reason the signal is so small is that the fish is still about 20 meters away from them. We were on spring low tides and this was as close as we could get the boat and the fish to the target area. The Hamster pointed his finger with great confidence and said "the target is there boys, about 20m off the starboard side in about -3m of water, in fact it looks like it's right smack bang in the middle of the huge flat rock which is a bit strange"

The Chiseller looks at I, and I looks at the Chiseller we are both grinning from cheek to cheek, are these the cannons in the painted mans cave, we believe it is? Which if it is would be bloody annoying as I am sure the Chiseller did a complete 360 degrees search around the rocky area.

The first good weather we get with the wind in the right direction and some half descent visibility, I and the Chiseller go out in my tiny rubber boat to check out our new cave target. We drop our anchor right next to the big rock and I dip in first. The water is nice and clear and I can see the bottom about 4meters before I hit it. I get myself sorted out and take out one of my two very sharp knives, I always like to dive with a knife in my hand if I am going up gullies where there is think kelp and a good chance of fishing line and crap washed in.

I slowly skirt the outside of the big rock about one metre off the sea bed looking for any possible clues or entrances to a cave or gullies. In the back of my mind on constant replay are words of the painted man. "Entrance hide by kelp, fallen rock blocking entrance, almost cut off on big spring tides, cannons and cannon balls" rewind replay, rewind replay!!

All I can see is the side of the rock meeting the sea bed, yeh there are some big chunks out of the rock and some caves but nothing I would call a gullies or a cave. Lots of kelp growing from the big rock and some small rocks near buy which makes it very difficult to make out any entrances.

I fin around a corner and spot a tiny piece of broken crockery laying on the sand, as I go to pick it up I see another small piece. Then I spot a bottom of a old glass bottle and the top of a old glass bottle, the bottle top is the widest I have ever seen, and believe me I have seen a few. Knowing what I know I instinctively follow the line of finds towards the big rock. With my knife I cut away all the kelp storks really low and brush them aside and as if my magic "open sesame" there is the entrance to what looks look like a long deep gullie.

I slowly make my way up the gully cutting some kelp away as I go, the painted mans words still on replay in my mind.

I travelled about six metres up the gullie and my ears are starting to pop and I can feel myself getting more buoyant. As I dive in a wet suit with a back pack and no bcd I have no air to dump to make me heavier. I definitely want to start floating up in case I get stuck up near the room of what was fast becoming a swim through so I revert to the old Indian trick and grab a big stone and put it inside my X-zip short john..Perfect nice and heavy. Eyes wide open I come to the fallen rock and I can see exactly what the painted man was describing, the cannons must have of got washed up inside the gully before this rock had fallen in.

The rock had got jammed about a half a metre above the sea bed at its highest point which was plenty of room to swim underneath. As I swam carefully underneath the fallen rock I turned over just to look up at where it was touching "as you do" just to check it wasn't going to fall. Mad thing to do I know it weighs tonnes and has been there for over twenty years, why should it fall when I am swimming underneath? It's just one of those things you need to do to put your mind at rest.

Once thought the other side I was now in what was more like a cave than a gully, there was some modern debris washed up inside the cave, a big old truck tyre, a fishing net and loads of fishing line uuumm not the place to get caught up in with no buddy. The bottom of the cave was stacked high with fist size pebbles not unlike the other swim through. But I could tell these where very mobile and move around with each big storm. Were there cannons underneath the pebbles? It was impossible to tell and if I started digging the visibility would go to zero, and with all this fishing line around it was a death trap waiting to happen.

I made my way out of the gully picking up some more shards of pottery as I swam, and surfaced to have a chat with the Chiseller.

I told him what I had found and said that I took back what I called him, being a donkey and as blind as a bat for not finding the cave when he looked. It was dammed hard to find. I explained to him the lay out and what we had found or not found. I told him that if he put the boat right over the top of the rock he would be able to see a very small entrance from through the top of the cave.

I told him that I wasn't sure where it was big enough to swim through, but at spring low water the top of the cave may be on the surface which would handy when it came to excavating the cannons.

We then had a conversation that went a little like this.

Right your move, put the boat right over the top of the rock and I will have another quick dip and see you in a minuet

"Ok! But don't you dare swim up through that gap back to the boat. Look at me Captain Black don't you bloody dare, you said it was small and you will really piss me off if you do. If you get stuck how will I know you're stuck? If you do Captain if you bloody do I swear"

As I looked up I could see the silhouette of the rubber boat and I could just about make out the Chisellers round bald head looking over the side of the boat. I had taken out the rock already and grabbed a spare lead weight from the boat so my buoyancy was good, and I had ditched the rock so I was a little more stream line. Kind of put my hands out to gauge the space and guestamated that I could fit through the gap fine, well at a squeeze any way. I checked my fin straps were clear of the fishing net and fishing lines, Check my knife sheaves where stowed away nicely. Din't have a spare second stage or any spare hoses flapping around as I only dived with one second stage and a contents gauge No big old clumsy BCD with all its buckles and toggles and crap hanging off it, just a simple back pack. My Shunto dive computer was tucked in nice up my glove, what could possible go wrong?

I looked up and gave a gentle fin kick and I was on my way, kept my neck extended and headed for the promised land all was peacefull and surreal until! clunk clunk clunk my cylinder was banging on the side of the small entrance oh shit its tighter than I thought, I wonder if the Chiseller had heard that, please God let me get through (its true what they say, there aint no atheist in a foxhole) even more, please don't let the Chiseller of heare this clunking.

I made it though and saw the Chisellers face, and then wished I hadn't.

A few weeks past and at last Mr Green, and more importantly his Aqupulse metal detector were able to dive. It was a beautiful day with great visibility and it was the first time in many months I could sit on the rubber boat and feel the warmth of the sun through my wet suit.

Mr Green kitted up and went over the side first, the plan was for him to do a more complete swim around and through the gully. I had drawn him a map of the gully so he should be fine. Well not really a map, more of a kids sketch with my finger on the dusty salt encrusted bonnet of my car. It was a bit like how my youngest kid counts, one, two miss a few ninety nine a hundred. A few lines here, a rock and cave there and there is the big lorry tyre.

He's a grown man he can work it out, don't want to make it too easy for him. After Mr Green had been in for about ten minutes which was enough time to get his bearings, I kitted up and joined him. Once again the rubber boat was going to be our big grey surface marker buoy, not exactly PADI drills but then we are not exactly PADI divers.

Mr Green started to point out targets to me and I started to dig, the problem once again was after a few minutes digging when you are up a gully the words turns black. The old saying "when you're in a hole stop digging came to mind a lot. Also the words "shit creek without a paddle" had been in my mind a lot lately. But only when I was diving, it was in my mind every time I thought about the money or when the wife asked me if we had paid the gas bill or electricity bill. In fact if I am honest it was even starting to enter my mind when I was supposed to be having fun with the kids. And that was the bit I hated about being a treasure hunter without any treasure most of all.

I signalled to Mr Green to surface for a chat and slowly we made our way up and had a pow wow. We decided we would concentrate on several target areas at the same time, some in the gully and some outside. By digging lots of targets it would give the ones that were too siltya chance to clear while we dug another target. It was slow hard work with very little results, the sand and pebbles were deep and there was very little tide or movement to take the sand we were hand fanning away and it just kept filling back in the holes. My cylinder was empty first and I got back in the boat, not the best dive ever and not very productive, couple of fishing weights and a very small copper nail about 20mm long. I just got myself sorted out, all comfortable with a cup of coffee in my hand when God damn it Mr green pops up, grabs the side of the boat and spills half my nice Luke warm cuppa. Once Mr Green was in and sorted we had a de-brief, OK a chat about the dive. He told me that under a very big rock near the end of the gully there was a massive signal from the detector, and also right up the cave end there was lots of big signals."Big enough signals to be cannons I questioned him" definitely! Was his reply.

After we were back on dry land and all the gear and boat was stowed away, we found a nice sheltered spot on the quay side at Fort Bovisands. The sun was high sky and we could actually eat our sandwiches with our T shirts off.

We must of looked like a couple of gay lovers, tucked away in a corner, shirts off eating out packed lunches. No prizes for guessing who had the best patch lunch, mine was second best by a mile. Mr Green had bought sandwiches, posh crisp, chockie bars and fresh fruit. I am surprised he didn't carry it in a hamper with serviettes and a glass of wine.

I am not going to tell you what was in mine, but the previous day, it was left over from my gorgeous daughters school packed lunch.

We heard footsteps approaching, and as we turned around there was good old Perky standing there. He had just finished taking some divers out on his nice big dive charter boat and was coming over to shoot the shit and see what we up to.

He asked us if we had found anything interesting and we got chatting about the area he had logged us diving in. Perky said that whilst waiting for the tide to get deep enough for him to bring his boat along side in Bovi harbour he did a bottom search with his fish finder where he has been noticing we have been diving lot. He said he had notice a anomaly on the sea bed and did I want to jump on his boat and go and look at it on the fish finder screen. I thought this was a very kind offer and jumped at the chance. Mr Green needed to get back home we kissed goodbye and off he went.

Perky being the good skipper that he is had marked the target on his GPS so we were able to steam straight to the exact spot. Up one side, down the other side, north to south, east to west we looked at it for all different angles.

Perky seem a little disappointed when I told him I thought it was nothing, possibly a small reef of some odd shaped rocks. We started to slowly head back to Bovi. I could see my Perkys face he was trying to work out weather I was telling the truth or throwing him a curve ball. No matter really because if Perky was half the pirate I know him to be he will go and the dive the target early one morning when no one is around.

Just as we where passing one of the many rocky sticky out points, Perky said, "do you remember about eighteen months ago, I mentioned to you that I once saw four cannons, and what I thought were ballast stones off one of these points."

Yep! You had some students on a compass dive with you."

"Well we are right over the spot now, where I think the cannons where, I have dived several time back here and I have never been able to find them again, they must get buried"

The location we had just steamed over and where he said the cannons lay, possibly buried, was about two hundred meters South of the painted mans cave.

We had been right over the exact spot with the Hamster whilst towing the magnetometer. I distinctly remember him saying wow wee! look at the big spike. Only then to say that on his chart plotter it showed there was under water cables crossing that spot. Probably laid during the Second World War, there are quite a few old cables laying on the sea bed around Plymouth. So we quickly disregarded this huge signal and put it down to cables.

But could it have been four cannons? They would certainly of given off a big signal, especially if they were close together or touching each other.

Driving home alone in my car, I slipped into a lonley poor place to be, I had been here before and it was nearly always when I was alone in my car on the way back from a dive. A dive that once again produced nothing I could call treasure. So we might have found the cannons in the Painted mans cave, big deal, and we might have possibly maybe found Perkys four cannons and some ballast stones whoopee my bank manager will be happy.

I remember an old treasure hunter saying to me one day, "if you can't eat it! It aint treasure" I know what he means now.

Some old iron cannons big deal, who cares, anyone going to buy them off me, I don't think so, anyone going to pay me to lift them or conserve them, I don't think so. Treasure definitely not! Pay the bills, put some food on the table oh no I don't think so!

I love the history behind things, I love trying to find out exactly how and where the ship sank. Trying to find each part of the ship is fantastic, putting all the bit of the puzzle together is so totally amazing. If I was on a salary working for some government body and an archaeologist working on pay for a University, the University of "go slow we are on pay" then I too would be happy to find some cannons. Mark them out, take some photos and video, dive with my paint brush and my time team trowel in my hand. Come up and spent a few hours drawing a little map, lovely jubbly, bank a few more hours on the old time sheet. Then let's go to the pub in our knitted jumpers and conduct a tougher de-brief, there's a few more hours logged. Few that was a hard day at this rate we will be here all summer:-)

Oh my God I am nearly home, for Gods sake Captain you need to pull over and have a word with yourself, nobody likes a miserable sad ass feeling sorry for themselves. So get a grip, hold the line, and be ready to greet the kids with a big smile .

Chapter Nineteen

The Shipwreck Conference

Here is…, look Mr Green the long lost Chiseller back from his winter Holidays.

Hi guys, I hope you been in the water lots and not slacking while I have been away in sunnier climes.

He's a cheeky dog isn't he Mr Green, goes off swanning around Australia and expects us to do all the ice diving here. I hope you have brought us both a nice present Chiseller.

No sorry guys I have brought you back sweet fa. Although you are welcome to look at my white bits if you want.

Arrr that is a god damn awful thought I think I'm going to throw up.

Well do it over there Mr Green, the long haired sergeant major will go nuts if you get any off your puke on her nice new table cloth.

Well come on lads get the booty box, lets see what you have found since I've been away on my hols.

Here you Chisler feast your eyes on that little lot while I make us all a nice cup of English tea, not that Ozzy shit you been drinking.

Wow you guys have been busy.

Yeh busy and bloody cold.

So what have we got here then guys talk me through it.

All different size off musket shots

A very cool fire and impacted musket shot

Small cannon balls

Large cannon balls

Another lead pipe flange

Some lead hinges

Our first shoe buckle

Some very nice tear drops with some kind of mark on them.

Two lead gold coin weights, which took a lot of time to research to find out exactly what they are.

Some very nice copper nails/pins

And a beautiful 4 pound lead weight, which if you look closely is made in three different sections.

I'm surprised you didn't find any crockery guys!

What! What did he say Captain Black?

Well I thought I heard him say, "Well done lads, great job, you guys are the best treasure hunters in the world"

Yeh that's what I thought he said.

Ok ok don't throw your toys out of pram, yes yes, the boys done good, what I meant to say is as you have done such a good job and found so much I am surprised there is no crockery in amongst your fantastic booty. Now before you get on my case let me make the next cuppa and then you can tell me all about the "Shipwreck Conference"

There you are guys and once again let me say well done.

Sit down fat boy and don't take the piss.

I'm not Captain I'm just saying well done.

Ha bloody ha.

Come on then Mr Green tell me all about the shipwreck conference and did your worst fears come true?

What fears Mr Green?

Oh didn't he tell you he was scared you wouldn't be able to hold all your excitement in and blag some secrets, you know how you get Captain Black it's always hard for you to keep tight lipped especially if you have a wee tickle of the black stuff.

He was actually very good this year, so good he looked in pain; I knew it was going to be painful for him as soon as I saw who one of the guest speakers was. And even more so when I read the title of his talk

An end to exploration and adventure? What more will we see of VOC shipwrecks? By Rex Cowan.

Ah my God that is so cool, I would love to have been there, not for the talk but just to see how much pain the Captain was in just having to keep his lips tightly closed.

Yeh! Just that alone was worth the £20 entry fee.

So come on then Captain what did Rex have to say?

Well you're not going to believe it but he was being introduced to the audience by none other than that good old boy Mr Richard Larn MBE. And Mr Larn was giving him the big lead in and said that Rex was a shipwreck hunter pioneer and had spent most of his life researching and looking for shipwrecks especially VOC shipwrecks. He said that he has been a good friend of Rex Cowan for longer than he could remember and had worked on my projects with him. He then named a few and then he said.

Correct me if I am wrong Mr Green.

"We both spent time together looking for the wreck of the "VOC ship Aakterkerka"

Mr Green if you please

Yep that is exactly what he said, the captain is correct word for word.

That must have been so cool to hear him say that.

Yes it was, not sure exactly why! As we have already read it in his own account of her sinking, but it was a sweet moment to hear him say it that was for sure. And too everyone else in the audience it was nothing but a tiny passing remark. A nothing ssswwiiiissshhhhhh there it goes right over their heads. Even Uncle Orange bless him ssswwiiiissshhhhhh over his head.

What about Dr Evil Pork Chop?

Don't know where he was seated so couldn't gauge his reaction.

English Heritage?

Ssswwiiiissshhhhhh

Receiver of Wrecks?

Ssswwiiiissshhhhhh

Short Red?

Ssswwiiiissshhhhh

I would love to have been there.

What instead of sunning yourself on some Ozzy beach checking out all those peaches?

Well now you mention it, it would have been a tough choice.

Tell the chiseler what Rex talked about.

Yes tell me Captain.

Ok! His talk was basically put forward the divers and adventures perspective on shipwreck hunting and how in today's time it would not be possible to do what he and his fellow treasure hunters did.

He has read the new MMO laws and the uniscon agreement that although we, the UK did not sign up to is being introduced through the back door.

He spoke some latin which I quite liked and then translated it "things are not what they were"

He spoke with passion and sorrow and spoke with fond memories in his eyes. He spoke of the days of adventure and adventures; he spoke of pioneers and times of bravery. When men were made of wood and men of steel. And now ships are made of steel and men of wood.

Rex is the man who put together teams and projects to go and search for ships that had been lost at sea and never ever found. He went where other men fear to tread. James Egan lane not a chance, an artificial reef, a ship that has been put there for people to find and dive on, wash your mouth out.

He talked of how his team found the shipwreck of the VOC Holandies of the Isles of Scilly, the wreck of the VOC Verhart off Holland and how he recovered the silver bars off the VOC Goodwin sand

Only four years diving and research is all it took them to find the Holinda. He talked of how they conserved all the items much of which is on show in the VOC museum in Holland.

He said that never has an archaeologist ever found a shipwreck, and whilst they have an important place on a team they only ever turn up when a wreck is found. He went through his slides which had a technical glitch, on his slides where bullet points of all the rules and regulations which believe now prohibit and deter any future adventures and treasure hunters. He showed slides of all the artefacts his team had found and the lessons and information that were gained from those finds. Without the prospect of financial reward, he did not believe any one was going to dive for four years looking for something they couldn't even touch if they found it. So he was kind of sticking it to the man, in this case the English Heritage man and if there had been one present the MMO man. I think even the English heritage man would of struggled to answer his last question.

"You find something on the sea bed, and whatever condition it's in its only going to get worse, there is very little knowledge to be gained from leaving it there. He asked for someone to tell him what possible good it can do to leave it there "

That was kind of the gist of it.

So if he was not so well educated and well mannered, he would have just said now days we are a bunch of pussies.

God your quick today Chiseller, must of been all that sun gone and grown your small brain. I told you to wear a hat.

Very funny ha ha. Was there chance for questions?

Yep

Well did you ask any?

Nope

I must say he was very good, I would have bet money he was going to stick his big fat hand in the air.

But you where stood on them? Right Mr Green

Something like that.

How was the rest of the day?

Saw Commander silver and his gorgeous wife Jill and she gave me a big hug which was nice. Allan was very busy catching up with old friends like Peter McBride and Rex so didn't get chance to talk to him

That was handy.

Would of liked to have had a chat with him, but like you say best stay under the radar. Professor Blue introduced to the Receiver of wrecks and the assistant receiver of wrecks. We had a nice long chat and I asked her about our Driots which are now 18months old. I asked her when we would hear about ownership of the cannon and other items on the Droits. She kind of just told us what we already knew; no one had come forward to claim the items within one year so all items now belong to the UK crown estate. She said she has been emailing museums and the like to see if anybody wants the cannon and would be able to undertake the five year conservation needed and as yet no one wanted it.

So how long before we get ownership?

She didn't say, she never gives me a date it's all very vague. She asked a few more questions about possible identity, and location. Her college asked if the site could be shore dived and I told her about that naked swimmer that came down the cliff last time me and you where diving there.

So we just sit tight and wait for her letter, is that the plan? Surely at some stage there must be and end game some type of closure.

I can assure you Mr Green nobody needs closure, the end game and hope fully pay dirt more than me. I have been giving it lots of thought and I have come up with a plan and a time table. The plan is to keep diving, keep filling in the Droits and if we find anything that has VOC on it a coin or something then that will be the end game and both us and the receiver of wrecks will have proof of the identity of the wreck site.

And if we don't find anything else or any "proof"

Then at the end of this summer 2012 we come out of the closet and say we believe we might have found the wreck of the VOC Aaktekerka sunk 1721.

How are we going to out? God I feel a little bit gay saying that.

We have always suspected you might be Mr Green and love you for it.

Piss off captain.

You have seen the great video on YouTube of Uncle Orange, well I have contacted the lady who made it and approached her to make an outing video for us.

So we are going to out on YouTube.

Yep and my kids will be proud and think there dad is hip and down with the times.

I think your mad, but let's just say it goes the way you say it will, what will happen next?

Not sure!

What do you mean you're not sure? You just can't say you're not sure for Gods sake.

Well I'm not, I can only guess.

Go on then guess.

I think the Receiver of wrecks or English Heritage will ask us why we believe it to be VOC, and then if they think we might be correct they will contact the Dutch Government and they will send over a archaeologist to say yes it is or no its not.

And what they say goes I suppose?

A big fat yes stamp or a big fat no stamp.

You're forgetting two things Captain.

What that Chiseller, speak up I thought you have been a bit quiet, what's that matter.

I have two things to say, because YouTube is global, it's as likely that someone in the Holland might see it before someone in the UK. Should we not give the Receiver the heads ups?

You are such a nice guy Chisler, but the answer is, I'm not sure. You said two points, what's the other one?

Well aren't we going to look like a right bunch of wankers if we are wrong, and it's not the Aktekerka?

You have certainly changed your tune, you have always agreed with all the research and our theories all along, sounds like you are getting cold feet?

I am just saying that maybe we should put our case forward in a bit less public way, maybe have a chat with the receiver of wrecks and English Heritage. Then if we are wrong we haven't been shot down on the World Wide Web.

What say you Mr Green, do you think he is right or should we just go for it?

I'm with you Captain; we have put in years of hard cold work and long hours of research into it. We've done things we have not been comfortable with, and risked things we should not have risked.

You have spent money you should not have spent and borrowed money you should not have borrowed. How you are still married and can pay the bills is be on beyond me, your wife deserves a medal. You need some pay back ten times more than me and Chiseller ever do. If it's not VOC if it's not the Aakterkerka then I don't think there will be any pay dirt. So for that reason I back your plan one hundred percent. I have been with you from the start and looked at all the evidence with you and unless we have put two and two together and got five, or we have been blinded by the finding sunken treasure I'm still in. Because if it's not what we think it is, then the ballast block is not VOC and there for its not "NAMBAN TETSU" and if it's not Namban Tetsu than there is no Samurai sword, and all the plans we had for that block have been just dreams.

So I say go for it in for a penny in for a pound. On a good note I have started electrolyses on the cannon and on the cannon balls etc.

Chapter Twenty

The Pen is Mightier Than The Sword

OK about 15 years ago I sold a shipwreck book to a mate of mine, and before I went away I phoned him up to ask if he still had it. He said he did and I could have it back if I wanted it. I think he forgot I sold it to him so I am now £10 up on the deal.

Well that £10 is the only money we have made from this wreck so far, so get your hands in your pocket and stick a tenner in the kitty you tight bastard. You know how skint I am, maybe I should stop treasure hunting and buy and sell old books like Frederick does. So what's so good about this book?

Now have either of you heard of the "Richard Larn UK Shipwreck Index?

Are you kidding? Mr Green has been after a copy for years, he has tried to get one everywhere, especially a Volume one.

Have you Mr Green

Sure have! The captain should have told you, it was a Richard Larns Article on the sinking of the "Aktekerka" that started our whole search. I have been looking for one to buy on the net but they never come up, and when they do they are silly money. Isn't there five in the set, one for different areas? The Volume one is for the south west of England. I have had a watch on that book on eBay for years now and they never come up, and every time I pass a second hand book shop I pop in to see if by some magic there is a copy there. Everyone I have spoken to swears by it, they basically say if it isn't in that book than it didn't sink. It's the definitive shipwreck list.

That's right five volumes and the volume that covers the South West of England is volume one! Which my learned friends have the volume I have in my van.

You sold your mate a shipwreck index for £10, you must have had a bad day, you're nuts. I will give you £200 for it here and now?

But you don't have £200 Captain, you would be lucky to raise 20 pence, any way it's not for sale.

I will give you £350

Like I said Mr Green it's not for sale.

I can't believe you have never mentioned this to us before Chiseller.

Just didn't think of it Captain, I had forgot all about it until I bumped into the guy the other day. Sorry.

Mr Green and I have been to several reference libraries trying to get access to a copy, we even asked them to get a loan copy for us to read but they couldn't even get hold of one from anywhere. We wanted to look through it so we could find some more possible targets

I will go to my van and fetch it in, the one thing that will surprise you is how many wrecks our listed in it, I mean like thousands. It must have taken him and his wife years of hard to work to complete. Richard and his wife did it together and I believe they had access to a huge amount of documents.

Isn't that what he got his MBE for, writing those shipwreck indexes?

I think your part right Mr Green; I think he got the MBE for service to maritime studies, archaeology and writing the books, kind of a life time achievement type of thing.

Go on then Chiseler go and get it chop chop.

Shall we go and get some lunch somewhere first; we can use that £10 I made from the book. How about it a nice all day breakfast down at Morrison's my treat.

Good idea, but later, after we have read the book, go and get it for Christ sake we have been wanting to see it for years. It's like you don't want me and Mr Green to see your precious new book. Go and get it, I am desperate to see it, stop trying to delay, what's wrong with you go and get it. We can eat afterwards.

Here it is boys and be a bit careful with it as it has seen better days.

Wow that is not what I was excepting, its much larger and heavier that I thought it would be.

Yeh that's what my wife says.

You wish Mr Green you wish.

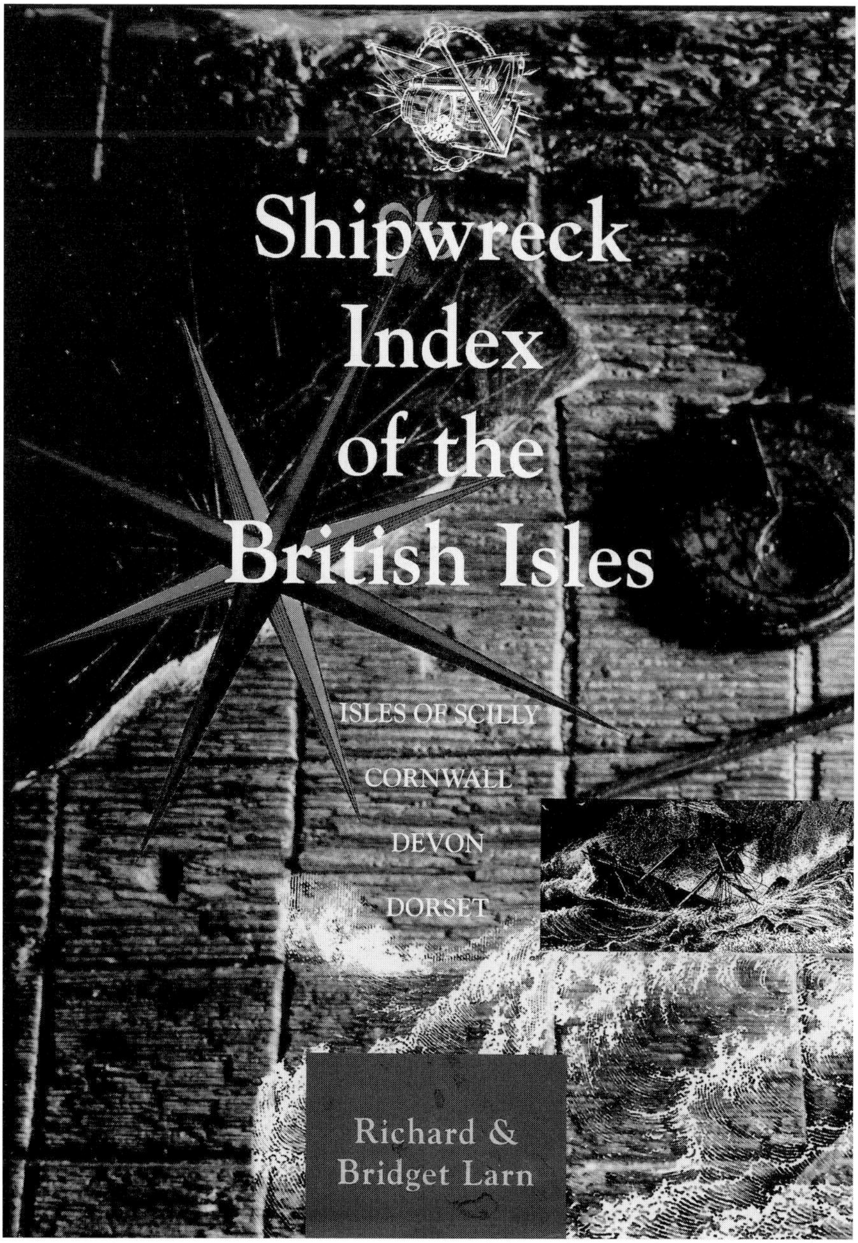

Pass it back to me a minute and take and a seat next to me I want to go through it with you both, and I don't want either of you turning the fragile pages.

First let's move to our area of interest South Devon. Now let's start right at the first entry Tarrit lost off Plymouth 1362, next John lost off

Exmouth 1573 next San Pedro Mayor lost off Bigbury 1588 and so it goes on giving a small piece of information on each ship lost. Sometimes it gives a long and lat sometimes just a rough area where it was reported to have sunk. On some entries there is more information than others which make sense as some wrecks have more data than others.

You can see that if the ships where carrying cannons there are a small symbol underneath and sometimes how many cannons. There are also small symbols for other stuff cargo etc.

Here take a look.

Volume 1 Section 5 *Shipwreck*

TARRIT (R) 00/00/1362

Plymouth *50.21.48N 04.08W*

ST Sailing vessel (unspecified); ***PN*** Sail

Stranded/Total Loss

C.SP.Dom.Select Pleas 1362 Vol.1 para.XLIV, Hugo de Courteneye

JOHN (R) 00/00/1573

Exmouth, Pole Sand *50.36.30N 03.25W*

VO Newfoundland - Exeter; ***ST*** Sailing vessel (unspecified); ***PT*** Lympston; ***FG*** England; ***CGO*** Fish unspecified; ***PN*** Sail

' - that the aforesaid Gilbert Peppet, Robert Vinton and John Hillman loaded a certain ship . . in parts beyond the sea with 70,000 salt fish called Newfoundland fish, and that the said ship with the aforesaid fish arrived safely off the port or river of Exmouth, and that the aforesaid John Parsons was hired as a pilot to conduct the aforesaid ship and fish into the port or river of Exmouth aforesaid. That he, Parsons hired his services . . in that behalf; taking upon himself the duty of conducting the ship and the rest of the premises into the aforesaid port, but by his craft, fault, ignorance, rashness and negligence caused the ship with the aforesaid fish to strike upon the sands and rocks of the sea and that in consequence the ship was wrecked, and that by reason thereof 18,000 of the fish were sunk in the sea and utterly perished and were lost, being valued at £200 . . by reason of the breaking up of the ship they sustained a loss to the amount of £66.13s.4d.'

Admiralty Court Miscellaneous Books & Exemplifications 1573 file 45 No. 301 p148

SAN PEDRO MAYOR 28/10/1588

Bigbury Bay, Hope Cove *50.14.34N 03.52W*

VO Lisbon - Cadiz; ***ST*** Hulk (wood); ***AR*** 29 x cannon; ***FG*** Spain; ***BM*** 581; ***CGO*** General cargo (unspecified); ***PN*** Sail; ***CR*** 28; ***PA*** 213; ***LO*** 40

One of two hospital ships or hulks which accompanied the 1588 Armada attempted invasion of England. Having circumnavigated the British Isles, this vessel was driven into the English channel to go ashore near Hope Cove. 'The crew, thoroughly dispirited, were taken prisoner and the ship plundered by the locals before the authorities could take measures to secure the wreck for the Queen. Of the drugs etc. on board, said to be 6,000 ducats worth, the greater part was spoiled by the sea. The prisoners were distributed amongst the villages, the officers being taken to Sir William Courtenay, at Ilton Castle, the wreck having occurred on his property.' The number of crew, soldiers and hospital personnel appear to vary with each reference, sometimes stated as 30 crew, 100 soldiers and 50 staff. Those crew captured included 123 Spaniards, 10 French, 10 Dutch, 2 Italians and 13 Portuguese. To date, the wreck site has never been located.

Devon Notes & Queries 1894; Maritime History of Devon, Oppenheim; Full Fathom Five, Martin, C. 1975

(Unidentified) 04/01/1596

Plymouth, harbour, rocks *50.21.48N 04.08W*

ST Sailing vessel (unspecified); ***CGO*** Tin ingots; ***PN*** Sail

'At about 12 o'clock, a ship belonging to a Mr. Superave was cast away and lost on the harbour by reason of the great storm, also another ship of the town lost at the same time. I hope to save the tin, because she came on the rocks in a full sea.'

C.SP.Dom.1596 Letter, James Bragg, merchant, and one time mayor of Plymouth

(Unidentified) (R) 06/01/1599

Plymouth, 'near the town' *50.21.48N 04.08W*

ST Sailing vessel (unspecified); ***PN*** Sail

'Although she has not taken any hurt, she may be lost.'

C.SP.Dom. Eliz. 1599 Vol.CCLXX p148

(Unidentified) (R) 00/00/1604

Plymouth, harbour, entrance *50.21.45N 04.08W*

ST Sailing vessel (unspecified); ***PN*** Sail

'Vessel wrecked in the harbour by tempest.'

C.SP.Dom. Add. James I 1604 Vol.XXXVI p454

(Unidentified) (R) 21/02/1625

Teignmouth, near *50.32.24N 03.30W*

ST Sailing vessel (unspecified); ***FG*** Netherlands; ***PN*** Sail

Stranded/Total Loss

C.SP.Dom.1625 James I Vol.CLXXXIV p480

BONAVENTURE (R) 04/12/1627

Plymouth, Cattewater *50.21.40N 04.07.30W*

ST Sailing vessel (unspecified); ***FG*** England; ***PN*** Sail

The reference details at some length the stranding of both this vessel and the RAINBOW, and the mode in which the latter vessel was salvaged and refloated.

C.SP.Dom.1627 Charles I Vol.LXXXVI p457 No's 11-12 & Vol.XC p517 No's 98-100

(Unidentified) (R) 16/01/1628

Plymouth *50.21.48N 04.08W*

VO Plymouth - La Rochelle; ***ST*** Sailing vessel (unspecified); ***CGO*** Lime unspecified, Stone unspecified; ***PN*** Sail

'Letters from Captain John Weddel to Commissioners of the Navy. Several of a fleet of ships have been cast away.'

C.SP.Dom. Charles I 1628 Vol.XC p517

(Unidentified) (R) 17/04/1628

Plymouth *50.21.30N 04.08.30W*

ST Barque (sail); ***PT*** Exeter; ***FG*** England; ***PN*** Sail

'A letter from Sir James Bagg, to Buckingham, from Plymouth.'

C.SP.Dom. Charles I 1628 Vol.CI p77 No.23

(Unidentified) (R) 20/02/1637

Bigbury Bay *50.16.30N 03.52.25W*

ST Sailing vessel (unspecified); ***PT*** St Malo; ***FG*** France; ***PN*** Sail

'Neither men nor goods were saved.'

C.SP.Dom.Charles I Vol.CCCLXXXII p270 No.54

(Unidentified) (R) 20/02/1637

Plymouth, Cattewater *50.21.40N 04.07.30W*

ST Sailing vessel (unspecified); ***PT*** Hamburg; ***FG*** Germany; ***PN*** Sail

'Letter from Sir John Eliot to Buckingham. Has attended with other gentlemen, about the removal of the ship sunk in the harbour of Cattewater.'

C.SP.Dom.(Sir John Pennington to the Lords of the Admiralty) Charles I Vol.CCCLXXXII p269 & Vol.

PAULSGROVE (R) 16/11/1637

Plymouth, St. Nicholas Isle *50.21.18N 04.09.12W*

VO Bantam - London; ***ST*** East Indiaman (sail); ***PT*** London; ***FG*** England; ***CGO*** General cargo (unspecified); ***PN*** Sail; ***CP*** Cluett

'East Indian Company versus Capt. Cluett. Witness Richard Robinson of the parish of St. Sepulchre, London, barber and surgeon, aged 34. When endeavouring to leave Plymouth, the weather upon the sudden grew exceeding violent that she could not with safety get out of the Sound. The pilot, purser and Thomas Monmouth, seeing the danger the ship was in, did entreat the defendant not to proceed but to return to her former moorings. Defendant being in a fretful mood and passionate humour, threw downe his staffe and stamping said, that he would not returne. That the company of the said ship, perceiving the great danger she was in, by prayer committed their Soules to God and about an hour later the carpenters were employed about, stopping her hawsers to

ACD Additional Construction Details; ***AR*** Armament; ***BL*** No. of Boilers; ***BM*** British Measurement Tonnage; ***BT*** Built; ***CGO*** Cargo(s); ***CL*** No. of crew lost; ***CN*** Construction; ***CP*** Captain; ***CR*** No. of Crew; ***FG*** Flag; ***GT*** Gross Tonnage

I think that is mad, how on earth did he get all the information on all those shipwrecks, it is so thorough and detailed it's fantastic.

I am glad you think so Captain Black and well worth the ten pounds I sold it to him for, would you not say. What about you Mr green you impressed?

Yeah I am! Very impressed indeed it's incredible; it's got all the wrecks listed in just one book. Ship ranging from a beaten up old tug to a First rate man of war. I think! if or when we come out of the closet, and say we think we have found a Dutch East Indianan, and which one we think we have found. The first thing the Dutch government, the Receiver of wrecks and all the sceptics will do is reach for a copy of this book. The only reservation I might have is that maybe I am just a little bit sceptical about how accurate the locations stated are. But yeah I am gob smacked it's the dogs bollocks. I just wonder if we should have tried a bit harder to get my hands on a copy before now. And if we have missed a trick, and perhaps, if we have missed this trick, what other tricks could we have missed.

Don't beat yourself up Mr Green we tried plenty hard enough to get a copy. Carry on Chiseller, let's cut to the chase, and then if we need to we can beat ourselves up later.

OK here we go, here is the money shot. Here we go start of the page we are looking form 1691-1732 South Devon.

Unidentified lost off Plymouth 1691, Next ship lost, CROWN PRINCE lost off Dartmouth 1692

Then as we come down we have DUNWICH lost off Plymouth 1714 then, MOOR lost off Plymouth 1716. And then we go to ASTREA lost off Plymouth 1725 and then it just carries on to 1732.

(Unidentified) 29/11/1691

Plymouth, E 10m 50.16N 03.52.30W

VO Jamaica - London; ***ST*** Sailing vessel (unspecified); ***PT*** London; ***FG*** England; ***PN*** Sail

Stranded/Total Loss

LG.07.12.1691

CROWN PRIZE 09/02/1692

Dartmouth, Start Point, near 50.13.25N 03.39W

ST Man o'War, sailing (unspecified) 6th Rate; ***AR*** 26 x cannon; ***LBD*** 25.60 x 7.62 x -; ***FG*** England; ***BM*** 223; ***BT*** France; ***PN*** Sail; ***CL*** 21; ***CP*** Tichborne, William

This 6th rate man o'war, captured from the French in 1691 as a prize, anchored off Dartmouth during very bad weather on the 7th, in an apparent effort to ride out the storm. Despite firing guns of distress, no help could reach the ship from the town because of the high seas and strong winds. The following day, her crew cut her anchor cables and attempted to stand out to sea. However, they were unable to weather Start Point, and during the early hours of the 9th she was driven ashore and wrecked. Her captain was drowned, along with what is generally believed to be twenty of the crew.

SRN Vol.1 p144; BWLS.p14; SRN Occ.Pub.No.5 Pt.1 p44 No.718; DS 1974 p125 & 251; Biographia Navalis

MERMAID 25/02/1693

Plymouth, Dockyard 50.22N 04.11.10W

ST Man o'War, sailing (unspecified) Fireship; ***AR*** 8 x cannon; ***FG*** England; ***BM*** 174; ***BT*** France; ***PN*** Sail; ***CP*** Rigby, Edward

Whilst fitting out at Plymouth Dockyard, the captain's servant dropped an unguarded candle in the store room, which started a fire and spread rapidly, burning her to the water line before sinking. N.B . Whilst reasonably certain that this accident took place in Plymouth(SRN & other accounts), BWLS states Portsmouth.

BWLS. p15; SRN Vol.1 p359; SRN Occ.Pub. No.5 Pt.1 p46 No.762; DS 1974 p21 & 260

(Unidentified) (R) 01/02/1695

Bigbury Bay 50.16.30N 03.52.25W

ST Sailing vessel (unspecified); ***FG*** France; ***CGO*** Salt; ***PN*** Sail; ***CR*** 20

'At the beginning of this week, by stress of weather, a vessel was driven on shore in the bay and staved to pieces, twenty crew, all saved and brought to Falmouth.'

C.SP.Dom.1695 p238; DS 1974 p269

MERMAID 05/01/1699

Plymouth, near 50.21.48N 04.08W

ST Man o'War, sailing (unspecified) 5th Rate; ***AR*** 32 x cannon; ***LBD*** 32.00 x 7.92 x -; ***FG*** England; ***BM*** 309; ***BT*** 1651 Graves, Limehouse; ***PN*** Sail

Vessel was rebuilt at Woolwich in 1689, when she was upgraded from a 24 gun 6th rate to 5th rate and 32 guns. Wrecked by accident near Plymouth.

SRN Vol.1 p359; DS 1974 p22-3 & 260; SRN Occ.Pub.No.5 Pt.1 p12 No.112

CORNELIUS 16/01/1700

Plymouth, Hamoaze 50.21.30N 04.11W

ST Sailing vessel (unspecified); ***PT*** Rotterdam; ***FG*** Netherlands; ***PN*** Sail

Stranded/Total Loss

SLL

(Unidentified) 29/12/1700

Dartmouth, harbour 50.20.30N 03.34W

ST Sailing vessel (unspecified); ***FG*** England; ***CGO*** Cannon as cargo; ***PN*** Sail

Stranded/Total Loss

The Flying Post 01.1701(R)

SEAHORSE 29/11/1711

Dartmouth, near 50.20.30N 03.34W

ST Man o'War, sailing (unspecified) 6th Rate; ***AR*** 14 x cannon; ***LBD*** 23.17 x 6.86 x -; ***FG*** Great Britain; ***BM*** 161; ***BT*** 1709 Yeames, Limehouse; ***PN*** Sail; ***CP*** Blower, Humphrey, Cdr' RN

Whilst lying at anchor off Dartmouth, the weather deteriorated, bringing in heavy rain and strong winds. The warship attempted to warp herself further up stream, however the wind shifting suddenly and increasing in squalls, caused her to go ashore on the rocks on the west side of the harbour, below Dartmouth Castle. Here she again anchored, but it was too late to prevent her stranding, being beaten to pieces on the rocks.

SRN Vol.1 p497; BWLS.p30; DS 1974 p125 & 265; SRN Occ.Pub.No.5 Pt.1 p49(826) nb.The date of loss q

SAUDADOES (R) 00/00/1712

Plymouth 50.21.48N 04.08W

ST Man o'War, sailing (unspecified) 5th Rate; ***AR*** 36 x cannon; ***LBD*** 31.55 x 8.84 x -; ***FG*** Great Britain; ***BM*** 385; ***BT*** France; ***PN*** Sail

A prize vessel captured from the French in September 1692, rebuilt at Deptford in 1673, was stripped of her armament and stores and sunk as a foundation at Plymouth, location unknown.

SRN Vol.1 p491; DS 1974 p23 & 265; SRN Occ.Pub.No.5 Pt.I p34 No. 534

DUNWICH (R) 00/00/1714

Plymouth 50.21.48N 04.08W

ST Man o'War, sailing (unspecified) 6th Rate; ***AR*** 24 x cannon; ***LBD*** 28.65 x 7.47 x -; ***FG*** Great Britain; ***BM*** 250; ***BT*** 1695 Collins & Chatfield, Shoreham; ***PN*** Sail

After being stripped of her guns, stores and upper deck fittings, was sunk as a breakwater at Plymouth.

SRN Vol.1 p177; DS 1974 p23 & 252; SRN Occ.Pub.No.5 p53 No.902

MOOR 07/03/1716

Plymouth 50.21.48N 04.08W

ST Man o'War, sailing (unspecified) 4th Rate; ***AR*** 54 x cannon; ***FG*** Great Britain; ***BM*** 811; ***BT*** France; ***PN*** Sail

Vessel was stripped of her guns, stores and upper deck fittings, before being sunk as a breakwater at Plymouth.

SRN Vol.1 p389; DS 1974 p23 & 261

ASTREA 09/10/1725

Plymouth, Cattewater 50.21.40N 04.07.30W

VO Texel - Batavia; ***ST*** East Indiaman (sail); ***AR*** 40 x cannon; ***PT*** Amsterdam; ***FG*** Netherlands; ***BM*** 800; ***CGO*** Gold coin/plate/specie, General cargo (unspecified); ***BT*** 1720, Delft; ***PN*** Sail; ***CR*** 200; ***CP*** t'Hoorn, Jakob

Outward bound as part of a convoy, the ASTREA was obliged to enter Plymouth, seeking shelter from a storm. Is believed to have been blown ashore on the rocks near Mount Batten where she was wrecked. Only a small portion of the gold specie carried was recovered.

Dutch-Asiatic Shipping, Vol.2 p386(Voyage No.2630.2); London Journal 10.1725(R)

POSTILION (R) 00/00/1732

Start Bay, Bee Sands 50.15N 03.39.18W

ST Sailing vessel (unspecified); ***FG*** Great Britain; ***PN*** Sail

Stranded/Total Loss

DNO Vol.27 p76

Hey! What are you on about! No way that can't that be right! it just can't be! You're pulling my chain!

Not I Captain not I, but I think someone else might have been pulling it all along!!

Give me that book, and move out of the way Chiseller you're as blind as a bat, Let me see that stupid book. **The End**

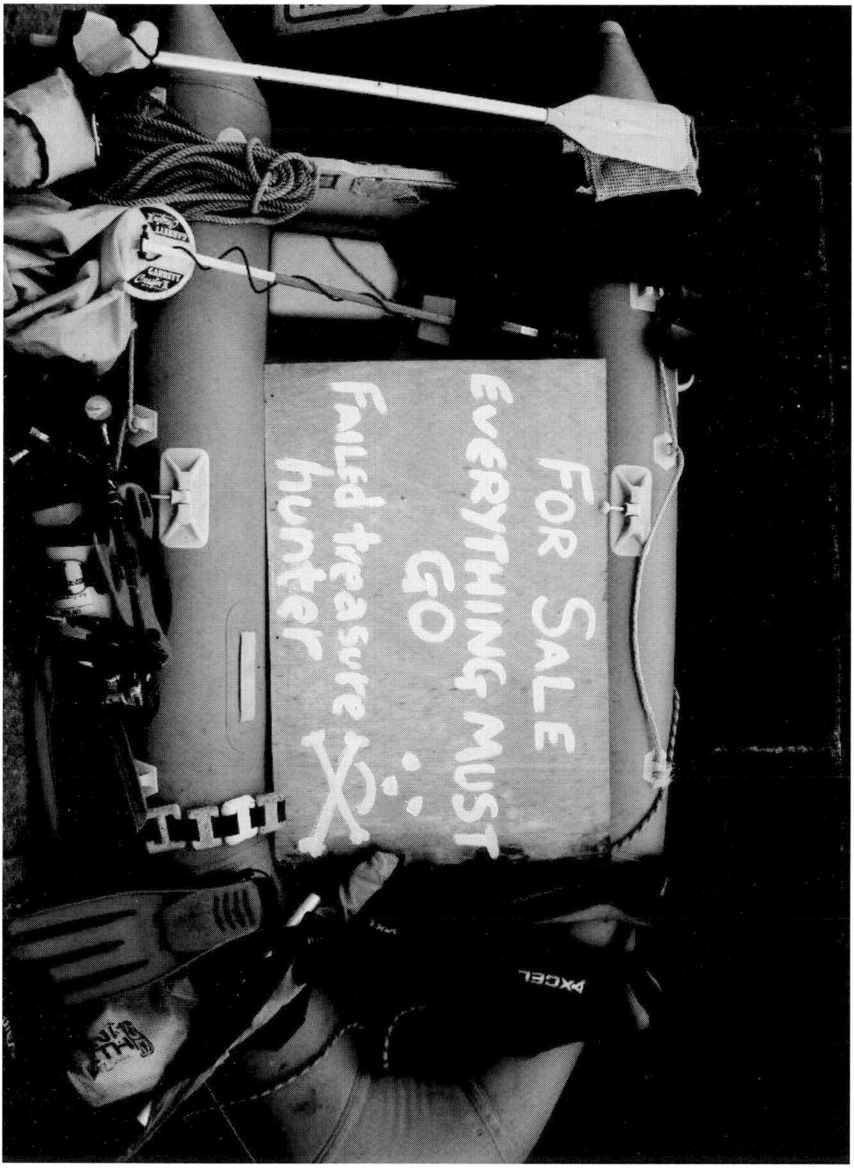
FOR SALE
EVERYTHING MUST
GO
Failed treasure
hunter

Epilogue

Have You Heard The One About The?

I can see his car in the drive

Chiseller I told you he would be in. I have heard he hasn't been diving for ages.

I know Mr Green; I even heard he had real money problems and all his dive kit was up for sale. I think he even wants to sell the Mk1 Rigid Raider. His wife is the most patient women in the world, but I guess even she knows when enough is enough. Park over there and we can give him some horn.

Beep Beep Hey Captain what you up to? Beep Beep.

Hi guys, nice to see you both, you're just in time to make the tea.

Better than that Captain we are going to take you to Yacht Haven cafe for a all day breakfast, you look like you could do with a good feed.

The full montie Captain Black, hash browns, fried bread, two eggs, bacon, sausages and unlimited T. What say you Captain?

How could I resist, Thanks guys.

What you up to with those iron blocks Captain?

I have been cleaning them and re examining them, I been knocking off some more crud and stuff. I cleaned up this one here I noticed the shape of a anchor. I think it has been put on the block after it was cast. Here have a look; it's got one side of its stock lower than the other.

That must have taken a long time to clean up.

Time is what I have got plenty of Mr Green, and while I am here cleaning these blocks I am not spending any money on petrol or my phone. Anyway I then spend hours on the internet searching for the same anchor logo. And the only one I can find is on a old weight found my a metal detectors in Norfolk, a small trading weight. And guess whose trade mark it was?

No idea!

Me neither, so tell us.

King George I.

So then I moved on to the other block, and I spent hours cleaning it but there was no anchor or any mark on the top. I turned it over and started work on the bottom and under on the really hard crud I found and lead plug. Just like the one on top of the Ballast block. Which as we know was used to make the blocks up to their exact weight 56 ponds. But this lead seal was much wider, about twice as wide actually. And there is a trade mark stamped on the seal. Here have a look.

You have a look first Mr Green I need to get my classes from the car.

What can you make out Mr Green?

I can see a crown, and then underneath I can see a C, no it could be a G, and then I think it's a R.

Pass it to Chiseller now he has his bins on. What can you make out there Chiseller?

A crown, Maybe a G and I'm not sure about the R but yeh it could be a R.

So there we have it both blocks date to King George I reign, I ran it to the computer and type in "when did King George I reign".

How's your history boys, is it better than mine, when did he reign?

Tell us Captain before you burst.

King of England 1714 -1727

So are you now saying the shipwreck was British and you now know which ship it was?

No, Mr Green I am not! Hold on a second while I line all three blocks up alongside each other. There now look at the difference in those block.

Ok clearly they are of vast different quality, the ballast block is clearly in much better condition.

You agree Chiseller?

I do Mr Green, far superior.

So if they have all been in the water for exactly the same time, why is one still almost still like new and the other two very in very bad condition? Not now Chiseller it's not a question. I tell you why, because one is made from Swedish Iron Ore. And the other two are made from English Iron Ore. Swedish Iron Ore as we know was then and still is now the highest quality Iron Ore in the world. "Namban Tetsu" made from the world's finest foreign steel.

So what were King George I English weights doing on the wreck site.

Good old reliable Mr Green, I knew you would ask that. They were used by the contemporary salvagers at the time. To hold down the rope ladders and mark the site. Just like dive boats would use them for shot weights today.

You're very quiet Mr Green.

Sorry Mr Green and sorry to you Captain, but I think we are grasping at straws. I don't mind keeping the faith, but this time I am with Mrs Black enough is enough. Keep the faith yes and God know we have done that, but blind faith that's what brings rags to your ass. I'm getting in the car and if anyone wants full English all day breakfast I am paying, but I leaving now.

How about you Mr Green, you've been here from the start, from day one, from sitting on the cliff while I told you of my mad idea too. To right here and now. Surely you can stay the course?

Let me ask you a question Captain, did you ever tell the Chiseller of "your blag it all idea", your "make it all up idea"? Your "Blair witch idea". I know you must have told Uncle Orange a little of it, as he is the gate keeper of all things lost and found, and he would of needed to know a reason.. And after all he is your Uncle.

No I didn't! what would have been the point in telling him about just an idea?

Then here is my answer Captain my Captain, I think I have been a loyal and trusted companion, I have done everything you have asked of me and more. I have kept my eyes wide open and my mouth tightly closed. We have dived in some shit awful holes. Blacker than I could of ever imagined the sea could get. We have been so cold we couldn't even start our outboard engine, and so hungry my tongue was crawling out of my ass looking for a feed. We have watched each other's back, and talked more than any gay couple on their honeymoon. Have I enjoyed the ride, the excitement the living on the edge and sailing close to the wind? I sure have. Have we been a little too close to breaking the law, breaking the pirate's code? Yes we have, but I believe I have kept you just on the right side, kept you from the dark side, but now for me

Captain it is over, it's been over for a while. And to keep your sanity it needs too be over for you to mate. I'm so sorry ****** you're not a Captain, I'm not Mr Green I am ****. You are my best mate and I love you to bits man. But it's over.

Lets pack away all this stuff and join **** for that all day breakfast.

Thanks Guys that was the best all day breakfast ever, I am so stuffed.

You are more than welcome Captain. What are your plans now? Any news or success in finding some work?

No luck yet, I will keep trying.

By the way! Have you heard the one about the Bronze Age slipway and The Hill Fort I have found?

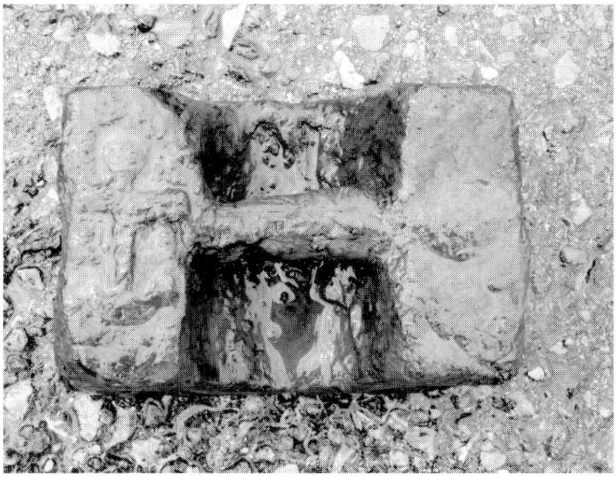

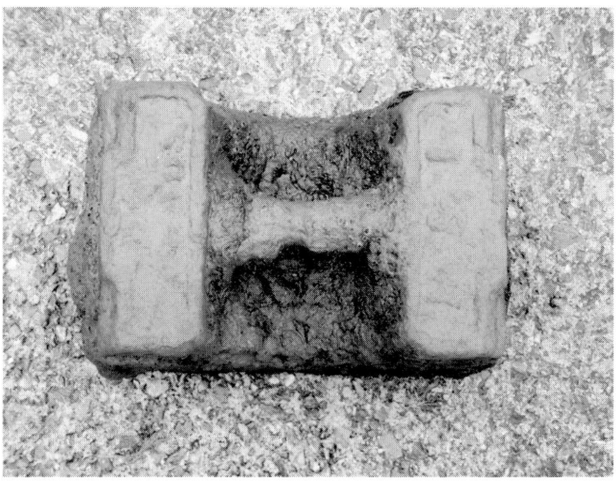

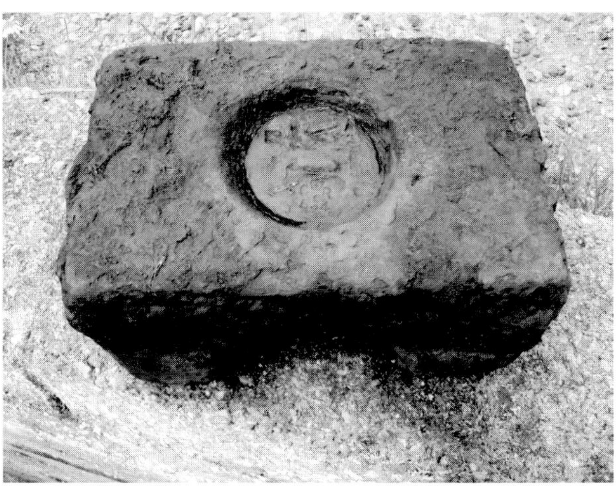

What Happens Next?

What happens now then Captain Black? Once the book is launched and we are out of the closet, what do you think will then happen?

Take a seat Mr Green, and you Chiseller.

Depending on what reaction the book receives and whether certain people think its Fiction or non Fiction. That will determine whether the shit hits the proverbial fan or not!

Three parties come immediately to mind when you say the worlds shit and fan.

And which three would that be Chiseller?

The Receiver of wrecks, English heritage and the Dutch Government (VOC)

You got any more to add to the list Mr Green?

Yes I do.

Well theres a surprise lets hear what you got.

Ok, people that might want to talk to us, or be pissed at us. Swedish science museum, Japanese Samurai sword museum, National Maritime museum, Evil Dr Pork Chop, Token society, nautical archaeology society, R.O.W and a whole lot more. I think English heritage will be all over us like a trap on chips. They will want to dive the site and close us down. Everyone will want to see if we really got the finds we say we have in the book. And someone will have to make a **decision** on

A) Is there a wreck site?
B) Is the wreck VOC.?
C) What is the name of the wreck?

Do you think we will ever get to own any of the finds?

Not sure Chiseller, I would like to think after two years of diving the site we get to keep some stuff. It would be nice if we get to keep it all as one collection for people to see for themselves. All I can say is batten down the hatches and enjoy the ride, come hell or high water we need to stick together and enjoy the ups and the downs. Let's stick to our story and watch each other's backs, just like the three meercats. Life's too Warwick Davis

All I can say to anyone who has read this book, you now get a chance to write your own sequel. Because we haven't got a clue what will happen next, not a clue. So you can put pen to paper and write your own sequel. And then when we publish "WHAT HAPPENED NEXT" you can see how close you where to getting it correct. The person who gets it the closest will get a free invite to come and play with our rusty balls :-) Remember what my dad always used to say, "Never let the truth spoil a good story"

Oh! Yeh, by the way.

Don't forget to include the small British cast iron swivel gun, a Bronze Age slipway and an 8000 year old hand axe.

Captain Black
Keep your head down, and your powder dry